普通高等教育“十一五”国家级规划教材

全国高等医药院校药学类专业第二轮实验双语教材

药剂学实验与指导

（第2版）

主　　编　周建平　蒋曙光
主　　审　平其能
副 主 编　吴正红　丁　杨
编　　者　（以姓氏笔画为序）
丁　杨　尹莉芳　吕慧侠　祁小乐
孙春萌　孙敏捷　苏志桂　杨　磊
吴正红　吴琼珠　何　伟　何东升
张建军　周建平　姚　静　秦　超
殷婷婕　高　缘　蒋曙光　韩晓鹏
霍美蓉

中国健康传媒集团
中国医药科技出版社 ·北京

内容提要

本教材是“全国高等医药院校药学类专业第二轮实验双语教材”之一，根据药剂学实验教学大纲的基本要求和课程特点编写而成。内容涵盖经典液体剂型、半固体剂型、固体剂型、注射剂、新剂型与新载体以及高端仪器设备操作等六大模块24个实验，每个实验均由目的与要求、基本概念与实验原理、仪器与材料、实验内容以及实验指导等五个部分组成，并附有思考题，具有强调基础理论、注重操作规范、激发创新思维、训练实验技能的特点，专门用于药学类专业及相关专业的药剂学实验设计与技能训练。本教材为书网融合教材，即纸质教材有机融合电子教材、配套资源（PPT）。

本教材供高等医药院校药学类专业及相关专业药剂学实验教学使用，也可供从事药学相关工作的科研人员参考。

图书在版编目（CIP）数据

药剂学实验与指导／周建平，蒋曙光主编．—2版．—北京：中国医药科技出版社，2020.1（2025.8重印）．

全国高等医药院校药学类专业第二轮实验双语教材

ISBN 978－7－5214－1406－6

Ⅰ.①药…　Ⅱ.①周…②蒋…　Ⅲ.①药剂学－实验－高等学校－教材－汉、英　Ⅳ.①R94－33

中国版本图书馆CIP数据核字（2019）第301303号

美术编辑　陈君杞
版式设计　南博文化

出版　**中国健康传媒集团**｜中国医药科技出版社
地址　北京市海淀区文慧园北路甲22号
邮编　100082
电话　发行：010－62227427　邮购：010－62236938
网址　www.cmstp.com
规格　889×1194mm 1/16
印张　13 3/4
字数　307千字
初版　2007年2月第1版
版次　2020年1月第2版
印次　2025年8月第4次印刷
印刷　河北环京美印刷有限公司
经销　全国各地新华书店
书号　ISBN 978－7－5214－1406－6
定价　40.00元

序

Preface

教学是学校人才培养的中心环节，实验教学是这一环节的重要组成部分。“全国高等医药院校药学类专业实验双语教材”是中国药科大学坚持药学实践教学改革，突出提高学生动手能力、创新思维，通过承担教育部“世行贷款21世纪初高等教育教学改革项目”等多项教改课题，逐步建设完善的一套与药学各专业学科理论课程紧密结合的高水平双语实验教材。

本轮修订，适逢“全国高等医药院校药学类专业第五轮规划教材”及《中国药典》（2020年版）、新版《国家执业药师资格考试大纲》出版，整套教材的修订强调了与新版理论教材知识的结合，与《中国药典》（2020年版）等新颁布的法典法规结合。为更好地服务于新时期高等院校药学教育与人才培养的需要，在上一版的基础上，进一步体现了各门实验课程自身独立性、系统性和科学性，又充分考虑到各门实验课程之间的联系与衔接，主要突出了以下特点。

1. 适应医药行业对人才的要求，体现行业特色，契合新时期药学人才需求的变化，使修订后的教材符合《中国药典》（2020年版）等国家标准及新版《国家执业药师资格考试大纲》等行业最新要求。

2. 更新完善内容，打造教材精品。在上版教材基础上进一步优化、精炼和充实内容。紧密结合“全国高等医药院校药学类专业第五轮规划教材”，强调与实际需求相结合，进一步提高教材质量。

3. 为适应信息化教学的需要，本轮教材全部打造成为书网融合教材，即纸质教材与数字教材、配套教学资源、题库系统、数字化教学服务有机融合，为读者提供全免费增值服务。

4. 坚持双语体系，强调素质培养教材以实践教学为突破口，采用双语体系编写有利于加快药学教育国际接轨，提高学生的科技英语水平，进一步提升学生整体素质。

“全国高等医药院校药学类专业第二轮实验双语教材”历经15年4次建设，在各个时期广大编者的努力下，在广大使用教材师生的支持下日臻完善。本轮教材的出版，必将对推动新时期我国高等药学教育的发展产生积极而深远的影响。希望广大师生在教学实践中对本套教材提出宝贵意见，以便今后进一步修订完善，共同打造精品教材。

吴晓明

全国高等医药院校药学类专业第五轮规划教材常务编委会主任委员

2019年10月

前言

Preface

根据高等医药院校对药剂学实验教学新的发展要求，我们本着强调基础理论、紧跟发展前沿、规范实验操作、训练实验技能的主旨编写了本教材。

本教材为药学类专业实验双语教材，供药学类院校药剂学实验教学使用，亦可为广大药剂工作者提供参考。实验内容涉及液体剂型、半固体剂型、固体剂型、注射剂、新剂型与新载体以及高端仪器设备操作等六大模块，每个实验均由目的与要求、基本概念与实验原理、仪器与材料、实验内容以及实验指导等五个部分组成。在“实验指导”中，提出了预习要求、操作要点和注意事项，并附有思考题，旨在培养学生根据实验现象及结果，结合理论知识，提高分析问题和解决问题的科研能力，养成独力思考的习惯。

本教材为书网融合教材，即纸质教材有机融合电子教材、教学配套资源（PTT）。

本教材是中国药科大学药剂系同仁多年教学实践的结晶。虽全体编者已努力做好本次教材的修订工作，但限于编者的水平，在实验内容编排和中英文表述方面恐有欠妥之处，诚请广大读者批评指正，以便修订时完善。

编　者

2019 年 10 月

目录

Contents

第一部分　液体制剂的制备

实验1　溶液型液体制剂的制备

【目的与要求】

1. 掌握　溶液型液体制剂的基本制备方法。溶解度的测定方法。
2. 熟悉　溶液剂中附加剂的使用方法。
3. 了解　增加药物溶解度的方法。

【基本概念与实验原理】

溶液型液体制剂系指药物以分子或离子状态分散于溶剂中制成的内服或外用的液体形态的制剂。常用溶媒有水、乙醇、甘油、丙二醇、聚乙二醇等。溶液剂通常采用溶解法、稀释法和化学反应法制备。属于溶液型液体制剂的有溶液剂、芳香水剂、糖浆剂等，最常用的是溶液剂和糖浆剂。

溶液剂系指小分子药物溶解于溶剂中所形成的澄明溶液，糖浆剂系指含有药物或芳香物质的浓蔗糖水溶液。纯蔗糖的近饱和水溶液称为单糖浆，其浓度为85%（g/ml）或64.7%（g/g），不含任何药物，除供制备含药糖浆外，还可作为矫味剂和混悬剂的助悬剂等。

在制备溶液型液体制剂时，首选水为溶剂，因而需要了解药物的水中溶解度。若药物在溶媒中溶解度不好，则常需采用一些方法，如成盐、增溶、助溶、潜溶等，以增加药物在溶媒中的溶解度。为了加速溶解进程，可将药物粉碎甚至微粉化处理，通常取溶媒处方量的1/2～3/4来溶解药物，必要时可加热，但受热不稳定的药物不宜加热。另外，根据需要还可加入抗氧剂、甜味剂、着色剂等附加剂。在制备流程中，一般先加入复合溶媒、助溶剂和稳定剂等附加剂。

胶体型液体制剂系指固体药物以1～500nm大小的粒子分散于适当的分散媒中制得的均相或非均相体系。一些胶体制品（如胃蛋白酶、胰蛋白酶、纤维素衍生物、右旋糖酐等），当遇水后都形成亲水的胶体溶液。亲水胶体溶液的制备与低分子溶液制备流程基本相同，但药物溶解时，首先要经过溶胀过程：分次撒布于水面，使之自然膨胀，然后搅拌或加热溶解。

增溶是药剂学中增加难溶性药物水中溶解度的常用方法。增溶是指某些难溶性药物在表面活性剂的作用下，在溶剂中的溶解度增大并形成澄明溶液的过程。具有增溶能力的表面活性剂称增溶剂，被增溶的物质称为增溶质。胶束的形成是增溶作用的基础。表面活性剂浓度达到临界胶束浓度以上，溶质的溶解度才显著提高。对于以水为溶剂溶解药物时，增溶剂的最适HLB值为15～18。常用的增溶剂为聚山梨酯（吐温）类和聚氧乙烯脂肪酸酯类。药物的增溶作用受诸多因素影响，如增溶剂的性质、增溶质的性质、增溶的温度、增溶质的加入顺序等。

【仪器与材料】

1. **仪器** 研钵，烧杯，量筒，量瓶，移液管，天平，玻璃棒，西林瓶，注射器，微孔滤膜，磁力搅拌器，紫外－可见分光光度计等。

2. **材料** 碘，碘化钾，胃蛋白酶，稀盐酸，甘油，蔗糖，布洛芬，聚山梨酯20（吐温20），聚山梨酯40（吐温40），聚山梨酯80（吐温80），甲醇，蒸馏水等。

【实验内容】

一、复方碘溶液的制备

1. **处方**

碘	2.5g
碘化钾	5g
蒸馏水	加至50ml

2. **制备工艺** 取5g碘化钾置研钵中，加约25ml蒸馏水，搅拌使溶解。再加2.5g碘，研磨使全部溶解，加水至50ml，搅匀，即得。工艺流程图见图1－1。

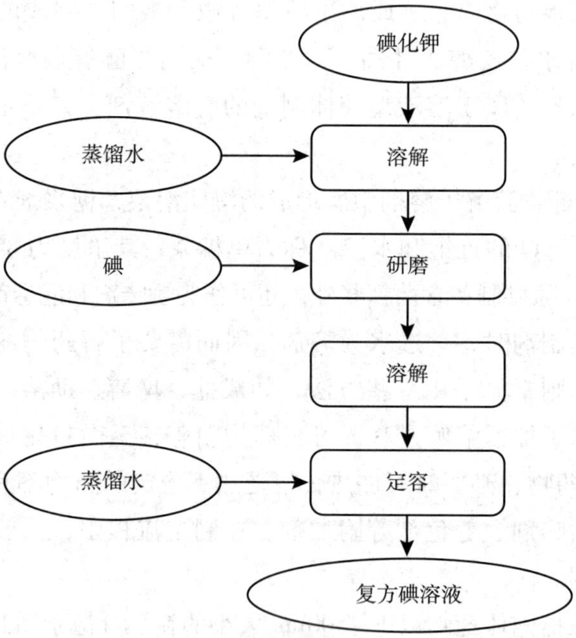

图1－1 复方碘溶液的制备工艺流程图

二、胃蛋白酶合剂的制备

1. **处方**

胃蛋白酶（1∶3000）	3g
稀盐酸	2ml
甘油	20ml
蒸馏水	加至100ml

2. **制备工艺** 取约70ml蒸馏水置烧杯中，加稀盐酸、甘油，搅拌溶解。将胃蛋白酶撒于液面上，使其自然膨胀后，轻轻搅拌使完全溶解。加水至足量，搅匀，即得。工艺流程图见图1－2。

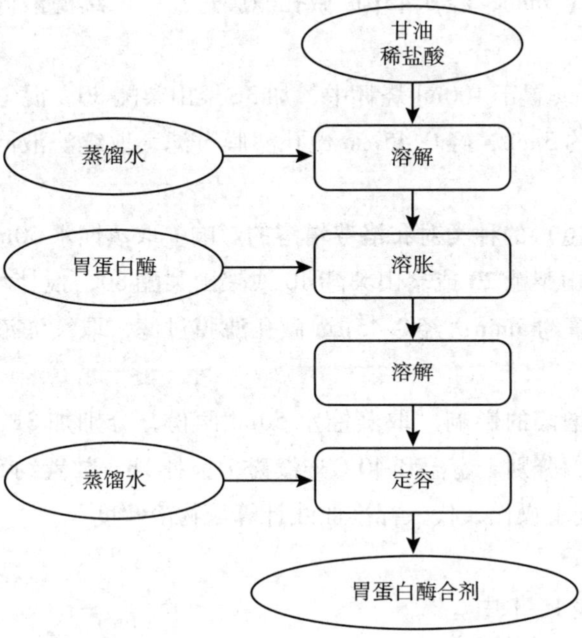

图 1-2　胃蛋白酶合剂的制备工艺流程图

三、单糖浆的制备

1. 处方

蔗糖	85g
蒸馏水	加至 100ml

2. 制备工艺　取约 80ml 蒸馏水，加蔗糖，加热煮沸，搅拌溶解，继续煮沸 5min，趁热用 0.8μm 微孔滤膜过滤，放冷，加水至足量，搅匀即得。

四、布洛芬在水中的溶解度测定

1. 标准曲线的绘制　取布洛芬对照品约 12mg，精密称定，置 10ml 量瓶中，加甲醇溶解并稀释至刻度，再分别精密量取 0.6，0.8，1.0，1.2 和 1.4ml 置 100ml 量瓶中，用水稀释至刻度，摇匀。以蒸馏水为空白，在 221nm 波长处测定吸光度。以浓度（C）为横坐标，吸光度（A）为纵坐标进行线性回归。

2. 溶解度试验及测定　取约 50mg 布洛芬置锥形瓶中，加水 250ml，具塞，置恒温水浴（25℃）中磁力搅拌，分别于 0.5，1，2，4h 取混悬液用 0.45μm 微孔滤膜过滤。精密量取续滤液 1ml 置 10ml 量瓶，用水稀释至刻度，摇匀，在 221nm 波长处测定吸光度，代入标准曲线计算，确定达到溶解平衡的时间，测定溶解度。

五、表面活性剂对布洛芬的增溶作用

1. 聚山梨酯 80（吐温 80）及其加入顺序对布洛芬增溶的影响

（1）取蒸馏水 50ml 置于 100ml 烧杯中，加布洛芬 50mg，持续磁力搅拌 1h，放置约 5min，经 0.45μm 微孔滤膜过滤，精密量取续滤液 0.5ml 置 100ml 量瓶，以蒸馏水稀释至刻度，摇匀，于 221nm 波长处采用紫外分光光度计测定吸光度，代入标准曲线计算药物溶解度。

（2）取蒸馏水 50ml 置于 100ml 烧杯中，加 3g 聚山梨酯 80 搅拌均匀，加布洛芬 50mg，持续磁力搅拌 1h，放置约 5min，经 0.45μm 微孔滤膜过滤，取续滤液同上操作，代入标准曲线计算药物溶解度。

（3）取蒸馏水 50ml 置于 100ml 烧杯中，加布洛芬 50mg，混匀，加 3g 聚山梨酯 80，持续磁力搅拌 1h，放置约 5min，经 0.45μm 微孔滤膜过滤，取续滤液同上操作，代入标准曲线计算药物溶解度。

（4）加布洛芬 50mg 置于 100ml 烧杯中，加 3g 聚山梨酯 80，混匀，加蒸馏水 50ml，持续磁力搅拌 1h，放置约 5min，经 0.45μm 微孔滤膜过滤，取续滤液同上操作，代入标准曲线计算药物溶解度。

2. 聚山梨酯（吐温）的种类对布洛芬增溶的影响 取蒸馏水 50ml 两份，分别置 100ml 烧杯中，分别加 3g 聚山梨酯 20 或聚山梨酯 40 或聚山梨酯 80，搅拌均匀，加布洛芬 50mg，持续磁力搅拌 1h，放置约 5min，经 0.45μm 微孔滤膜过滤，取续滤液同上操作，代入标准曲线计算药物溶解度。

3. 温度对布洛芬增溶的影响 取蒸馏水 50ml 两份，分别加 3g 聚山梨酯 80，搅拌均匀，各加布洛芬 50mg，分别于室温和 40℃ 连续磁力搅拌 1h，放置约 5min，经 0.45μm 微孔滤膜过滤，取续滤液同上操作，代入标准曲线计算药物溶解度。

4. 实验结果

实验结果记录在表 1－1 中。

表 1－1 实验结果

考察因素	试验内容	体系的外观状态	药物浓度（g/100ml）
聚山梨酯加入顺序	不加表面活性剂		
	先加聚山梨酯 80，后加药物		
	先加药物，后加聚山梨酯 80		
	聚山梨酯与药物先混合，再加水		
聚山梨酯类型	聚山梨酯 20 室温		
	聚山梨酯 40 室温		
	聚山梨酯 80 室温		
实验温度	聚山梨酯 80 40℃		

实验指导

一、预习要求

1. **掌握** 溶液剂的分类。
2. **熟悉** 增加药物溶解度的方法。
3. **了解** 表面活性剂的类型及使用方法。

二、操作要点和注意事项

1. 碘在水中的溶解度为 1∶2950，碘化钾作为助溶剂可与碘生成易溶于水的络合物，同时使碘稳定不易挥发，并减少其刺激性。制备复方碘溶液时应注意加入次序：先加入碘化钾溶解后再投入难溶性碘。

2. 溶解碘化钾时所用的蒸馏水为处方量的 50%，既能使碘化钾溶解，又能使碘化钾具有较高浓度，以利于碘的溶解。

3. 碘溶液为氧化剂，应贮存于密闭玻璃瓶内，不得与木塞、橡皮塞及金属塞接触。试验所得样品应统一回收。

4. 测定溶解度时要确定好药物溶解度达到平衡的时间：在不同时间点时取样过滤，根据溶液浓度变化来判断。

5. 增溶试验操作中各项条件应尽可能保持一致，如加药量、搅拌时间等。增溶操作中，样品搅拌后应放置一段时间，以利于气泡的消除和药物充分进入胶团。

6. 胃蛋白酶易吸潮，称取时宜迅速。胃蛋白酶在 pH 1.5～2.0 时活性最强，但盐酸的量若超过0.5%时，会破坏其活性，亦不可直接将其加至未经稀释的盐酸中。处方中 20% 的甘油具有保持胃蛋白酶活力和调味的作用。强力搅拌及用棉花、滤纸过滤等均会影响本品的活性和稳定性。

三、思考题

1. 制备复方碘溶液时有哪些注意事项？
2. 影响药物溶解度的因素有哪些？
3. 如何确定药物达到平衡溶解度所需要的时间？
4. 影响表面活性剂对难溶性药物增溶效果的主要因素有哪些？
5. 制备胃蛋白酶合剂时，如何选择盐酸溶液的加入顺序？
6. 简述增加药物溶解度的方法。

Experiment 1　Preparation of Solutions

扫码“学一学”

Objectives and Requirements

1. To master the basic preparation methods of solutions.
2. To master the determination of solubility.
3. To be familiar with the usage of inactive ingredients in solution.
4. To understand the ways to increase the solubility.

Introduction

Solution preparations are liquid preparations containing active pharmaceutical ingredients (API) dissolved in liquid dispersion medium in molecular or ionic state. They are usually prepared by the technical of solution, dilution and chemical reaction method. Water, alcohol, glycerol, propylene glycol and polyethylene glycol are the most frequently used solvent. Solution preparations include solutions, aromatic waters, syrups, etc.

While solutions (liquid preparations containing small molecular API dissolved in a suitable solvent to form a clear solution) and syrups (concentrated aqueous solutions of sucrose containing extracts of crude drugs or aromatic materials) are more commonly used. Nearly saturated pure sucrose aqueous solution is known as simple syrup and its concentration is 85% (g/ml) or 64.7% (g/g) without containing any drugs. Except for using to prepare medicated syrup, it can also act as a flavoring agent and mixed suspension agent, suspending agent.

To prepare a solution, water is the solvent which is the first choice. It requires the understanding of the drug's solubility in water. If the drug's solubility in the solvent is poor, some methods are used to increase the solubility of the drug, such as the most important respect is the approaches to improvement of aqueous solubility. Feasible methods include: salt formation, solubilization, hydrotropy and cosolvency. Pulverization and micronization can be applied to accelerate the process of drug dissolution. It usually takes 1/2 - 3/4 of the solvent to dissolve the drug. Heating is often used if the drug is not heat - sensitive. In addition, antioxidants, sweeteners, coloring agent can be added if needed. During the preparation, composite solvent, cosolvent, stabilizer and other additives are added before the insoluble ingredients.

A colloidal solution is a homogeneous or heterogeneous liquid system containing 1 - 500nm solid particles. Some colloidal materials, such as pepsin, trypsin, cellulose derivatives, dextran, can form hydrophilic colloidal solution in water. The preparation of colloidal solutions is similar to low molecular solution. However, the drug should be swollen in water before completely dissolved with the help of stirring or heat.

Solubilization is a commonly used method in pharmaceutics to increase the solubility of insoluble drugs in water. Solubilization refers to the process that under the action of surface active agent, the solubility of some insoluble drugs increases to form a transparent solution. The formation of micelles is the basis of solubilization. When the concentration of surface active agent reaches the critical micelleconcentration, the solubility of the solute is significantly improved. When water is used as the solvent, the optimum HLB value is 15 - 18. The commonly used solubilizers include polysorbates (Tween) and polyoxyethylene fatty acid ester. The solubilization is generally influenced by a variety of factors, such as the properties of the solvent and the solute, the temperature and the addition order of the solute.

Equipment and Materials

1. Equipment

Mortar, beaker, measuring cylinder, measuring cylinder, balance, glass stick, pipettes, vials, syringes, porous membrane, magnetic stirrer, UV spectrophotometer.

2. Materials

Iodine, potassium iodide, pepsin, diluted hydrochloric acid solution, glycerol, sucrose, ibuprofen, polysorbate 20 (Tween 20), polysorbate 40 (Tween 40), polysorbate 80 (Tween 80), methanol, distilled water.

Experimental Methods

1. Preparation of Compound Iodide Solution

(1) Formulation

Iodine	2.5g
Potassium iodide	5g
Distilled water	add to 50ml

(2) Manufacturing process

Place potassium iodide into a mortar, and add about 25ml water and stir to dissolve. Add 2.5g iodine to the solution and grind to make it dissolve completely. Then add water to 50ml and mix well. The flow chart is shown in Figure 1－1.

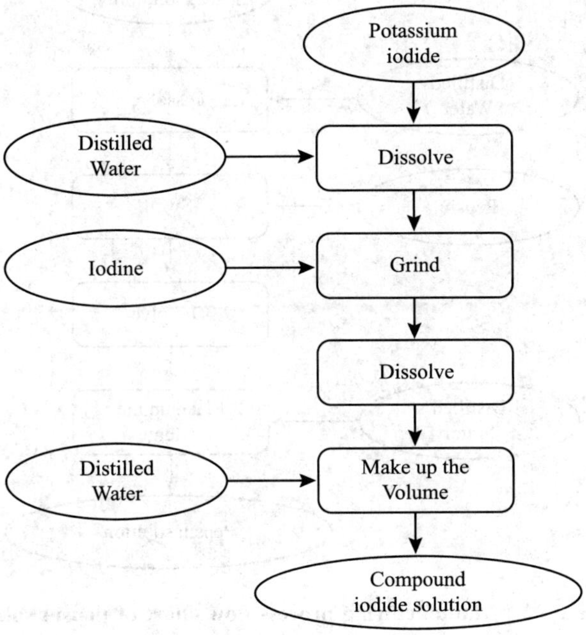

Figure 1－1　Manufacturing process flowchart of compound iodide solution.

2. Preparation of Pepsin Solution

(1) Formulation

Pepsin	3g
Diluted hydrochloric acid solution	2ml
Glycerin	20ml
Distilled water	add to 100ml

(2) Manufacturing process

Add 70ml distilled water to a beaker, add diluted hydrochloric acid solution and glycerin and stir to get a solution. Disperse pepsin onto the solution surface and let pepsin swell for about 10－30min. Stir gently to dissolve. Add water to 100ml and mix well. The flow chart is shown in Figure 1－2.

3. Preparation of Simple Syrup

(1) Formulation

Sucrose	85g
Distilled water	add to 100ml

(2) Manufacturing process

Boil 80ml of water and sucrose, and stir until they dissolve. Continue to boil for 5min. Filter the solution using 0.8μm membrane. Add the remaining water to the filtrate and mix well.

4. Determination of Solubility of Ibuprofen in Water

(1) Preparation of the standard curve

Weigh about 12mg of ibuprofen standard accurately and place in 10ml volumetric flask. Dissolve and dilute to volume with methanol. Measure accurately 0.6, 0.8, 1.0, 1.2 and 1.4ml into 100ml volumetric flask and dilute to the mark with distilled water and shake. Measure the absorbance of

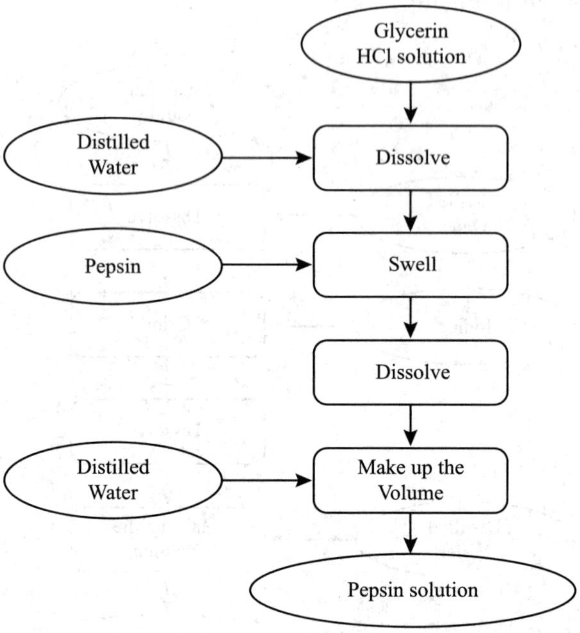

Figure 1 – 2 Manufacturing process flow chart of pepsin solution.

each solution at 221nm, using distilled water as the blank. Make linear regression using concentration (C) as the horizontal coordinate, and the absorbance (A) as the vertical coordinate.

(2) Determination of the solubility

Weigh about 50mg of ibuprofen and place in an Erlenmeyer flask. Add 250ml of water. Seal the flask. Place it in the water bath (25℃) and stir until reach the solubility equilibrium. Take suspension at 0.5, 1, 2, 4h and filter. Measure the absorbance of the solution at 221nm after dilution of 1ml of filtrate in 10ml. Put the absorbance data into the standard curve to determine the time to achieve dissolution equilibrium and to calculate the solubility of ibuprofen.

5. Solubilization of Surfactants on Ibuprofen

The effect of polysorbate 80 (Tween 80) and its adding sequence on the solubilization of ibuprofen

(1) Put 50ml distilled water into 100ml beaker and add 50mg ibuprofen. Stir for 1h. Filter through 0.45μm membrane filter. Measure accurately 0.5ml to 100ml volumetric flask and dilute to the mark with water and then measure the absorbance of the solution at 221nm. Calculate the solubility of the drug.

(2) Put 50ml distilled water into 100ml beaker and add 3g polysorbate 80 mixing well. Add 50mg ibuprofen and stir for 1h. Filter through 0.45μm membrane filter. Operate as the above procedure. Calculate the solubility of the drug.

(3) Put 50ml distilled water and 50mg ibuprofen into 100ml beaker, then add 3g polysorbate 80 mixing well. Stir for 1h. Filter through 0.45μm membrane filter. Operate as the above procedure. Calculate the solubility of the drug.

(4) Put 50mg ibuprofen into 100ml beaker and add 3g polysorbate 80 mixing well. Add 50ml distilled water and stir for 1h. Filter through 0.45μm membrane filter. Operate as the above procedure. Calculate the solubility of the drug.

Effects of the type of polysorbates(Tween) on the solubilization of ibuprofen

Take 50ml distilled water into 100ml beaker. Add 3g polysorbate 20 and mix well. Add 50mg ibuprofen and stir for 1h. Filter through 0.45μm membrane filter. Operate as the above procedure. Calculate the solubility of ibuprofen. The solubilization of polysorbate 40 and polysorbate 80 on ibuprofen shall be done as the same procedure.

Effect of the temperature on the solubilization of ibuprofen

Take 50ml distilled water, add 3g polysorbate 80 and mix well. Add 50mg ibuprofen. Stir for 1h at room temperature. Filter through 0.45μm membrane filter. Operate as the above procedure. Calculate the solubility of the drug. This experiment will also be done 40℃.

Results

The results are recorded in Table 1 - 1.

Table 1 - 1　Solubilization of polysorbates and temperature on ibuprofen

Factors investigated	Tests	Appearance of the system	Solubility(g/100ml)
Adding order	Without surfactant		
	Polysorbate 80 first, then add drug		
	Drug first, then add polysorbate 80		
	Mix polysorbate 80 with drug, then add water		
Types of polysorbates	Polysorbate 20(RT)		
	Polysorbate 40(RT)		
	Polysorbate 80(RT)		
Effect of temperature	Polysorbate 80 40℃		

Experimental Instructions

Requirements for Preview

1. To master the classification of solution.
2. To be familiar with the ways to increase the solubility of insoluble drugs.
3. To understand the types and use of surfactants.

Procedures and Precautions

1. The solubility of iodine in water is 1∶2950. Potassium iodide may effectively enhance the solubility of iodine by interacting with iodine to form a soluble complex, meanwhile, potassium iodide may reduce the volatility and irritation of Iodine. When preparing compound iodine solution, the adding order of the material should be cared. Potassium iodide should be dissolve first before insoluble iodine is added.

2. The volume of water to dissolve potassium iodide should better be 50%, which may dissolve potassium iodide rapidly and keep the higher concentration of potassium iodide beneficial to the dissolution of iodine.

3. Compound iodine solution should be preserved in airtight glass bottle without any contact with cork, rubber or metal stopper due to its oxidation character. The sample got in the experiment should be recovered in uniform.

4. The time for ibuprofen to reach dissolution equilibrium should be determined before determining the solubility. The equilibrium can be decided by the change of concentration at different time points.

5. Conditions in the solubilization test should be as consistent as possible, such as addition of active ingredient and stirring time. During solubilization experiment, the samples should be placed still for some time to facilitate the elimination of bubbles and drugs into the micelles fully.

6. The weighing process should be quick in high humidity conditions due to the ability of pepsin to absorb moisture. Pepsin can keep its activity at pH 1.5 – 2.0; however, more than 0.5% HCl may destroy its activity. Direct mixing of pepsin with HCl was not allowed for the stability concern. 20% of glycerol may adjust the taste of this preparation and help maintain the stability of pepsin. Vigorous stirring and filter with cotton or filter paper may undermine the activity and stability of pepsin.

Questions

1. What precautions should be taken in the preparation of compound iodine solution?

2. What are the factors that influence the solubility of the drug?

3. How to determine the time for the insoluble drug to reach the dissolution equilibrium?

4. What are the main factors that influence the effect of surfactants on the solubilization of insoluble drugs?

5. How to determine the adding order of diluted hydrochloric acid during the preparation of pepsin solution?

6. What are the ways to increase the solubility of drugs?

实验 2　混悬型液体制剂的制备

【目的与要求】

1. **掌握**　混悬剂和纳米混悬剂的基本制备方法。
2. **熟悉**　混悬剂中的附加剂及其粒径测定法。
3. **了解**　混悬剂的质量评定方法。

【基本概念与实验原理】

混悬剂系指难溶性固体药物分散在液体介质中所形成的非均相分散体系。混悬剂应分散均匀，放置后若有沉淀物，经振摇应易再分散。

混悬剂的物理不稳定性包括：微粒的沉降、微粒的成长与晶型转变、微粒间的斥力和范德华引力、微粒的荷电与水化等。为改善混悬剂的稳定性，常须在混悬剂中加入如下三类稳定剂。助悬剂：可增大介质黏度，降低微粒聚集速度；或被药物微粒表面吸附，形成保护膜，防止微粒间聚集或晶型转变；或使混悬剂具有触变性，增加稳定性。絮凝剂和反絮凝剂：使微粒间的斥力和引力保持一定的平衡，形成疏松的絮状沉淀，其沉降体积大，不结块，重分散性好。某些有临床特殊要求的混悬剂，其混悬粒子应细腻无絮凝，以免影响诊断的准确性，为此可加电解质减少絮凝，称为反絮凝。此类物质一般为电解质。润湿剂：使混悬剂中有较好的固－液两相结合状态。常用聚山梨酯（吐温）类、油酸山梨醇酯（司盘）类、泊洛沙姆等表面活性剂。

混悬剂的制备方法有分散法（如研磨粉碎）和凝聚法（微粒结晶法和化学反应法）。

纳米混悬剂是由纯药物粒子加入少量表面活性剂作为稳定剂，在分散介质中高度分散，形成亚微粒分散系统，粒径一般在 10～1000nm。纳米混悬剂可提高难溶性药物的饱和溶解度和溶出速率，提高生物利用度，减少用药剂量，降低不良反应，增加临床用药安全性和顺应性。制备纳米混悬剂的方法主要有高压匀质法、乳化法等。

【仪器与材料】

1. 仪器　研钵，烧杯，量筒，天平，超声仪，高压均质机，粒径及 Zeta 电位测定仪。

2. 材料　沉降硫黄，硫酸锌，聚山梨酯 80（吐温 80），樟脑醑，甘油，酮洛芬，泊洛沙姆 188，卵磷脂，蒸馏水等。

【实验内容】

一、复方硫黄洗剂的制备

1. 处方

沉降硫黄	1.5g
硫酸锌	1.5g
樟脑醑	2.5ml
聚山梨酯 80	0.2g
甘油	2g
蒸馏水	加至 50ml

2. 制备工艺　取 1.5g 沉降硫黄，置研钵中，加聚山梨酯 80 及 1ml 水，研磨 15min。加硫酸锌水溶液（1.5g 硫酸锌溶于 12.5ml 水中，摇匀即得）和甘油，同时研磨。再缓缓加入樟脑醑同时研磨，加余水，研匀即得。工艺流程图见图 2－1。

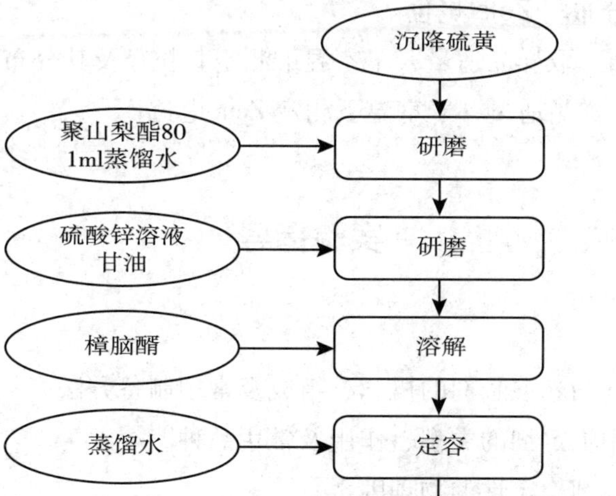

图 2－1　复方硫黄洗剂的制备工艺流程图

3. 沉降体积比 F 的测定 将配制好的洗剂置 50ml 具塞量筒中，闭塞，强力振摇 1min，记录初高度 H_0，静置 3h 后记录沉降物高度 H，按照 $F = H/H_0$ 计算沉降体积比。

二、酮洛芬纳米混悬剂的制备

1. 处方

酮洛芬	50mg
泊洛沙姆 188	0. 1g
卵磷脂	0. 1g
蒸馏水	50ml

2. 制备工艺 取泊洛沙姆 188 和卵磷脂置烧杯中，加 50ml 蒸馏水，置冰水浴中超声 15min，使均匀分散。加微粉化酮洛芬原料，超声分散 10min。将得到的粗混悬剂转入高压均质机，在 40psi 下均质 2 个循环，再在 70psi 压力下均质 10 个循环，即得。工艺流程图见图 2 - 2。

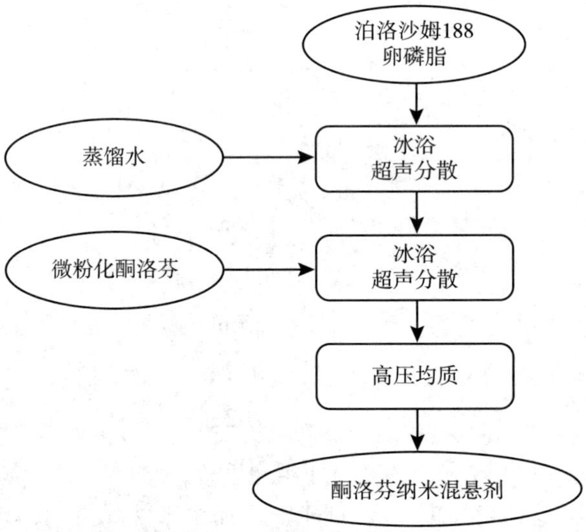

图 2 - 2 酮洛芬纳米混悬液的制备工艺流程图

3. 测定粒径及其分布与 Zeta 电位

（1）粒径及其分布 取样品适量，于室温下测定其粒径及其分布范围。

（2）Zeta 电位 取样品适量，于室温下测定 Zeta 电位。

实验指导

一、预习要求

1. 掌握 混悬剂和纳米混悬剂的概念、组成及常用制备方法。

2. 熟悉 混悬剂中稳定剂的类型、作用及常用品种。

3. 了解 影响混悬剂稳定性的物理因素。

二、操作要点和注意事项

1. 硫黄有升华硫、精制硫和沉降硫三种，其中沉降硫颗粒最细，故本品选用沉降硫。硫黄为疏水性强的物质，不易被水润湿，且表面吸附有空气，给制备混悬剂带来困难。但能被甘油所润湿，故应加入润湿剂甘油，充分研磨，使其吸附于微粒表面，增加亲水性，利于硫黄的分散。樟脑醑中含有乙醇，能使硫黄润湿，故亦可将硫黄先用樟脑醑润湿。加入樟脑醑时，应以细流慢慢加入至水中并急速搅拌，以防止樟脑醑因骤然改变溶媒而析出大颗粒。

2. 沉降体积比是判断混悬剂处方设计优劣的一个重要指标。口服混悬剂沉降体积比应不低于0.90。

3. 纳米混悬剂在进行高压均质前应尽量降低固体粒子的粒径。单一的稳定剂作用效果往往有限，可采用联合使用稳定剂。另外，高压均质应控制均质压力和均质时间。

三、思考题

1. 分析本实验中各处方中各种组分的作用。
2. 影响混悬剂物理稳定性的因素有哪些？
3. 试举一例上市口服混悬剂，说明其处方中各组分的作用。
4. 口服纳米混悬剂中可以选择哪些稳定剂？
5. 使用高压均质机时有哪些注意事项？
6. 请阐述纳米混悬液的应用。

Experiment 2　Preparation of Suspensions

扫码“学一学”

Objectives and Requirements

1. To master basic preparation methods of suspensions and nanosuspensions.
2. To be familiar with the use of additives in suspensions and the determination of the particle size.
3. To understand the quality evaluation of suspensions.

Introduction

Suspension systems are non－homogeneous dispersion system containing solid API which has difficult solubility dispersed in a liquid dispersing medium. The suspensions should disperse uniformly. If there is a precipitate after placing, the precipitate should be easy to disperse after shaking.

The physical instability of the suspensions includes: sedimentation of particles, growth of particles and polymorph transformation, the repulsion force and the van der Waals force, the charge and hydration of the particles. To improve the stability of suspensions, three kinds of stabilizers are usually used in formulations of suspensions: Suspending agent: it can increase the viscosity of the medium and therefore to decrease the rate of particle aggregation; or it can be absorbed by the surface of the drug particle to form a protection film, so that it can prevent the particle aggregation and polymorph transformations. Meanwhile, it can also make the suspension exhibit thixotropy which also helps increase the stability. Flocculation agent or deflocculation agent: it can balance the repulsion and attraction forces be polysorbate particles and can form loose floc. Its sedimentation volume is large enough to prevent agglomeration and improve the redispersibility of suspensions. In order not to affect the accuracy of the diagnosis, some kinds of suspensions have special clinical requirements that the particles should be fine and has no flocculation. For this purpose, the electrolyte can be added to reduce the flocculation, the so - called anti - flocculation. Wetting agent: it can make the suspension to have a good combination state be polysorbate solid and liquid phase. The commonly used surfactants include polysorbate (Tween), sorbitan oleate (span) and Poloxamer.

Preparation methods of suspension include dispersing method (such as grinding) and coacervation method (such as microparticle recrystallization and chemical reaction).

Nanosuspension isa submicron dispersion system containing pure drug highly dispersed by small amounts of surfactants. The size of nanosuspension is generally about 10 - 1000nm. Nanosuspension can improve the solubility and dissolution rate of insoluble drugs, improve the bioavailability, reduce the dosage, reduce adverse reactions, increase the safety and compliance. The two methods mainly used for nanosuspension preparations include high pressure homogenization method and emulsification method.

Equipment and Materials

1. Equipment

Mortar and pestle, beaker, measuring cylinder, balance, Ultra - sonifier, high pressure homogenizers, Particle size and zeta potential determination machine.

2. Materials

Precipitated sulfur, zinc sulfate, polysorbate 80 (Tween 80), camphor spiritus, glycerol, ibuprofen, sodium carboxymethyl cellulose, citric acid, simple syrup, ketoprofen, poloxamer 188, lecithin, distilled water.

Experimental Methods

1. Preparation of Compound Sulfur Lotion

(1) Formulation

Precipitated sulfur	1.5g
Zinc sulfate	1.5g
Camphor spiritus	2.5ml
Polysorbate 80	0.2g
Glycerol	2g
Distilled water	add to 50ml

(2) Manufacturing process

Add precipitated sulfur in a mortar, add polysorbate 80 and 1ml distilled water, grind for 15min. Add zinc sulfate solution (dissolve 1.5g zinc sulfate in 12.5ml water) and glycerol while grinding. Slowly add camphor spirits while grinding. Finally, add the remaining water and grind well. The flow chart is shown in Figure 2 - 1.

(3) Determination of sedimentation volume (F) of compound sulfur lotion

Place the lotion into 50ml measuring cylinders with stopper respectively. Stopper the measuring cylinders and shake for 1min. Write down the original height H_0. After 3h specified interval, the height of sedimentation H was written down, then make out the F according to $F = H/H_0$.

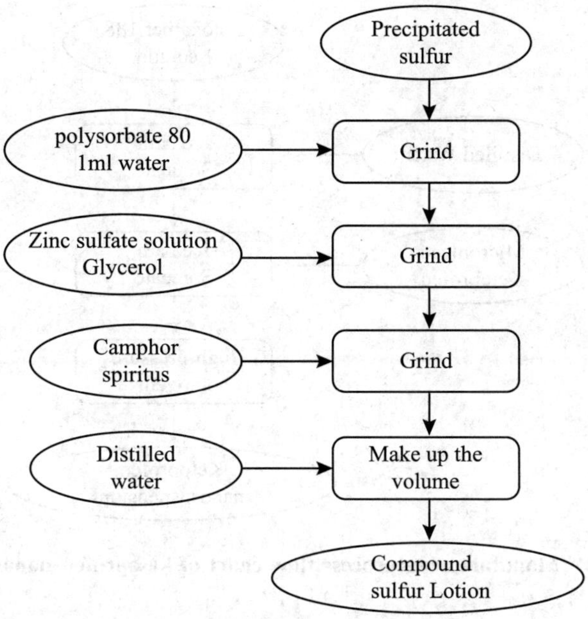

Figure 2 - 1　Manufacturing process flow chart of compound sulfur lotion.

2. Preparation of Ketoprofen Nanosuspensions

(1) Formulation

Ketoprofen	50mg
Poloxamer188	0. 1g
Lecithin	0. 1g
Distilled water	50ml

(2) Manufacturing process

Add poloxamer F68, lecithin and 50ml distilled water into a beaker. Sonicate the mixture for 15min in the ice bath to get a homogeneous dispersion. Add micronized ketoprofen and sonicate for 10min. Transfer the raw suspension into a high - pressure homogenizer. Homogenize 2 cycles at 40 psi and 10 cycles at 70psi. The flow chart is shown in Figure 2 - 2.

(3) Determine the particle size and its distribution and zeta potential

Particle size and distribution: Take the sample and measure the particle size and distribution of the sample at room temperature.

Zeta potential: Take the sample and measure the zeta potential of the sample at room temperature.

Experimental Instructions

Requirements for Preview

1. To master the concept, composition and preparation methods of the suspensions and nanosuspensions.

2. To be familiar with the types, functions of stabilizers in suspensions.

3. To understand the physical factors which influence the stability of suspensions.

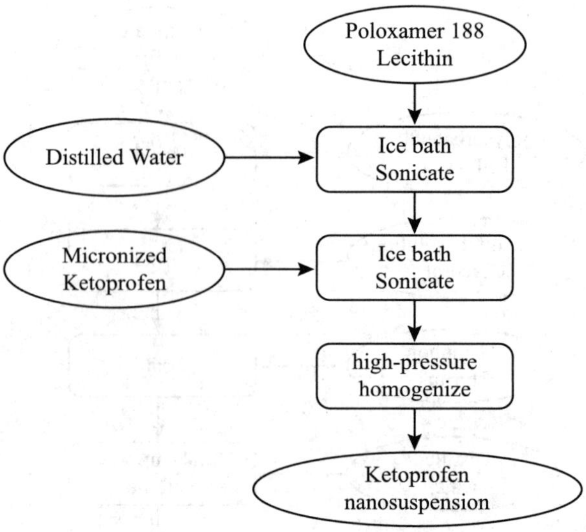

Figure 2 - 2 Manufacturing process flow chart of ketoprofen nanosuspension.

Procedures and Precautions

1. Among the three types of sulphur (sublimation sulphur, refined sulphur and precipitated sulfur), the particle size of precipitated sulfur is the finest. Therefore, it was chosen as the material to prepare the sulphur lotion. As a hydrophobic substance, sulphur cannot be wetted easily by water and its surface adsorbs lots of air, which makes it difficult for us to prepare the sulphur suspensions. However, sulphur can be wetted by glycerol serving as a wetting agent which can be adsorbed on the surface of sulphur particles to increase the hydrophilicity and facilitate the dispersion of sulphur. Camphor spiritus contains ethanol which can also wet sulphur.

2. Sedimentation volume is an important index to judge the quality of the formulation of the suspension. The sedimentation volume of the oral suspension should be no less than 0. 90.

3. Before high pressure homogenization, the size of the solid particles in nanosuspensions should be reduced as small as possible. The effect of single stabilizer is often limited, so stabilizer combination is usually used. In addition, the homogeneous pressure and homogeneous time of the high pressure homogenization should be controlled.

Questions

1. What are the functions of inactive ingredients in the formulations of this experiment?

2. What are the factors that affect the physical stability of suspensions?

3. Give an example of oral suspensions on the market and illustrate the functions of inactive ingredients in the formulation.

4. Which stabilizer can be selected in the production of oral nanosuspension?

5. What are the precautions when using the high - pressure homogenization equipment?

6. Please describe the application of nanosuspension.

实验3 乳剂型液体制剂的制备

【目的与要求】

1. **掌握** 乳剂的一般制备方法。

2. **熟悉** 测定油相乳化所需 HLB 值的方法。

3. **了解** 复乳的特点、类型及制备方法。

【基本概念与实验原理】

乳剂系指一相液体（分散相）以细小液滴的形式分散于另一相互不相溶的液体（连续相）中得到的一种非均相液体制剂。根据连续相和分散相不同分为 O/W 型或 W/O 型，常采用稀释法和染色镜检法进行鉴别。除此之外，还有复合乳剂，是由普通乳剂进一步乳化而形成的复杂乳剂体系，粒径一般在 50μm 以下，根据内外水相的组成可分为二组分二级乳（W/O/W 或 O/W/O）和三组分二级乳（$W_1/O/W_2$ 或 $O_1/W/O_2$）。目前研究最多的是 W/O/W 型复乳。

乳剂中需加入乳化剂使乳剂稳定。乳化剂类型有表面活性剂（阴离子型乳化剂、非离子型乳化剂、两性离子型乳化剂）、天然乳化剂（如阿拉伯胶、西黄蓍胶、明胶等）、固体微粒乳化剂（如氢氧化镁、氢氧化铝、氢氧化钙等）和辅助乳化剂（如十八醇、单硬脂酸甘油酯、硬脂酸等）。乳化剂的选择应根据乳剂的类型、乳化剂性能及给药途径等综合考虑，适当选择。通常将乳化剂组成混合乳化剂来使用，以防止单独使用乳化剂所产生的不稳定性。

普通乳剂的制备方法有油中乳化剂法（干胶法）、水中乳化剂法（湿胶法）、新生皂法及两相交替加入法等。复乳的制备有一步乳化法和二步乳化法。小量制备时可用乳钵，大量生产可用搅拌机、乳匀机、胶体磨、超声波乳化器完成。

【仪器与材料】

1. **仪器** 三角瓶，研钵，具塞量筒，天平，高压均质机，磁力恒温搅拌器等。

2. **材料** 氢氧化钙，花生油，液状石蜡，阿拉伯胶，西黄蓍胶，1% 糖精钠溶液，5% 羟苯乙酯乙醇溶液，聚山梨酯 80（吐温 80），油酸山梨坦（司盘 80），蒸馏水，茶多酚，豆磷脂，单硬脂酸甘油酯，大豆油，蔗糖酯等。

【实验内容】

一、W/O 型乳剂石灰搽剂的制备

1. 处方

氢氧化钙溶液	10ml
花生油	10ml

2. 制备工艺 采用新生皂法制备。取氢氧化钙溶液与花生油，置具塞三角瓶中，加塞，强力振摇约 5min，至乳剂形成，即得。

二、O/W 型液状石蜡乳的制备

1. 处方

液状石蜡	12ml

阿拉伯胶	4g
西黄蓍胶	0.5g
1%糖精钠溶液	0.1ml
5%羟苯乙酯乙醇溶液	0.1ml
香精	适量
蒸馏水	加至30ml

2. **制备工艺** 采用干胶法制备。取阿拉伯胶与西黄蓍胶粉，置干燥研钵中，加液状石蜡，充分研磨直至充分分散。加8ml蒸馏水，持续研磨直至形成初乳。加糖精钠溶液、羟苯乙酯乙醇溶液、香精及剩余量的蒸馏水，持续研磨直至乳剂形成，即得。工艺流程图见图3-1。

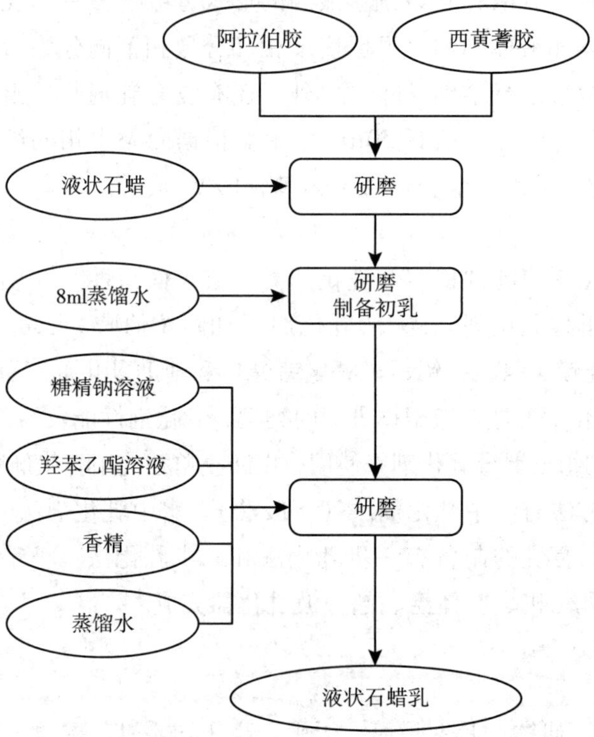

图3-1 O/W型液状石蜡乳的制备工艺流程图

三、W/O/W型茶多酚复乳的制备

1. **处方**

茶多酚	1.5g
豆磷脂	5g
单硬脂酸甘油酯	2g
大豆油	13g
蔗糖酯	1g
水	80g

2. **制备工艺** 采用二步乳化法制备。

取茶多酚溶于30g水中，作为内水相。取豆磷脂和单硬脂酸甘油酯溶于大豆油中，作为油相。取蔗糖酯，溶于50g水中，作为外水相。

在室温下持续搅拌油相（采用高剪切乳化机乳化更佳），缓慢加入内水相，继续搅拌

1min，再用高压均质机或高剪切乳化机乳化制备得到 W/O 型初乳。另搅拌外水相（500 ~ 1000r/min），加入上述初乳，搅拌 5min，即得 W/O/W 型复乳。

四、液状石蜡乳化所需 HLB 值的测定

1. 处方

处方见表 3 - 1。

表 3 - 1　液状石蜡乳处方组成

原辅料组成	处方 1	处方 2	处方 3	处方 4	处方 5
液状石蜡（ml）	8	8	8	8	8
聚山梨酯 80（吐温 80）（g）	0.3	0.6	0.9	1.3	1.6
油酸山梨坦（司盘 80）（g）	1.5	1.2	0.9	0.5	0.2
蒸馏水 加至（ml）	25	25	25	25	25

其中，$HLB_{Tween80}=15$，$HLB_{Span80}=4.3$。

2. 制备工艺　取聚山梨酯 80、油酸山梨坦，置研钵中，加液状石蜡，研磨 5min 形成均匀分散物。加水，持续研磨 5 分钟，即得。工艺流程图见图 3 - 2。

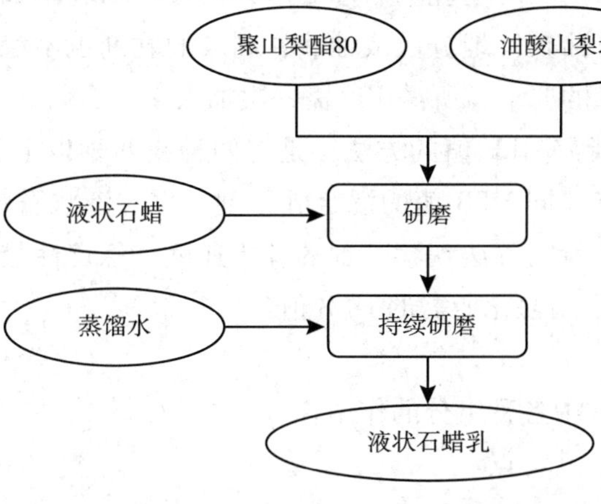

图 3 - 2　液状石蜡乳的制备工艺流程图

将所制备的乳剂转移至具塞量筒中，分别于第 5、10、30 和 45min 测量水层高度，记录于表 3 - 2 中，判断液状石蜡乳化所需 HLB 值（判断依据：分层速度最慢者为最稳定乳化剂，该 HLB 值即为液状石蜡所需 HLB 值）。

$$HLB_{AB}=W_A\cdot HLB_A+W_B\cdot HLB_B$$

式中，W_A、W_B分别为两种乳化剂的质量分数。

结果记录在表 3 - 2 中。

表 3 - 2　不同处方液状石蜡乳分层速率数据

处方号	混合乳化剂的 HLB 值	时间（min）			
		5	10	30	45
1					
2					
3					
4					
5					

实验指导

一、预习要求

1. **掌握** 常用的乳化剂。

2. **熟悉** 干胶法、湿胶法、新生皂法及二步乳化法。

3. **了解** 制备乳剂常用的设备。

二、操作要点和注意事项

1. 石灰搽剂 W/O 型乳剂。其中的乳化剂系氢氧化钙与花生油中所含的少量游离脂肪酸经皂化反应所形成的钙皂，此钙皂可再乳化花生油而生成 W/O 型乳剂。其他植物油（如菜油、麻油等）也含有少量游离脂肪酸，可替代本品中的花生油。制备石灰搽剂时，容器内不可装量太多，最好不超过容器体积的 2/3，振摇时用力要大，时间要较长，不要看到乳化剂一产生就不振摇了，一般 3 ~ 5 分钟。

2. 液状石蜡乳系 O/W 型乳剂，在制备初乳时，添加的水量不足或加水过慢时，易形成 W/O 型初乳，且难以转变成 O/W 型乳剂，形成后易破裂；初乳中如果添加水量过多，因外相水液黏度较低，不能将油较好地分散成油滴，制成的乳剂也不稳定和易破裂。故操作上应遵守用干胶法制备初乳的要求，所需用水需一次加入。

3. 测定液状石蜡乳化所需 HLB 值的方法，是将两种或两种以上已知 HLB 值的乳化剂按不同重量比例，配成具有不同 HLB 值的混合乳化剂，再与液状石蜡制备成一系列乳剂，在室温条件下或采用加速试验的方法观察乳剂的乳析速度。稳定性最佳的乳剂所用混合乳化剂的 HLB 值，即为液状石蜡乳化所需的 HLB 值。

三、思考题

1. 分析本实验中各处方中各种组分的作用。

2. 请叙述乳剂的类型及其特点。

3. 如何提高乳剂的稳定性？

4. 试举一例上市口服乳剂，说明其处方中各组分的作用。

5. 乳剂的制备方法有哪些？各有什么特点？

6. 请设计维生素 E 皮肤用乳剂的处方与制备工艺。

扫码“学一学”

Experiment 3 Preparation of Emulsions

Objectives and Requirements

1. To master the commonly used preparation methods of emulsions.

2. To be familiar with the methods of determining the required HLB value to emulsify the oil.

3. To understand the characteristics, types and preparation methods of multiple emulsions.

Introduction

Emulsions is defined as a phase of liquid (the dispersed phase) in the form of tiny droplets dispersed in another mutually immiscible liquid (the continuous phase) of a heterogeneous phase liquid preparation. According to the different continuous phase and dispersed phase, emulsions can be divided into O/W type or W/O type. Dilution method and staining microscopic method are often used to identify the types of emulsions. In addition to the primary emulsion, there is a multiple emulsion with the droplet size less than 50μm, which is a complex emulsion system formed through further emulsification of the primary emulsion. The multiple emulsion could be divided into two two-component secondary emulsion (W/O/W or O/W/O) and three-component secondary emulsion (W_1/O/W_2 or O_1/W/O_2), depending on the composition of the inner and outer water phase. At present, the W/O/W type multiple emulsion is well studied.

Emulsifying agents are indispensable for stabilizing the emulsion. There are various types of emulsifiers including surfactants (e.g. anionic emulsifiers, nonionic emulsifiers, amphoteric ionic emulsifiers), natural emulsifiers (such as acacia, tragacanth, gelatin), solid particles emulsifiers and auxiliary emulsifiers (such as octadecanol, glycerin monostearate, stearic acid). The choice of emulsifying agents should be based on comprehensive consideration of the type emulsions, emulsifiers' performance and route of administration. The emulsifiers are often mixed to use in order to prevent instability.

There are various methods to prepare emulsions, such as emulsifier-in-oil method, emulsifier-in-water method, nascent soap method and two-phase alternating join method. Preparation of the multiple emulsions has one-step emulsification method and two-step emulsification method. Mortar can be used when preparing small amount of emulsions, while mixer, milk mix machine, colloid mill, and ultrasonic emulsification are employed in large-scale preparation.

Equipment and Materials

1. Equipment

Flasks, mortar, cylinder with a stopper, balance, high-pressure homogenization machine, magnetic stirrer.

2. Materials

Calcium hydroxide, peanut oil, liquid paraffin, acacia, tragacanth, 1% sodium saccharin, 5% ethylparaben alcohol solution, polysorbate 80 (Tween 80), sorbitan oleate (span 80), distilled water, tea polyphenols, soy lecithin, glycerin monostearate, soybean oil, sucrose esters.

Experimental Methods

1. Preparation of Lime Liniment (W/O Type Emulsion)

(1) Formulation

Calcium hydroxide solution	10ml
Peanut oil	10ml

(2) Manufacturing process

Nascent soap method is used. Add calcium hydroxide solution and peanut oil into a flask, stopper, strongly shake for several minutes until the emulsion is formed.

2. Preparation of Liquid Paraffin Emulsion (O/W Type Emulsion)

(1) Formulation

Liquid paraffin	12ml

Acacia	4g
Tragacanth	0. 5g
1% Sodium saccharin solution	QS
5% Ethylparaben alcohol solution	0. 1ml
Flavor	QS
Distilled water	add to 30ml

(2) Manufacturing process

Emulsifier – in – oil method is employed. Add acacia and tragacanth gum in a dry mortar and mix, add liquid paraffin and grind until the two gums dispersed completely. Add 8ml water and grind continuously until formation of a primary emulsion. Add sodium saccharin solution, ethylparaben alcohol solution, flavor and residuary water. Keep grinding until the emulsion is formed. The flow is shown in Figure 3 – 1.

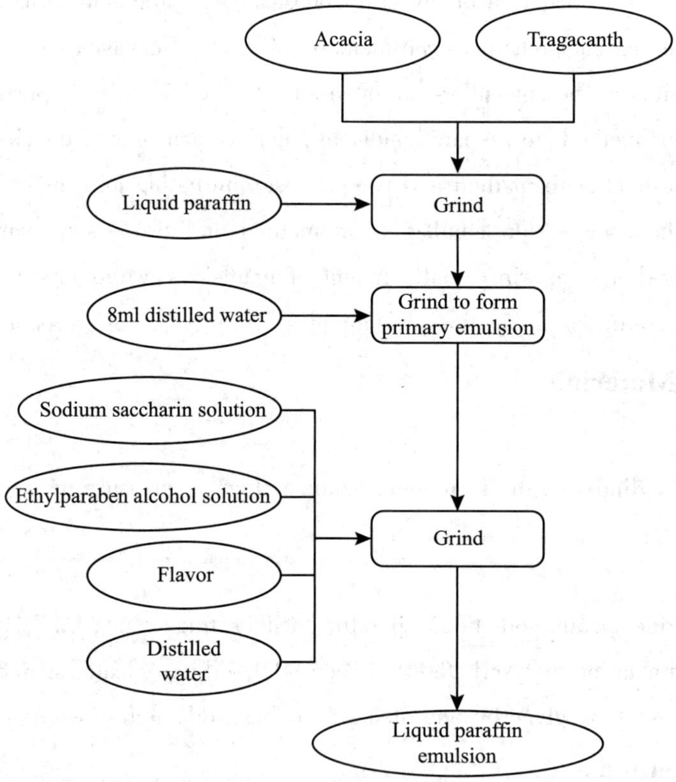

Figure 3 – 1 Manufacturing process flow chart of liquid paraffin emulsion.

3. Preparation of W/O/W Type Multiple Emulsion

(1) Formulation

Tea polyphenols	1. 5g
Soybean lecithin	5g
Glycerinmonostearate	2g
Soybean oil	13g
Sucrose esters	1g
Water	80g

(2) Manufacturing process

Two-step emulsification method is used.

Dissolve the polyphenols in 30g water as the internal water phase. Dissolve bean phospholipids and glycerin monostearate in soybean oil as oil phase. Dissolve sucrose ester in 50g water as external water phase.

Stir the oil phase at room temperature (high shear emulsifying machine would be better), add internal water phase slowly with continuous stirring for another 1min, then, transfer it into high-pressure homogenizer (or high shear emulsifying machine) to prepare W/O primary emulsion. Stir the external water phase (500-1000r/min), add the primary emulsion slowly into the external water phase with continuous stirring for another 5min, and W/O/W emulsion would be obtained.

4. Determination of Required HLB to Emulsify Liquid Paraffin

(1) Formulations

As shown in Table 3-1.

Table 3-1　Composition of five groups of liquid paraffin emulsion

Composition	Group 1	Group 2	Group 3	Group 4	Group 5
Liquid paraffin (ml)	8	8	8	8	8
Polysorbate 80 (Tween 80) (g)	0.3	0.6	0.9	1.3	1.6
Sorbitan oleate (Span 80) (g)	1.5	1.2	0.9	0.5	0.2
Distilled water (ml)	add to 25	add to 25	add to 25	add to 25	add to 25

$HLB_{Tween80} = 15$, $HLB_{Span80} = 4.3$.

(2) Manufacturing process

Add polysorbate 80 and sorbitan oleate into a dry mortar, add liquid paraffin, grind for 5min to form a uniform dispersion. Add distilled water under grinding. Then grind for another 5minutes. The flow chart is shown in Figure 3-2.

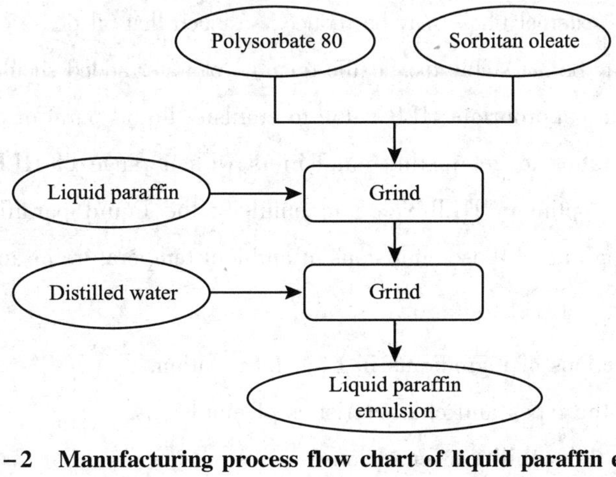

Figure 3-2　Manufacturing process flow chart of liquid paraffin emulsion.

Transfer emulsion into measuring cylinders and record the height of water layer at time 5, 10, 15 and 45min. The results are recorded in Table 3-2. Judge the HLB value for liquid paraffin emulsification. The slowest stratification speed is the most stable emulsifier, and the HLB value is the value required for liquid paraffin.

Table 3 – 2 Data recorded for the stability of liquid paraffin emulsion

Group	HLB Value	Time(min)			
		5	10	30	45
1					
2					
3					
4					
5					

Experimental Instructions

Requirements for Preview

1. To master the emulsifying agent commonly used.

2. To be familiar with the emulsifying – in – oil method, emulsifier – in – water method, emulsifier – in – water method and nascent soap method.

3. To understand the equipment used in the preparation of the emulsions.

Procedures and Precautions

1. This W/O type of lime liniment was made by nascent soap method. The emulsifier in the formulation is a nascent calcium soap generated from reaction between calcium hydroxide solution and free fatty acid in peanut oil. Other vegetable oil, such as rape oil and benne oil also contain a small amount of free fatty acid, so the peanut oil in the formulation can be replaced by them. When preparing lime liniment, container should not install too many ingredients (no more than 2/3 of container volume). The shaking force should be strong enough for a long period (generally 3 – 5min).

2. In preparing this O/W type of liquid paraffin emulsion, inadequate water or too low adding speed may result in W/O primary emulsion and emulsion cracking. If primary emulsion contains too much water, the viscosity of the external phase may be reduced so much that oil phase cannot be dispersed well; the resulting emulsion may be not stable too. So, the quantity of water added should be well controlled.

3. In determining the appropriate HLB value to emulsify liquid paraffin, we should combine two emulsifiers at different ratios to get mixing emulsifiers with a range of HLB value and prepare a series of emulsions. The optimum HLB value to emulsify the liquid paraffin can be obtained by determining the creaming rate of those emulsions at ambient temperature or accelerated experiments.

Questions

1. Analyze the functions of ingredients in each formulation.

2. Please describe the types and characteristics of emulsions.

3. How to improve the stability of emulsions?

4. Give an example of oral emulsions on the market and illustrate the functions of inactive ingredients in the formulation.

5. What are the preparation methods of emulsions? What are their characteristics?

6. Please design the formulation and preparation process of vitamin E emulsion for skin use.

第二部分　半固体制剂的制备

实验 4　软膏剂与乳膏剂的制备

【目的与要求】

1. **掌握**　不同类型软膏和乳膏基质的制备方法。
2. **熟悉**　药物、基质的性质及药物的加入方法。
3. **了解**　软膏剂和乳膏剂的质量评价方法。

【基本概念与实验原理】

软膏剂系指药物与油脂性或水溶性基质混合制成的均匀的半固体外用制剂。因药物在基质中分散状态不同，有溶液型软膏剂和混悬型软膏剂之分。溶液型软膏剂为药物溶解（或共熔）于基质或基质组分中制成的软膏剂；混悬型软膏剂为药物细粉均匀分散于基质中制成的软膏剂。

乳膏剂系指药物溶解或分散于乳状液型基质中形成的均匀的半固体外用制剂。乳膏剂由于基质不同，可分为水包油型乳膏剂与油包水型乳膏剂。

眼用软膏剂的基质一般由凡士林、羊毛脂及液状石蜡组成。眼用基质应纯净、均匀、细腻、对眼无刺激性，并在150℃干热灭菌1h以上，过滤后备用。

【仪器与材料】

1. **仪器**　蒸发皿，烧杯，玻璃棒，水浴装置，电炉，温度计，显微镜等。
2. **材料**　硬脂酸，单硬脂酸甘油酯，白凡士林，甘油，液状石蜡，羊毛脂，三乙醇胺，氢氧化钙，羧甲基纤维素钠，油酸山梨坦（司盘80），蒸馏水等。

【实验内容】

一、油/水型乳剂基质的制备

1. 处方

硬脂酸	4.8g
单硬脂酸甘油酯	1.4g
液状石蜡	2.4g
白凡士林	0.4g
羊毛脂	2.0g
三乙醇胺	0.16g
蒸馏水	加至40.0g

2. 制备工艺 按处方，称取硬脂酸、单硬脂酸甘油酯、液状石蜡、白凡士林及羊毛脂，置蒸发皿中，于水浴上加热至80℃左右混合熔化，得到A液。另将三乙醇胺和蒸馏水置烧杯中，于水浴上亦加热至80℃左右，得到B液。在加温下（80℃左右）将B液缓缓倾入A液中，边加边搅拌，直到冷凝，即得乳白色细腻的基质。

3. 用途 本品为雪花膏的一种基质。

二、水/油型乳剂基质Ⅰ的制备

1. 处方

单硬脂酸甘油酯	0.85g
蜂蜡	0.25g
石蜡	3.75g
硬脂酸	0.625g
液状石蜡	20.5g
白凡士林	3.35g
油酸山梨坦	0.5g
氢氧化钙	0.05g
羟苯乙酯	0.1g
香精	适量
蒸馏水	20.0g

2. 制备工艺 按处方，称取单硬脂酸甘油酯、蜂蜡、石蜡、硬脂酸置蒸发皿中，于水浴上加热熔化，再加入白凡士林、液状石蜡、油酸山梨坦，加热至80℃左右，得到A液。另将氢氧化钙、羟苯乙酯、香精溶于蒸馏水中加热至80℃，得到B液。将B液缓缓倾入A液中，边加边搅拌，直到冷凝，即得乳白色细腻的基质。

3. 用途 本品为冷霜的一种基质。

三、水/油型乳剂基质Ⅱ的制备

1. 处方

		HLB值
单硬脂酸甘油酯	4.0g	3.8
石蜡	4.0g	4.0
液状石蜡（重质）	20.0g	4.0
白凡士林	2.0g	5.0
油酸山梨坦	0.1g	4.3
OP乳化剂	0.2g	15.0
氯甲酚	0.04g	
蒸馏水	10.0g	

2. 制备工艺 按处方，称取单硬脂酸甘油酯、石蜡置蒸发皿中，于水浴上加热熔化，再加入白凡士林、液状石蜡、油酸山梨坦，至完全熔化后保持温度80℃，得到A液。将同温的OP乳化剂和氯甲酚水溶液（B液）加入上述A液中，边加边不断顺向搅拌，至呈乳白色稠厚状，凝固，即得。

3. 用途 本品为冷霜的一种基质。

四、水溶性基质的制备

1. 处方

羧甲基纤维素钠	1.2g
甘油	3.0g
羟苯乙酯	0.04g
蒸馏水	加至 20.0g

2. **制备工艺**　将羧甲基纤维素钠与甘油在乳钵中研匀，加入适量蒸馏水使溶解，加入溶有防腐剂的水溶液研匀，加蒸馏水至全量，即得。

3. **用途**　本品为水凝胶基质。

五、软膏剂质量评价方法

1. **乳剂型软膏基质类型鉴别**　有染色法和显微镜观察法等。染色法的鉴别方法是：加苏丹红油溶液，若连续相呈红色则为 W/O 型乳剂；加亚甲蓝水溶液，若连续相呈蓝色则为 O/W 型乳剂。

2. **稳定性试验**　将各基质均匀装入密闭容器中，编号后分别置烘箱（39±1℃）、室温（25±3℃）和冰箱（5±2℃）中 1 个月，检查其稠度、失水、pH、色泽、均匀性以及霉败等现象。

3. **基质配伍试验**　将 5g 基质与主药按常用浓度制成软膏后，置密闭容器中，贮存一定时间，观察基质是否被破坏。

实验指导

一、预习要求

1. **掌握**　常用软膏基质的主要性质，肥皂类乳化剂的主要特征。

2. **熟悉**　常用非离子型表面活性剂的性质、应用等方面的区别。

3. **了解**　软膏剂的一般制法以及用乳化法制备乳剂型基质的注意事项。

二、操作要点和注意事项

1. 采用乳化法制备 W/O 型或 O/W 型乳剂基质时，油相和水相应分别于水浴上加热并保持温度 80℃，然后将水相缓缓加入油相中，边加边不断顺向搅拌。若不是沿一个方向搅拌，往往难以制得合格的乳剂基质。

2. 乳剂基质处方中，有时存在少量辅助乳化剂，目的在于增加乳剂的稳定性。例如处方一中的单硬脂酸甘油酯即为辅助乳化剂。

3. 乳剂基质的类型决定于乳化剂的类型、水相与油相的比例等因素。例如，乳化剂虽为 O/W 型，但处方中水相的量比油相量少时，即使使用了 O/W 型乳化剂，往往也难以得到稳定的 O/W 型乳剂，会转相而生成 W/O 型乳剂基质或破乳。

4. OP 乳化剂商品名为 0340 乳化剂 OP［烷基芳基聚乙二醇醚］，系非离子型表面活性剂，HLB 值 15.0，为 O/W 型乳化剂。易溶于水，1% 水溶液的 pH 为 5～7，遇酸、碱、重金属、盐类和硬水均较稳定，但遇大量铁、镁、铝、铜等离子时，表面活性有所降低。

5. CMC－Na 等水溶性高分子物质制备溶液时，可先将其撒在水面上，静置数小时，使其慢慢吸水充分膨胀后，再加热即溶解。若搅动则易成团块，水分难以进入而很难得到溶液。若先用甘油研磨分散开后，再加入水时则不会结成团块，能较快溶解。

三、思考题

1. 在 O/W 型乳剂基质的处方中，乳化剂应满足什么要求？

2. 根据实验结果，含一价新生皂的乳剂基质的外观、稳定性如何？

3. W/O 型乳剂基质第一个处方中的乳化剂是什么？

4. W/O 型乳剂基质第二个处方中油相被乳化所需的 HLB 值为多少？混合乳化剂的 HLB 值为多少？该乳剂基质属于哪种类型？为什么？

5. 水溶性基质的常用辅料有哪些？

6. 乳膏剂中药物的加入方法有哪些，分别适用于哪种类型的药物？

扫码“学一学”

Experiment 4　Preparation of Ointments and Creams

Objective and Requirements

1. To master preparation of different types of bases for ointments and creams.

2. To be familiar with the methods of adding drugs into bases.

3. To understand the evaluation of ointments and creams.

Introduction

Ointments are semisolid preparations made of medicaments with water soluble base or oleaginous bases, which are intended for external application to the skin. Depended on the dispersed state of drug in the matrix, ointments could be divided into two types: solution type ointments and a suspension type ointments. For a solution type ointment, drugs are dissolved in the base or one ingredient of the base, while drug powder is uniformly dispersed in the base of a suspension type ointments.

Creams are semi - solid preparations, in which drugs are dissolved or uniformly dispersed in a emulsion base. According to the types of emulsion base, creams could be divided into water - in - oil type creams and oil type - in - water creams.

Ophthalmic ointments are ointments for application to the eye. Special precautions must be taken in the preparation of ophthalmic ointments. Ophthalmic bases should be pure, uniform and exquisite. They are manufactured from sterilized ingredients under rigidly aseptic conditions. Usually, the ointment base is composed of vaseline, lanolin and liquid paraffin, which should be dry sterilized under 150℃ for more than 1h and filtered.

Equipment and Materials

1. Equipment

Evaporating dish, water bath, electric hot plate, analytical balance, thermometer, microscope etc.

2. Materials

Stearic acid, glycerol monostearate, glycerol, liquid paraffin, vaseline, wool fat, triethanolamine, beeswax, calcium hydroxide, CMC – Na, sorbitan oleate (Span 80), nonoxynol – 10, distilled water etc.

Experimental Methods

1. Preparation of O/W Emulsion Base

(1) Formulation

Stearic acid	4.8g
Glycerolmonostearate	1.4g
Liquid paraffin	2.4g
Whitevaseline	0.4g
Wool fat	2.0g
Triethanolamine	0.16g
Distilled water	add to 40.0g

(2) Manufacturing process

Weigh and add stearic acid, glycerol monostearate, liquid paraffin, vaseline and wool fat into evaporating dish, which the mixture is used as A solution. Add triethanolamine and distilled water into a beaker, which the solution is used as B solution. The two containers are heated to 80℃ in a water bath and kept until melting completely. Pour A solution into B solution slowly, and stir them fully. Cool at room temperature, then the O/W emulsion base can be got.

(3) Application

This product is a base that belongs to face cream.

2. Preparation of W/O Emulsion Base Ⅰ

(1) Formulation

Glycerolmonostearate	0.85g
Beeswax	0.25g
Paraffin	3.75g
Stearic Acid	0.625g
Liquid paraffin	20.5g
Whitevaseline	3.35g
Sorbitan oleate (Span 80)	0.5g
Calcium hydroxide	0.05g
Ethylparaben	0.1g
Essence	QS
Distilled water	20.0g

(2) Manufacturing process

Weigh and add glycerol monostearate, beeswax, paraffin and stearic acid into the evaporating dish which is above water bath. When the mixture is melted, add vaseline, liquid paraffin and aluminum distearate into it. The above mixture is used as the A solution. Calcium hydroxide and ethylparaben are dissolved in distilled water. The degree of water is about 80℃. The solution is used as the B solution. A stir is needed when add B solution into A solution. Cool the base to the room temperature, then the W/O emulsion base can be got.

(3) Application

This product is a base that belongs to sober.

3. Preparation of W/O Emulsion Base Ⅱ

(1) Formulation

		HLB Value
Glycerolmonostearate	4. 0g	3. 8
Paraffin	4. 0g	4. 0
Liquid paraffin (heavy)	20. 0g	4. 0
Whitevaseline	2. 0g	5. 0
Span 80	0. 1g	4. 3
Nonoxynol – 10	0. 2g	15. 0
Chlorocresol	0. 04g	
Distilled water	10. 0g	

(2) Manufacturing process

Weigh and add glycerol monostearate and paraffin into the evaporating dish which is above the water bath. Then add vaseline, liquid paraffin, span 80 into this evaporating dish. This mixture is used as the A solution. Nonoxynol – 10 and chlorocresol are dissolved in distilled water. This solution is used as the B solution. The degree of water is about 80℃. Add the B solution into the A solution with clockwise stirring Cool the mixture, then the W/O emulsion base can be got.

(3) Application

This product is a base that belongs to sober.

4. Preparation of Water Soluble Bases

(1) Formulation

CMC – Na	1. 2g
Glycerol	3. 0g
Ethylparaben	0. 04g
Distilled water	add to 20. 0g

(2) Manufacturing process

Weigh and add CMC – Na and glycerol into a mortar, grind and mix them. Then add distilled water and preservatives into it. Grind and mix them fully, the water – soluble bases can be got.

(3) Application

This product is a hydrogel base.

5. Evaluation or Determination on Ointments and Creams

(1) Identification of the styles of the emulsion base

Add sudan red solution or methylene blue solution into the ointment, and observe the color of the base. The type is W/O if the continuous phase shows red while O/W if blue.

(2) Stability test

Exam the pH, moisture content, color, viscosity and uniformity etc. of ointments after one month's storage in oven (39 ± 1℃), room temperature (25 ± 3℃), refrigerator (5 ± 2℃)

respectively.

(3) Base compatibility test

Prepare ointment with 5g of base and drug according to general concentration. Keep in closed container for some time, and then observe the base's change.

Experimental Instructions

Requirements for Preview

1. To preview the character of general bases of ointments and creams, and master the characteristics of the emulsifying agent.

2. To be familiar with the difference of characters and applications of general nonionic surfactant.

3. To know the general preparation of ointments and the precautions of emulsification.

Procedures and Precautions

1. Oil phase and water phase should be kept at 80℃ respectively when prepared by emulsification. Then add the water phase into oil phase slowly in the clockwise agitation. Otherwise, qualified bases cannot be got.

2. Auxiliary emulsifying agents, such as glycerol monostearate, can help emulsifying agents to stabilize the bases.

3. The styles of emulsions are decided by styles of emulsifying agents, the amounts of the oil phase and the water phase. For example, stable O/W emulsions cannot be prepared if the proportion of the water phase is low although O/W emulsifiers are used, which will only convert to W/O emulsion bases or demulsification.

4. Nonoxynol – 10 is a nonionic surfactant that has a HLB value of 15.0. It is a O/W emulsifier, soluble in water and pH 5 – 7 with a concentration of 1%, stable when contact with acid, base, heavy metals, salts and hard water. But its surface activity decreases if meet with considerable iron, magnesium, aluminium or copper ion.

5. CMC – Na is a kind of macromolecules. There are two processes in the dissolution of macromolecule. The first step is the process of swelling. The second step is the process of dissolving. They will be aggregate if stirring water at the beginning step of dissolution, which prevents water from permeating into the inside of the macromolecules. The problem can be solved if grinding with glycerol completely first.

Questions

1. What is the emulsifying agent in O/W emulsioncream base?

2. How about the appearance and stability of the cream base containing monatomic soap according to the experimental results?

3. What is the emulsifying agent in the first formulation of W/O emulsioncream base?

4. Calculate the HLB value of the oil phase in the second formulation of W/O. What is the HLB value of the multi – emulsifying agent? Does the cream base refer to the type of O/W or W/O?

5. What are the common excipients for water - soluble substrates?

6. What are the methods of adding drugs into creams, and which type of drugs are applied separately?

实验 5　不同类型软膏剂和乳膏剂的制备及透皮吸收实验

【目的与要求】

1. **掌握**　不同类型软膏剂和乳膏剂基质的制备方法。
2. **熟悉**　不同类型软膏剂和乳膏剂基质对药物释放的影响。
3. **了解**　经皮渗透实验用皮肤的处理及药物释放速率参数的测定。

【基本概念与实验原理】

经皮渗透法是研究软膏中药物释放的体外测定方法。该法是将软膏涂在离体皮肤表面，置于扩散池中，在维持动态条件下，测定单位时间内通过皮肤的药量。通过比较药物透皮速率及时滞可分析基质对药物渗透的影响。

药物的经皮渗透是被动扩散过程，本实验把皮肤看作简单的膜，在维持皮肤两侧浓度梯度条件下，当皮肤扩散达到伪稳态时，单位面积累积渗透量 Q（$\mu g/cm^2$）与扩散时间 t 有如下关系：

$$Q = kt$$

式中，k 是渗透系数，可以从稳态时 Q 对 t 作图所得直线斜率计算。该直线在横轴 t 上的截距即为时滞 T_1（图 5-1）。

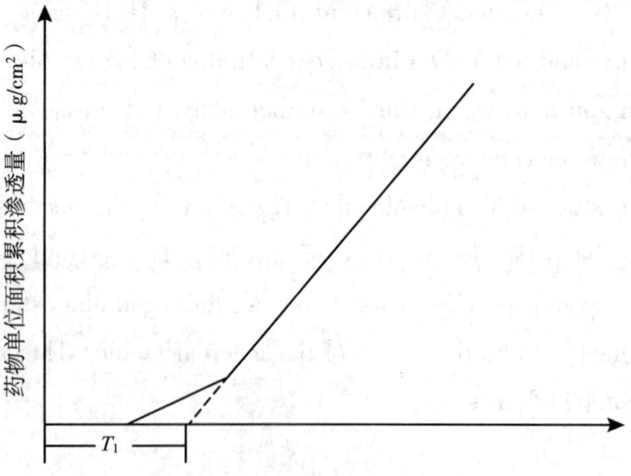

图 5-1　药物单位面积累积渗透量-时间曲线

软膏剂系指药物与油脂性或水溶性基质混合制成的均匀的半固体外用制剂。乳膏剂系指药物溶解或分散于乳状液型基质中形成的均匀的半固体外用制剂。乳膏剂由于基质不同，可分为水包油型乳膏剂与油包水型乳膏剂。基质除起赋形剂的作用外，对软膏质量起重要作用。基质在一定程度上影响药物的释放、穿透和吸收。由于实验条件的不同，得到的结果有时也不一致。释药速度顺序依次为：水溶性基质 > O/W 型基质 > W/O 型基质 > 油溶性基质。故水溶性基质中的药物释放、穿透、吸收最快，油脂溶性基质中最差。

【仪器与材料】

1. 仪器　紫外 - 可见分光光度计，电热恒温水浴，多功能磁力搅拌器，改进 Franz 扩散池，微孔滤膜（Φ25mm × 0.45μm），试管（10ml），注射器（5ml），吸量管（1ml），量瓶（10ml，250ml），烧杯（50ml，100ml），刮刀，手术剪，手术镊，蒸发皿，研钵等。

2. 材料　小白鼠（18 ~ 22g），水杨酸，脱毛剂（6% Na_2S 水溶液），显色剂（硫酸铁铵溶液），硬脂酸，单硬脂酸甘油酯，液状石蜡，白凡士林，羊毛脂，三乙醇胺，聚山梨酯 80（吐温 80），蜂蜡，石蜡，油酸山梨坦 80（司盘 80），氢氧化钙，羧甲基纤维素钠，甘油，蒸馏水等。

【实验内容】

一、油/水型水杨酸乳膏的制备

1. 处方

水杨酸	2.0g
硬脂酸	4.8g
单硬脂酸甘油酯	1.4g
白凡士林	2.4g
羊毛脂	0.4g
三乙醇胺	0.16g
聚山梨酯 80	0.04g
蒸馏水	加至 40g

2. 制备工艺　将水杨酸研细后过 80 目筛，备用。按处方，称取硬脂酸、单硬脂酸甘油酯、白凡士林及羊毛脂，置蒸发皿中，于水浴加热至 80℃左右，得到 A 液；另将三乙醇胺、聚山梨酯 80、蒸馏水置烧杯中，于水浴加热至 80℃左右，得到 B 液。在等温下将 B 液缓缓倒入 A 液中，边加边搅拌，直至冷凝，即得乳白色细腻的基质。将以上备用的水杨酸加入基质，搅拌均匀，即得。

二、水/油型水杨酸乳膏的制备

1. 处方

水杨酸	2.5g
单硬脂酸甘油酯	0.85g
蜂蜡	0.25g
石蜡	3.75g
硬脂酸	0.625g
液状石蜡	20.5g
白凡士林	3.35g
油酸山梨坦	0.5g
氢氧化钙	0.05g
蒸馏水	20.0g

2. **制备工艺** 将水杨酸研细后过 80 目筛，备用。称取处方量的单硬脂酸甘油酯、蜂蜡、石蜡及硬脂酸置于蒸发皿中，于水浴上加热熔化，再加入白凡士林、液状石蜡、油酸山梨坦，加热至 80℃左右，得到 A 液。将氢氧化钙与水混悬好后，得到 B 液。在等温下将 B 液缓缓倒入 A 液中，边加边搅拌，直至冷凝，即得乳白色细腻的基质。将以上备用的水杨酸加入基质，搅拌均匀，即得。

三、水溶性基质水杨酸软膏制备

1. **处方**

水杨酸	1.3g
羧甲基纤维素钠	3.0g
甘油	3.0g
蒸馏水	加至 20g

2. **制备工艺** 将水杨酸研细后过 80 目筛，备用。将羧甲基纤维素钠与甘油在研钵中研匀，加入适量蒸馏水使溶解，加入水溶液研匀，加蒸馏水至全量，分次少量加入以上备用的水杨酸，混匀，即得。

四、油脂性基质水杨酸软膏的制备

1. **处方**

水杨酸	0.25g
白凡士林	5.0g

2. **制备工艺** 将水杨酸研细后过 80 目筛，备用。将凡士林置于蒸发皿中，在水浴上熔化，待温度降至 60℃左右加入以上备用的水杨酸，边加边研至凝固即可。

五、离体小鼠皮肤的制备

取体重 18 ~ 22g 的小鼠，断颈处死，剪去腹部绒毛，用脱毛剂（含 7% 硫化钠、1% 肥皂粉、2% 淀粉）涂抹均匀脱毛，3min 后用生理盐水冲洗干净，剥离皮肤，除去皮下脂肪组织，用生理盐水洗净，备用。

六、标准曲线的制备

精密称取水杨酸对照品 125.0mg，置 250ml 量瓶中，加水适量，振摇，待全溶后，加水至刻度。吸取上述溶液 1.0，2.0，3.0，4.0，5.0，6.0 和 7.0ml 置 25ml 量瓶中，加水定容，分别吸取 2.5ml 置试管中，加 8% 硫酸铁铵显色剂 0.5ml，混匀，于波长 530nm 处测定吸光度 A。

七、渗透扩散装置

智能透皮实验仪 TP - 6 型如图 5 - 2 所示，由温度控制、电机转速控制、时间控制三部分组成，包括恒温水浴箱、控制箱、操作台、透皮扩散池、补液瓶和连接管等。其中渗透扩散装置由上下两筒状玻璃对合而成，皮肤夹于上下两室之间，上室为扩散室，下室为接受室，在接受室底部有一取样管，供取液用。渗透扩散面积约 2.00cm^2。渗透扩散装置置恒温水浴中，温度维持 37 ± 1℃，并以多功能搅拌器维持接受室动态环境。

八、透皮吸收实验

1. **实验操作** 将预处理好的小鼠皮肤固定在两室之间，扩散室中加入软膏 2g，固定。接受室中加满生理盐水，记录体积，持续搅拌，分别于 1，2，3，4，6，8，12h 定时取样 5.0ml（立即补充 5.0ml 生理盐水），过滤。取续滤液 2.5ml 置于试管中，加入 0.5ml 硫酸铁铵显色剂，混匀。另吸取空白皮肤浸泡滤液 2.5ml，加入 0.5ml 硫酸铁铵显色剂作为空白，测定样品在 530nm 波长处吸光度 A_n。

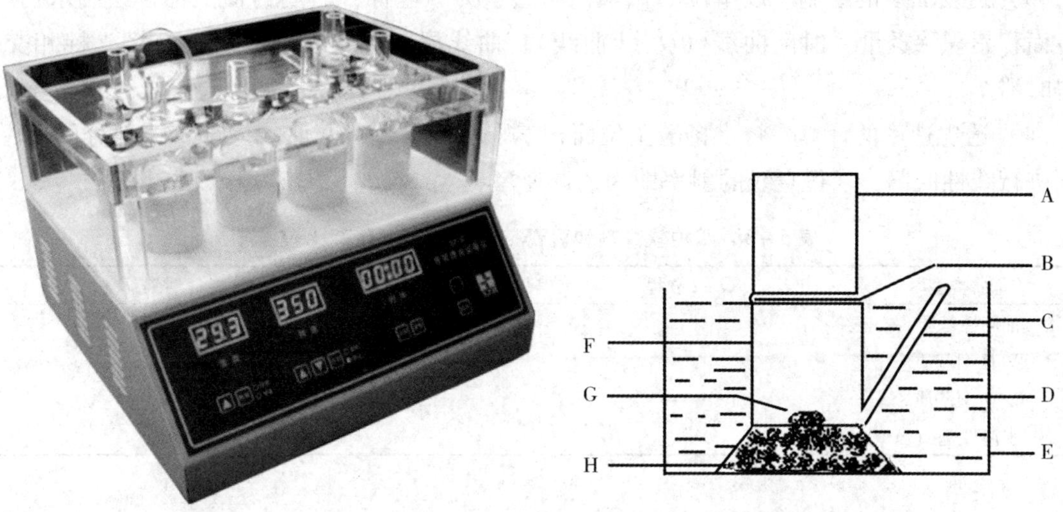

图5-2　智能透皮试验仪及渗透扩散装置

A. 扩散室；B. 皮肤；C. 取样管；D. 水；E. 水浴；F. 接受室；G. 搅拌子；H. 磁力搅拌器

2. 实验结果与数据处理

（1）标准曲线的绘制　将上述对照品溶液测得的浓度（C）与吸光度（A）进行线性回归，即得标准曲线方程为 $C=$　（$r=$　），线性范围：　μg/ml。数据记录于表5-1中。

表5-1　水杨酸标准曲线数据

浓度 C（μg/ml）	
吸光度 A	

（2）单位面积累积渗透量的计算　将各取样时间点（$n=1\sim7$）测定的吸光度 A_n 代入标准曲线方程，计算不同取样时间接受室中水杨酸浓度 C_n。

按照下式计算不同取样时间的单位面积累积渗透量 Q_n，并将数据与结果填入表5-2。

$$Q_n=(C_n\times V+\sum_{i=1}^{n-i}C_i\times V_s)/S$$

式中，Q_n 为单位面积累积渗透量（$\mu g/cm^2$）；C_n 为第 n 个时间点测得的药物浓度（μg/ml）；C_i 为第 i 个时间点测得的药物浓度（μg/ml）；V 为接受池的总体积（ml）；V_s 为每次取样体积（5ml）；S 为渗透扩散面积（cm^2）。

表5-2　软膏基质对水杨酸透皮速率的影响

时间（h）	油脂性基质			W/O 型基质			O/W 型基质			水溶性基质		
	A_n	C_n	Q_n	A_n	C_n	Q_n	A_n	C_n	Q_n	A_n	C_n	Q_n
1												
2												
3												
4												
6												
8												
12												

（3）透皮曲线的绘制　以单位面积累积渗透量为纵坐标，时间为横坐标，绘制水杨酸单位面积累积渗透量－时间曲线（$Q-t$ 曲线），曲线尾部的直线部分外推与横坐标相交，求得时滞 T。

（4）透皮速率的计算　将水杨酸单位面积累积渗透量－时间曲线尾部直线部分的 $Q-t$ 数据进行线性回归，求得直线的斜率即为渗透速率 J（$\mu g/cm^2 \cdot h$），填入表 5－3。

表 5－3　四种软膏剂和乳膏剂基质的透皮速率比较

基质类型	$Q-t$ 方程	J（$\mu g/cm^2 \cdot h$）	时滞 T（h）
油脂性基质			
W/O 型基质			
O/W 型基质			
水溶性基质			

实验指导

一、预习要求

1. **掌握**　软膏剂和乳膏剂的基质与药物释放的关系。
2. **熟悉**　菲克扩散定律及有关扩散的基本理论。
3. **了解**　透皮给药研究的概况及进展。

二、操作要点和注意事项

1. 制备离体动物皮肤时，使用的脱毛剂应新鲜配制，并严格控制脱毛时间，脱毛后应立即用生理盐水冲洗干净，防止损伤角质层。

2. 同一组软膏剂或乳膏剂的扩散实验尽量使用相同部位的皮肤（即使用背部皮肤或腹部皮肤），因为皮肤部位不同，角质层厚度不同（药物渗透与厚度成正比）。

3. 装上扩散池后在旋紧螺丝之前，应用镊子将皮肤拉紧，否则会增大扩散面积。

4. 在装填软膏剂或乳膏剂时，可先取少量涂在皮肤表面，然后继续装填，以保证软膏与皮肤紧密接触，以免软膏与皮肤间形成气室。装好扩散室后，应轻拍几下使软膏均匀涂布于皮肤上。

5. 接受室灌注生理盐水后，应将室内空气全部排除。磁力搅拌转速以能均匀混合液体为宜，转速太快会形成旋涡，减少扩散面积，转速太小接受室上、下层溶液难以混匀。

6. 理想的透皮量－时间曲线如图 5－1 所示，其直线为伪稳态，直线段延长线与横轴的截距为时滞。

7. 水杨酸浓度过高时，应定量稀释，然后吸取 5ml，精密加入 1ml 硫酸铁铵。硫酸铁铵显色剂本身有吸收，它的用量对吸光度有影响，应作空白对照。

三、思考题

1. 透皮给药剂型有何优缺点？
2. 试说明各类软膏剂和乳膏剂释药能力不同的原因。
3. 影响药物经皮渗透的剂型因素和生理因素有哪些？
4. 除本实验所用的扩散池外，你还知道有哪些扩散池，各有何优缺点？
5. 试说明不同类型乳膏剂的基质种类对药物释放行为的影响。
6. 试说明离体动物皮肤制备的注意事项。

Experiment 5　Preparation and Transdermal Absorption Experiment of Different Types of Ointments and Creams

扫码“学一学”

Objective and Requirements

1. To master the preparation procedure of different types of ointments and creams.

2. To be familiar with the influence of the types of bases on the drug release from ointments and creams.

3. To understand the preparation of the skin and the parameters of drug release rate in the experiment.

Introduction

The method of percutaneous penetration is a classical method in vitro to study the drug release in the ointments. This method includes placing the ointments on the surface of the hairless skin in vitro, setting the skin into Franz diffusion cells and measuring the permeated cumulative amount of drug on the steady state of this system. At last, you can compare the rates and the lag time of percutaneous penetration to analyze the influence of bases on the percutaneous penetration of a drug.

Generally, the percutaneous penetration of a drug is a procedure of passive diffusion. In this experiment, we use hairless skin as a simple membrane. On the condition of keeping the concentration gradient of the two sides of the membrane, when a steady state arrives in the procedure of percutaneous penetration, the relationship of Q (the accumulated permeation amount per unit area) with t (the time of diffusion) is as follows:

$$Q = kt$$

Where k is the permeability coefficient. On a steady state of the system, you can have a line when plot the permeated cumulative amount per unit area as a function of the diffusion time and k is the slop of the line. The lag time (T_1) is the x - intercept of the line (Figure 5 - 1).

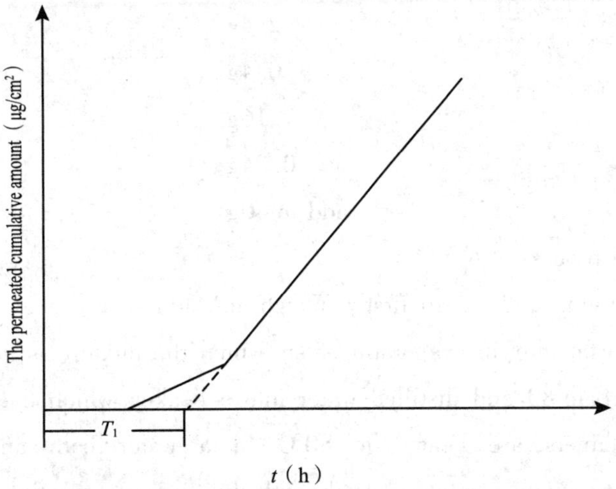

Figure 5 - 1　The curve of the accumulated permeation amount per unit area - time.

Ointments are uniform semisolid preparations for external application, which are consisted of medicaments and water soluble or oleaginous bases. Creams refer to semisolid preparations, while medicaments are dissolved or dispersed in emulsion bases uniformly for external application. According to the types of bases, creams could be divided into O/W creams or W/O creams. A large part of the ointments is the bases, which not only have the function of excipients, but also have important influence on the release, penetration and absorption of a drug at a certain extent. The results of the experiments rely on the conditions of the experiments. Generally, the order of the rate of drug release: the water soluble bases > O/W emulsion bases > W/O emulsion bases > the oleaginous bases. That is to say, the rate of release, penetration and absorption of a drug will be the fastest in the water soluble bases and the rate will be the slowest in the oleaginous bases.

Equipment and Materials

1. Equipment

752 UV - vis spectrometer, thermostatic waterbath, magnetic force whisk, improved Franz diffusion cells, filter membrane(Φ25mm × 0.45μm), test tube(10ml), injector(5ml), pipet(1ml), scraper, operating scissors, surgical tweezers, evaporating dish, mortar.

2. Materials

Salicylic acid, 6% Na_2S(depilatory), ammonium ferric sulfate color developing reagent, stearic acid, glycerol monostearate, liquid paraffin, white vaseline, wool fat, triethanolamine, polysorbate 80 (Tween 80), beeswax, paraffin, sorbitan oleate(Span 80), calcium hydroxide, CMC - Na, glycerol, mice(18 - 22g).

Experimental Methods

1. Formulations and Preparations of Salicylic Acid Containing Ointments of O/W Emulsion Base

(1) Formulation

Salicylic acid	2.0g
Stearic acid	4.8g
Glycerol monostearate	1.4g
White Vaseline	2.4g
Wool fat	0.4g
Triethanolamine	0.16g
Sorbitan oleate	0.04g
Distilled water	add to 40g

(2) Manufacturing process

Salicylic acid is ground and sieved firstly. Weigh and add stearic acid, glycerol monostearate, white vaseline and wool fat into an evaporating dish, which the mixture is used as A solution. Add triethanolamine, polysorbate 80 and distilled water into a beaker, which the solution is used as B solution. The two containers are heated to 80℃ in a water bath and kept until melting completely. Add B solution into A solution slowly with the same temperature of the two phases and stir fully on water bath. Stir and cool at room temperature until the mixture condensates. Add salicylic acid(after grinding) to the ice - cream semisolid in batches and stir fully, then the ointment of O/W emulsion base containing salicylic acid can be got.

2. Formulations and Preparations of Salicylic Acid Containing Ointments of W/O Emulsion Base

(1) Formulation

Salicylic acid	2.5g
Stearic acid	0.625g
Glycerol monostearate	0.85g
White vaseline	3.35g
Beeswax	0.25g
Paraffin	3.75g
Liquid paraffin	20.5g
Sorbitan oleate (Span 80)	0.5g
Calcium hydroxide	0.05g
Distilled water	20.0g

(2) Manufacturing process

Salicylic acid is ground and sieved firstly. Weigh and add glycerol monostearate, beeswax, paraffin and stearic acid into an evaporating dish. Heat the mixture on water bath until dissolved. Add white vaseline, liquid paraffin and sorbitan oleate, and then heat this mixture at about 80℃. The above mixture is used as the A solution. Add calcium hydroxide and the distilled water into a beaker, heat the mixture at about 80℃. The solution is used as the B solution. Clockwise stirring is needed when add B solution into A solution at the same temperature. An ice - cream semisolid is got when stir and cool at room temperature. Add salicylic acid (after grinding) to the semisolid in batches and stir fully, then the ointment of W/O emulsion base containing salicylic acid can be got.

3. Formulations and Preparations of Salicylic Acid Containing Ointments of Water Soluble Base

(1) Formulation

Salicylic acid	1.3g
Glycerol	3.0g
CMC - Na	3.0g
Distilled water	add to 20g

(2) Manufacturing process

Salicylic acid is ground and sieved firstly. Weigh and add CMC - Na and glycerol into a mortar, grind and mix them, then add distilled water to dissolve the mixture, grind continuously, then add the residual distilled water. Grind and mix them fully, the water soluble ointment can be got. Add salicylic acid (after grinding) to the mixture and stir fully until the mixture condensates, then the ointment of water soluble base containing salicylic acid can be got.

4. Formulations and Preparations of Salicylic Acid Containing Ointments of Oleaginous Base

(1) Formulation

Salicylic acid	0.25g

White vaseline 5. 0g

(2) Manufacturing process

Salicylic acid is ground and sieved firstly. Weigh and dissolve the white vaseline on water bath, and then cool the mixture at about 60℃, add salicylic acid (after grinding) to the mixture in batches and stir fully until the mixture condensates, then the ointment of oleaginous base containing salicylic acid can be got.

5. Preparation of Hairless Skin of Mouse *in vitro*

Mice, weighting 18 – 22g, are killed by neck dislocation. Clip off the ventral hair, wipe off the hair with depilatory 6% Na_2S and 3min later wash the skin with physiological saline solution. Peel off the skin, remove the fat tissue and wash the skin with physiological saline solution, then the hairless skin of mice can be got.

6. Preparation of the Standard Curve

Weigh precisely reference substance (salicylic acid) 125. 00mg, put it into 250ml volumetric flask, and add proper volume of water to dissolve salicylic acid, shake thoroughly. After dissolved, dilute to volume with water. Withdraw 1. 0, 2. 0, 3. 0, 4. 0, 5. 0, 6. 0 and 7. 0ml of the above solution, place in 25ml volumetric flask, dilute to volume with water. Withdraw 5ml of the solution and place in 5ml test tube, add 1ml of ammonium ferric sulfate color developing reagent and mix fully. Measure the absorbance at 530nm by ultraviolet spectrophotometer.

7. The Introduction of Improved Franz Diffusion Cells

The intelligent transdermal tester TP – 6 is shown in Figure 5 – 2. It consists of temperature control, motor speed control and time control, including: constant temperature water bath, control box, console, transdermal diffusion tank, rehydration bottle and connection. Tube and so on. The Franz diffusion cells are joined with two tubular glasses and the above and lower compartment are respectively the diffusion compartment and the receptor compartment. The skin is placed in the joint of the two compartments. A sampling tube is at the bottom of the receptor compartment, where you can sample and supply receptor fluid. The diffusion area is 2. 00cm^2. The diffusion cells are placed in a thermostatic water bath at a constant temperature of 37 ± 1℃. The receptor compartment is stirred with a magnetic stir bar to keep a dynamic condition.

8. Transdermal Absorption Experiments

(1) Experimental operation

Fix the above skin in the two compartments and add 2g ointment into the diffusion compartment. Fill the receptor compartment with physiological saline solution, note the volume and stir continuously. Withdraw a sample of 5ml of the solution at 1, 2, 3, 4, 6, 8, 12h, respectively, filter through 0. 45μm membrane filter and supply 5ml of physiological saline solution immediately to maintain the volume constant. To gain sample solution, measure accurately 2. 5ml of the filtrate solution into a 10ml test tube, add 0. 5ml of the color developing reagent and mix fully. To gain blank solution, measure accurately 5ml of the solution immersed with blank skin, add 1ml of the color developing reagent and mix fully. Then, measure the absorbance (A) of the sample solutions at 530nm using a spectrometer. According to the standard curve, concentrations of salicylic acid can be got.

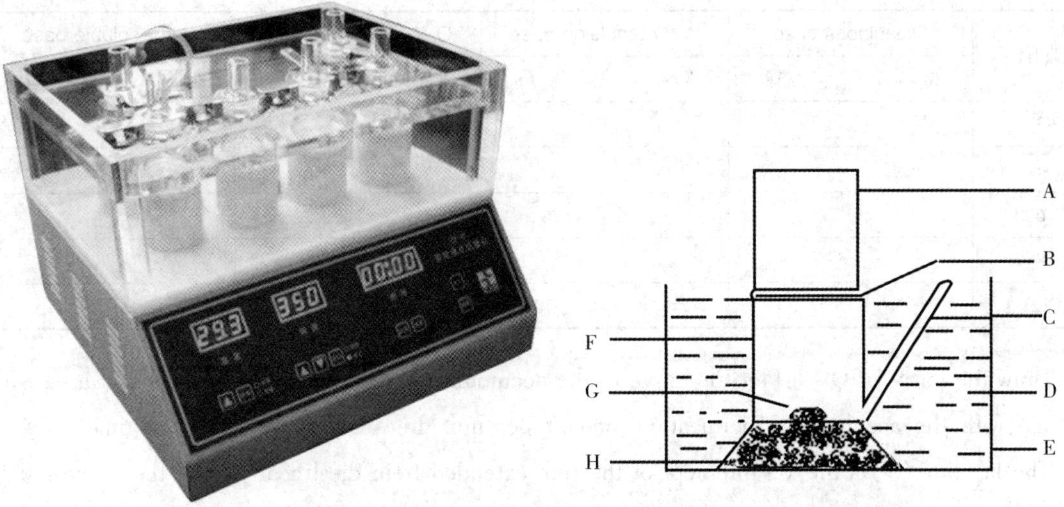

Figure 5 – 2　The intelligent transdermal tester TP – 6 and Franz diffusion cells

A. diffusion compartment; B. skin; C. sampling tube; D. water; E. water bath;

F. receptor compartment; G. magnetic stir bar; H. magnetic stirrer

(2) Data processing and experimental results

Draw the standard curve: Fill the Table 5 – 1 and establish a standard curve by plotting the concentration (C) of the reference solution above versus absorption (A).

Table 5 – 1　Data of the standard curve of salicylic acid

C (μg/ml)							
A							
Equation	(Range of linearity is　　μg/ml)						

Calculate the accumulated permeation amount per unit area: Calculate the drug concentration (C_n) in the receptor compartment at different time point ($n = 1 - 7$), by the standard curve and the A_n.

According to the following formula, calculate the accumulated permeation amount per unit area (Q_n) at different time, and fill the data in Table 5 – 2.

$$Q_n = (C_n \times V + \sum_{i=1}^{n-i} C_i \times V_s)/S$$

Where Q_n is the accumulated permeation amount per unit area (μg/cm^2), C_n (μg/ml) is the drug concentration at different time point(n), C_i (μg/ml) is the drug concentration at different time point(i), V is the total volume of receptor compartment (ml), V_s is the sampling volume (5ml), S is the permeation area (cm^2).

Table 5 – 2　Influence of bases to the percutaneous penetration of salicylic acid.

T(h)	Oleaginous base			W/O emulsion base			O/W emulsion base			Water soluble base		
	A_n	C_n	Q_n	A_n	C_n	Q_n	A_n	C_n	Q_n	A_n	C_n	Q_n
1												
2												

续表

T(h)	Oleaginous base			W/O emulsion base			O/W emulsion base			Water soluble base		
	A_n	C_n	Q_n	A_n	C_n	Q_n	A_n	C_n	Q_n	A_n	C_n	Q_n
3												
4												
6												
8												
12												

Draw the curve of Q – t: Plot the curve of the accumulated permeation amount per unit area with the time, with the accumulated permeation amount per unit area as Y – axis and the time as X – axis. The lag time(T) is the x – intercept of the line extended from the linear part of the curve tail.

Calculate the rate of percutaneous penetration: Carry out the linear regression of the data of the accumulated permeation amount per unit area at the tail of the curve of $Q-t$ with the diffusion time (t), and then J(μg/cm^2 · h) is the slop of the line. Fill in the Table 5 – 3.

Table 5 – 3 Compare about the percutaneous penetration of the four bases.

Kind of bases	Equation($Q-t$)	J(μg/cm^2 · h)	Lag, T(h)
Oleaginous base			
W/O emulsion base			
O/W emulsion base			
Water soluble base			

Experimental Instructions

Requirements for Preview

1. To preview the relationship between the drug release and the bases types of ointments or creams.

2. To be familiar with the basic theory of Fick's law and related diffusion theory.

3. To know the development of transdermal drug delivery systems.

Procedures and Precautions

1. When you prepare the skin of the mouse, depilatory must be prepared freshly. The time to wipe off the hair with depilatory must be controlled strictly. Immediately wash the skin with physiological saline solution to avoid the damage of stratum corneum after wipe off the hair with depilatory.

2. Using the skin in the same position of the mouse is necessary for the same ointments or creams because the thickness of the skin in different position is different resulting in different rate of penetration.

3. Use tweezers to strain the skin before tighten the screw of the diffusion cells, or else the diffusion area will be larger.

4. When place the ointments or creams onto the skin, firstly place small amount of the ointments or creams onto the skin, then fill the diffusion compartment continuously to keep the tight contact and avoid an air－cell be polysorbate the skin and the ointment.

5. When the receptor compartment has been filled with physiological saline solution, drain away the air in this compartment. It is better for the rotation speed of the magnetic force whisk to keep the solution mixed fully. If the rotation speed of the magnetic force is too fast, the diffusion area will be deceased. If the rotation speed of the magnetic force is too slow, it is difficult to keep the solution of the receptor compartment mix fully.

6. An ideal curve of the percutaneous penetration is showed as Figure 5－1.

7. If the concentration of salicylic acid in the solution is too high, dilution is necessary. Because ammonium ferric color developing reagent also has ultraviolet absorption, it will affect the measurement of absorption of sample solutions. To avoid that, blank test is needed.

Questions

1. What are the advantages and disadvantages of transdermal drug delivery?

2. Try to explain the reasons for the different drug－release of various ointments or creams.

3. What are the formulational and physiological factors influencing percutaneous penetration of a drug?

4. Besides Franz diffusion cells, what else diffusion cells do you know? Please list their advantages and disadvantages respectively.

5. Explain the effects of different types of cream base on drug release behavior.

6. Explain the precautions for the preparation of isolated animal skin.

实验 6　膜剂的制备

【目的与要求】

1. **掌握**　水溶性膜剂的一般制法。
2. **熟悉**　膜剂的一般处方组成。
3. **了解**　聚乙烯醇等成膜材料的性能。

【基本概念与实验原理】

膜剂系指药物溶解或均匀分散在成膜材料中加工制成的膜状制剂。大量生产膜剂时常用流延法，即配制成膜材料的浆液，加入药物和着色剂等，脱泡后经涂膜、干燥、脱模和包装制得。小量制备膜剂一般采用涂膜法，具体操作可采取下面两种方法。

1. **浇铸法**　将浆液倒入培养皿中，在适宜温度下干燥后剥离即得。膜的厚度可由浆液加入量控制。此外，可用带有小方凹槽的铝合金板浇铸。如取厚 15mm、宽 135mm、长 165mm 铝合金板一块，加工铣平成材，再加工铣成宽 12mm、长 15mm、深0. 3mm 的小方凹槽共 100 个。浇铸浆液后，用刮板刮平。用此板浇铸的膜剂，主药含量准确、膜片整齐、撕下容易、剂型美观、使用方便。

2. **刮板法** 选择大小适宜的光洁玻璃板或不锈钢板，洗净，擦干，涂上少许液状石蜡，再用清洁的纱布擦净。然后将浆液倒上，用有一定间距的刮刀将其刮平后，置烘箱干燥，即得。

其中，液状石蜡是脱模剂，能有利于膜的剥离。此外，尚有用聚乙烯薄膜为垫材者，效果较佳。该法先将玻璃板以75%乙醇涂擦，趁湿铺上一张两边宽于玻璃板的一块塑料薄膜，驱除残留的气泡，使薄膜紧贴在玻璃上，即可在薄膜上制膜。此法不但容易揭膜，且可把塑料膜作为药膜的衬材一起剪裁，防止药膜在包装中相互粘连，可于临用前揭膜。

【仪器与材料】

1. **仪器** 光洁玻璃板（30cm×45cm），圆铜棒（1cm×45cm），烧杯（50ml、100ml），量瓶（50ml），秒表，小铁夹，吸管（5ml），测厚仪，尼龙筛网（100 目），分析天平，752型紫外-可见分光光度计等。

2. **材料** 聚乙烯醇（0486、0588、1788），壬苯基聚乙二醇醚，丙二醇，甘露醇，羧甲基纤维素钠，甘油，糖精钠，地塞米松磷酸钠，蒸馏水等。

【实验内容】

一、壬苯基聚乙二醇醚膜剂的制备

1. **处方**

壬苯基聚乙二醇醚	5g
聚乙烯醇（0486）	7.5g
甘油	1g
蒸馏水	20g

2. **制备工艺** 称取聚乙烯醇（0486）7.5g，置50ml烧杯中，加水20g，搅拌1min，放置过夜。取完全溶胀的聚乙烯醇置水溶（70℃）中，搅拌使溶解，加壬苯基聚乙二醇醚5g、甘油1g，搅拌均匀，保温静置（70℃）或超声波脱泡。将膜料倒入同温度的玻璃板下沿，用推杆（调至需要厚度）向前推动膜料，移置烘箱经70～80℃鼓风干燥5～10min后立即脱模，冷却，切成5cm×5cm薄膜，包装，即得。

3. **用途** 本品具有杀精子作用，外用避孕。送入阴道深处后不超过50s即可溶解，接触面较栓剂大，显效迅速。

二、地塞米松磷酸钠膜剂的制备

1. **处方**

地塞米松磷酸钠	0.2g
羧甲基纤维素钠	1.5g
甘油	2.0g
聚乙烯醇	1.5g
糖精钠	0.3g
蒸馏水	加至100ml

2. 制备工艺　将聚乙烯醇、羧甲基纤维素钠加于适量蒸馏水中，浸泡过夜，使其溶解。将地塞米松磷酸钠、甘油、糖精钠溶于蒸馏水中，再加至 PVA 和 CMC - Na 的胶浆中，用蒸馏水补至 100ml。放置除泡后，将膜料倒入玻璃板下沿，用推杆向前推动。移置 50℃干燥箱中干燥脱模。将膜切成 1cm × 2cm 面积的片，包装即得。

3. 用途　本品具有口腔消炎的作用，常用于治疗口腔溃疡。

三、盐酸丙卡特罗速溶膜剂的制备

1. 处方

盐酸丙卡特罗	0.13g
丙二醇	20.0g
聚乙烯醇（0588）	52.5g
聚乙烯醇（1788）	17.5g
甘露醇	10.0g
蒸馏水	加至 1000ml

2. 制备工艺　将聚乙烯醇加于适量蒸馏水中，浸泡过夜，使其溶解。将盐酸丙卡特罗、丙二醇、甘露醇溶于蒸馏水中，再加至 PVA 的胶浆中，用蒸馏水补至 100ml。放置除泡后，将膜料倒入玻璃板下沿，用推杆向前推动。移置 50℃干燥箱中干燥脱模。将膜切片，包装即得。

3. 用途　本品对于过敏原引起的支气管哮喘具有较好的疗效。

四、膜剂的质量控制

1. 溶解时限的测定　取药膜 1 片，上端用小铁夹固定后将其浸入 37 ± 0.5℃的蒸馏水浴中，同时开启秒表，记录药膜从夹子上脱落的时间，应不超过 30s。

2. 厚度　用测厚仪测定。一般厚度为 0.065 ± 0.015mm。

3. 重量差异检查　除另有规定外，取膜 24 片，精密称定总重量，求得平均重量后，再分别精密称定各片的重量。每片重量与平均重量相比较，超出重量差异限度的膜片不得多于 2 片，并不得有 1 片超出限度的 1 倍。

膜剂重量差异限度要求：0.02g 以下或 0.02g 是 ± 15%；0.02g 以上至 0.2g 是 ± 10%；0.2g 以上是 ± 7.5%。

4. 含量测定　取药膜 1 片，置 50ml 烧杯中，加适量蒸馏水浸泡，待溶解后转移至 50ml 量瓶中，加水至刻度，摇匀，精密量取 5ml 置 50ml 量瓶中，加水至刻度，于波长 273nm 处测定吸光度，再计算出含量。

实验指导

一、预习要求

1. 掌握　成膜材料的质量要求。

2. 熟悉　聚乙烯醇的特性。

3. 了解　膜剂的制备工艺。

二、操作要点和注意事项

1. 聚乙烯醇（PVA）是目前常用的较为理想的成膜材料，是水溶性多羟基高分子聚合物，由聚醋酸乙烯（酯类）经醇解而得。醇解度（聚醋酸乙烯醇解百分率）大小与产品水溶性有关（表6－1）。

表6－1　PVA的醇解度与水溶性

醇解度（%）	残留醋酸根（%）	水溶性
>99.5	<0.5	仅溶于95℃水中
95～99.5	0.5～5	溶于65～70℃水中
88	12	水中溶解度最大
50	50	水中不溶

聚乙烯醇在水中溶解过程与亲水胶体相似，即经与水亲和、湿润、渗透、膨胀和溶解等阶段。浸泡溶胀时间应充分，否则溶解不完全。

2. 配料、涂膜和干燥的温度不宜过高，时间不宜过长。若配料时超过70℃，主药中聚氧乙烯基与水形成的氢键被拆开，使主药在膜料中起浊而不能均匀混合。若涂膜时，温度过高可造成膜中发泡，成膜和脱模发生困难，膜还发脆，且因膜料中失水过度，膜料收缩，主药载量降低。

3. 保温静置时，要使膜料中空气逸尽，则涂膜时不得搅拌，否则成膜后，膜中形成气泡。

4. 成膜后要注意控制干燥温度和时间。干燥不足或干燥过度，均可发生脱模困难。

5. 玻璃板要光洁，加热前可先涂抹少量液状石蜡，以免脱模困难。但因成膜材料不同，对膜板的亲和力也不同。亲和力太小，浆液铺展困难，容易聚结成块；亲和力太大，则不易脱模。一般可以通过改变膜板、改换垫层或改换润滑剂改善之。

6. 制备膜剂中常见的问题与解决办法。

常见问题	产生原因	解决办法
药膜不易剥离或浆液不易铺展	①干燥温度太高；②模板未清洗或润滑剂不足；③模板不适宜	①降低干燥温度；②涂润滑剂适量；③改换模板或垫层
药膜表面有不均匀的气泡	开始干燥温度太高	①开始干燥温度应在溶媒沸点以下；②通风
药膜“走油”	①油的含量太高；②成膜材料选择不当	①降低含油量；②用填料吸收油后再制膜；③更换成膜材料
药粉从药膜中“脱落”	固体成分含量太多	①减少粉末含量；②增加增塑剂含量
药膜太脆或太柔软	①增塑剂太少或太多；②药物与成膜材料发生化学反应	①增加或减少增塑剂用量；②更换成膜材料
药膜中有粗大颗粒	①未经过滤；②制膜时已溶的药物从浆液中析出结晶	①制膜前浆液应过滤；②采用研磨法等促进药物溶解
药膜中药物含量不均匀	①浆液久置，药物沉淀；②不溶性成分粒子太大	①浆液混匀，排除气泡后即应制膜，不宜久置；②应研细

本实验所用壬苯基聚乙二醇醚系一种非离子型表面活性剂，其结构式为：

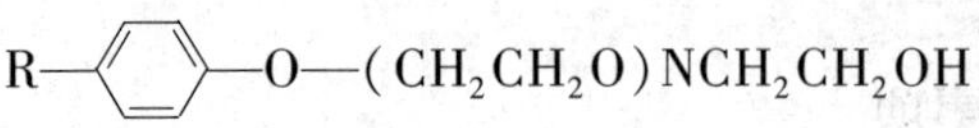

氧乙烯聚合度在9%～10%，熔点65～70℃，羟基84，HLB值13.2，在275nm波长处的紫外吸收系数$E_{1cm}^{1\%}=23.7\pm1$。

三、思考题

1. 聚乙烯醇的性质与其分子量和醇解度有何关系？
2. 何谓聚合度、醇解度？PVA 05－88、17－88 的聚合度和醇解度各为多少？
3. 除聚乙烯醇外，较常用的成膜材料还有哪几种？
4. 速溶膜的处方组成特点是什么？
5. 常用的增塑剂种类有哪些？
6. 刮板法制备膜剂过程中的注意事项有哪些？

Experiment 6　Preparation of Films

扫码“学一学”

Objectives and Requirements

1. To master the basic methods of water－soluble films preparation.
2. To be familiar with the formulation of films.
3. To understand the function of film－forming materials such as polyvinyl alcohol.

Introduction

Films refer to the film－likepreparations that are made by dissolving or dispersing the drug to the film－forming materials uniformly. Mass production of films is through flow casting method. The procedure of this method is as follows：First，preparing the slurry of the film－forming material. Then drugs，colorants and preservatives are added. After defoaming the slurry，painting and dying it，we can detach it and get the product that is ready to be packed. However，coating method is used when small amount production is needed. There are two concrete methods to achieve this.

1. Casting/pouring method

Pour the slurry to the culture dish，and dry it at the proper temperature，at last detach it. The thickness of the film can be controlled by the amount of the slurry. Besides，aluminum alloy plate with a little square groove can be used in the process. For example，an aluminum alloy plate with the dimension of 165mm × 135mm × 15mm is manufactured by milling and adding 100 little square groove with the dimension of 15mm × 12mm × 0. 3mm. After pouring the slurry，scrape the plate to the flat condition. Films prepared by this method have an accurate drug content，regular shape，good appearance and can be easily split.

2. Scraping method

Choose appropriate clean glass or stainless steel plate，then wash and dry it. After that，spread some liquid paraffin on it and then wipe it with clean gauze. Pour the slurry on it，and scrap it to flat using a scraper with a definite distance and then dry it in the oven. By doing so，the films will be made.

Liquid paraffin is a release agent，which could make the detachment easier. Also，polyethylene film can be used as a cushion material to get better effect. The process of this method is as follows：①Wipe the glass plate with 75% alcohol. ②Put a piece of plastic film on the glass when it is still wet. (the film should be wider than the glass on both sides). ③Expel the remaining bubble to make the film stick on the glass tightly and the process of film - making can be started. This method is not only prone to detach the films easily but also prevent the mutual adherence between the drug films and the package, because the drug films can be cut together with the plastic films. It is convenient for us to split the film just before the use.

Equipment and Materials

1. Equipment

Smooth and purity glass plate (30cm × 45cm), circle copper stick (1cm × 45cm), beaker (50ml, 100ml), volumetric flask(50ml), seconds - counter, little iron folder, haustorial tube(5ml), thickness tester, nylon sieve(100mesh), analytic balance, 752 UV - vis spectrometer, etc.

2. Materials

Polyvinyl alcohol (0486, 0588, 1788), nonylphenyl polyethyleneglycol ether, CMC - Na, glycerol, saccharin sodium, dexamethasone sodium phosphate, distilled water, etc.

Experimental Methods

1. Preparation of Nonylphenyl Polyethyleneglycol Ether Films

(1) Formulation

Nonylphenyl polyethyleneglycol ether	5.0g
Glycerol	1.0g
Polyvinyl alcohol 0486	7.5g
Distilled water	about 20.0g

(2) Manufacturing process

Weigh 7.5g of polyvinyl alcohol, put it into a 50ml beaker, add 20g of water, stir for 1min, and place overnight. Take the fully expanded polyvinyl alcohol, place it in a water bath (70 ℃), stir it to make it dissolve, add nonylpolyglycol ether and glycerin, stir evenly, and leave it at a temperature of 70 ℃ or ultrasonic for defoaming. Then pour the film material to the lower edge of the glass plate with the same temperature, push the material forward with a push rod, put it in the oven of 70 - 80℃ for 5 - 10min and detach the film immediately. After cooling, cut it into small films of 5cm × 5cm. The finished product can be got after package.

(3) Usage

The product can kill sperms as an external drug for contraception. It can dissolve within 50 sec after it is administered into the deep part of the vagina. It has a larger contact area comparing with suppository and has an apparent and instant effect.

2. Preparation of Dexamethasone Sodium Phosphate Films

(1) Formulation

Dexamethasone sodium phosphate	0.2g
Glycerol	2.0g
CMC - Na	1.5g
Saccharin sodium	0.3g
Polyvinyl alcohol	1.5g

Distilled water	add to 100ml

(2) Manufacturing process

Weigh 1.5g of polyvinyl alcohol, 1.5g of CMC – Na, and put them into distilled water. Keep it still overnight until it dissolves. Add dexamethasone sodium phosphate, glycerol, saccharin alcohol and distilled water into the container and dissolve it. The solution was then put into the mixed liquid of PVA and CMC – Na. Finally, add the remaining water. Defoam by standing for a certain length of time. Then pour the film material to the lower edge of the glass plate, push the material forward with a push rod, put it in the oven of 50℃ and detach the film. After cooling, cut it into small films of 1cm × 2cm. The finished product can be got after package.

(3) Usage

The product can relieve oral inflammation, so it is commonly used in dental ulcer.

3. Preparation of Procaterol Hydrochloride Instant Films

(1) Formulation

Procaterol hydrochloride	0.13g
Propylene glycol	20.0g
Polyvinyl alcohol 0588	52.5g
Polyvinyl alcohol 1788	17.5g
Mannitol	10.0g
Distilled water	add to 1000ml

(2) Manufacturing process

Weigh polyvinyl alcohol 0588 and 1788, and put them into distilled water. Keep it still overnight until it dissolves. Add procaterol hydrochloride, propylene glycol, mannitol and distilled water into the container and dissolve it. The solution was then put into the mixed liquid of PVA and CMC – Na. Finally, add the remaining water. Defoam by standing for a certain length of time. Then pour the film material to the lower edge of the glass plate, push the material forward with a push rod, put it in the oven of 50℃ and detach the film. After cooling, cut it. The finished product can be got after package.

(3) Usage

This product has a good effect on bronchial asthma caused by allergens.

4. Quality Control of Films

(1) Dissolution time

Take a piece of film, immerse it into a distilled water bath of 37 ± 0.5℃ with its upper side fixed by a little iron clamp. At the same time open the stopwatch. Record the time when the film falls off the clamp. The time should not exceed 30 sec.

(2) Thickness

It is determined by a thickness gauge. Usually the thickness should be 0.065 ± 0.015mm.

(3) Weight variation test

Take 24 pieces of films (except for special regulations), weigh accurately the total weight and calculate the mean weight, then weigh accurately every piece, comparing the results with the mean weight. There should be less than 2 pieces of films whose weight are beyond the limitation of weight variation and at the same time none of them could exceed twice the limitation of weight variation.

Weight variation requirement of films: ±15%, when the weight of films is 0.02g or lower than 0.02g; ±10%, when the weight of films is between 0.02g and 0.2g; ±7.5% when the weight of films is higher than 0.2g.

(4) Content determination

Put a piece of film into a beaker of 50ml, add some distilled water to dissolve it and transfer it to a volumetric flask of 50ml, add water to scale and shake evenly. Accurately measure 5ml to a volumetric flask of 50ml, add water to scale and determine its absorbance at the wavelength of 273nm. The content can be got by calculation.

Experimental Instructions

Requirements for Preview

1. To preview the quality requirements for film – forming material.
2. To be familiar with the properties of PVA.
3. To understand the procedures of the preparation of films.

Procedures and Precautions

1. Polyvinyl alcohol is a kind of ideal and common film – forming material. It is a water – soluble multi – hydroxyl polymer which is got by the alcoholysis of polyvinyl acetate. The alcoholysis degree is affected by the solubility of the product (Table 6 – 1).

Table 6 – 1 The alcoholysis degree and the solubility of PVA.

Alcoholysis degree (%)	Residual acetate (%)	Solubility
>99.5	< 0.5	Only soluble in water at T 95℃
95 – 99.5	0.5 – 5	Soluble in water with at 65 – 70℃
88	12	Having the maximum solubility in water
50	50	Cannot dissolve in water

The dissolving process of polyvinyl alcohol in water is similar to that of hydrophilic colloid. It must go through several stages which include affinity with water, wetting, permeation, expansion and dissolving. The time for PVA to swell should be enough or it will not dissolve completely.

2. During the process of arranging the ingredients, spreading the slurry and drying, the temperature should not be too high and the time should not be too long. If temperature is higher than 70℃ when preparing the slurry, the hydrogen bonds between the polyethenyl and water are easily broken which may lead to non – uniformity of the drug in the film. If temperature is too high when spreading the slurry, bubbles can be found in the film which makes the process of film – forming and detachment difficult and the product would be brittle and have a low drug load.

3. When keeping the slurry still, try to wait until the bubbles completely disappear. In order to avoid the formation of the bubbles, do not stir before spreading the slurry.

4. Try to control the temperature and time of drying after the film is formed. Less or over drying

will both lead to detaching difficulty.

5. The glass should be clean and smooth. Spread some liquid paraffin before heating to avoid detaching difficulty. Different film – forming materials show different degrees of affinity to the glass plate. Too little affinity would make the spreading process hard to perform and the film uneven. Too much affinity would make the detachment difficult. Usually it can be improved by changing the plate or cushion layer or lubricant.

6. Common problems and solutions

Problems	Reasons	Solutions
The film is hard to detach or the slurry is hard to spread	1. Drying temperature is too high 2. Insufficient lubricant or the plate is not cleaned 3. The plate is not appropriate	1. Lower the drying temperature 2. Add sufficient lubricant 3. Change the plate or cushion layer
There are uneven bubbles on the surface of the films	The temperature is too high at the beginning of the drying	1. Keep the drying temperature below the boiling point of the solvent 2. Ventilation
Oil overflows from films	1. Oil content is too high 2. Film – forming material is not appropriate	1. Reduce the oil content 2. Use fillers to absorb the oil before preparing the film 3. Change the film – forming material
The drug powder ' shed ' from the film	There are too many solid ingredient	1. Reduce the content of solid ingredient 2. Add more plasticizer
The film is too brittle or too soft	1. There are too much or too little plasticizer 2. There is chemical reaction between the drug and the film – forming material	1. Add or reduce the quantity of plasticizer 2. Change the film – forming material
There are coarse particles in the films	1. No filtration 2. The drug precipitates from the slurry during preparation	1. Filtration 2. Promote the dissolving of the drug by grinding method
Unevenness of the drug in the films	1. The drug precipitates because of storing for too much time 2. The insoluble particles of the components are too big	1. Do not store for too much time after the slurry is prepared 2. Grinding into smaller particles

Nonylphenyl polyethyleneglycol ether which is used in this experiment is a kind of non – ionic surfactant. Its structural formula is:

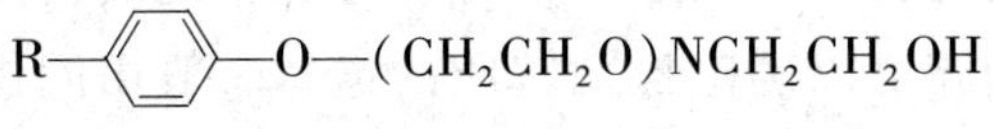

The polymerization degree of polyethylene is about 9% – 10%, the clouding point is 65 – 70℃, hydroxyl value is 84. HLB value is 13.2, and ultraviolet absorption coefficient at the wavelength of 275nm is 23.7 ± 1.

Questions

1. What are relationships between the characteristics and the alcoholysis degree or molecular weight of PVA?

2. What is the meaning of the polymerization degree and the alcoholysis degree? What is the polymerization degree and the alcoholysis degree of PVA 05 – 88, 17 – 88, respectively?

3. Besides PVA, how many kinds of film – forming materials commonly used are there?

4. What are the characteristics of the prescription of instant films?

5. What are the common types of plasticizers?

6. What are the precautions in the process of preparing the film by the scraper method?

实验 7　栓剂的制备

【目的与要求】

1. **掌握**　熔融法制备栓剂的特点及适用情况。
2. **熟悉**　置换价的换算。
3. **了解**　各类栓剂基质的特点及适用情况。

【基本概念与实验原理】

栓剂系指药物与适宜基质制成的供腔道给药的固体制剂。栓剂因使用腔道部位和作用的不同，其大小和形状各不相同。常用的有阴道栓和肛门栓，实验用栓剂模具如图 7－1。

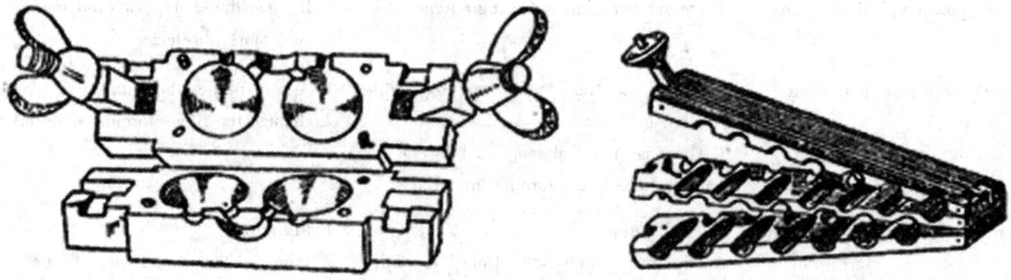

A　　B

图 7－1　栓剂实验模具

A. 阴道栓；B. 肛门栓

栓剂中药物与基质应混合均匀，栓剂外形要完整光滑；塞入腔道后应无刺激性，应能融化、软化或溶化，并与分泌液混合，逐渐释放出药物，产生局部作用；并应有适宜的硬度，以免在包装或贮藏时变形。

通常情况下栓剂模型的容积是固定的，由于药物和基质密度的不同，可容纳的质量也不同。通过置换价的计算可以确定栓剂基质的量。一般用同体积药物和可可豆脂的重量比表示置换价。如鞣酸的置换价为 1.6，即表示 1.6g 鞣酸和 1g 可可豆脂所占的容积相等。

栓剂常用脂溶性基质和水溶性或亲水性基质。一般采用热熔法制备栓剂。

【仪器与材料】

1. **仪器**　阴道栓模具，肛门栓模具，蒸发皿，水浴，冰浴，电炉，分析天平，崩解度测定仪等。

2. **材料**　可可豆脂，甘油，明胶，硬脂酸，碳酸钠，鞣酸，醋酸氯己定，聚山梨酯 80（吐温 80），枸橼酸，冰片乙醇溶液（2%），蒸馏水。

【实验内容】

一、甘油栓的制备

1. 处方

甘油	10.0g
干燥碳酸钠	0.2g
硬脂酸	0.8g
蒸馏水	2.0g
制成	4枚

2. 制备工艺 取干燥碳酸钠与蒸馏水置蒸发皿中，搅拌溶解，加甘油混匀，加热(100℃水浴)，搅拌下缓缓加入硬脂酸细粉。待泡沸停止、溶液澄明，立刻将溶液倒入涂过润滑剂（液状石蜡）的栓模中，共注3枚。放冷、整理，启模，取出，即得。制备工艺流程图见图7-2。

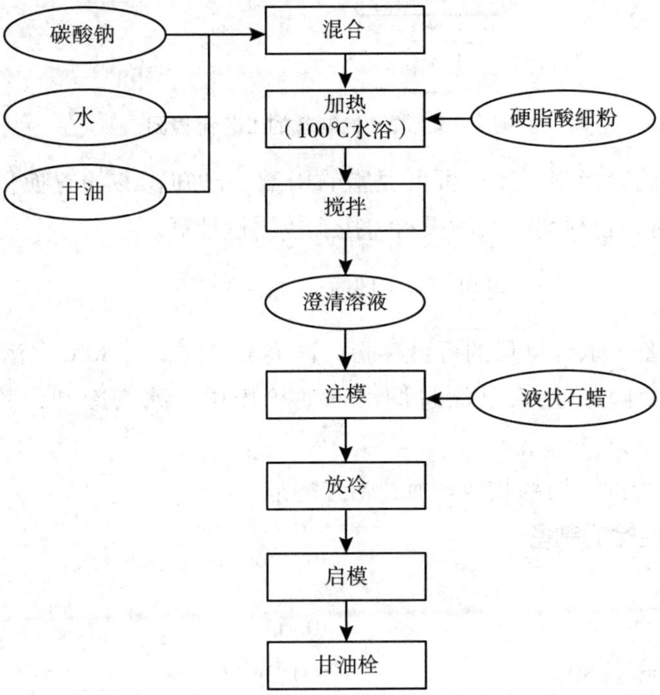

图7-2 甘油栓制备的工艺流程图

二、鞣酸栓的制备

1. 处方

鞣酸	0.8g
可可豆脂	4.0g
制成	3枚

2. 制备工艺

（1）测空白栓重量（栓模大小） 取可可豆脂约4g置蒸发皿内，加热（80℃水浴）至可可豆脂约2/3熔融时立即取下蒸发皿，搅拌使全部熔融，注入涂过润滑剂（肥皂醑）的栓模中，共注3枚。冰浴冷却，整理、启模、取出，称重，其平均值即为该空白栓重量

（或栓模大小），制备工艺流程见图 7－3。

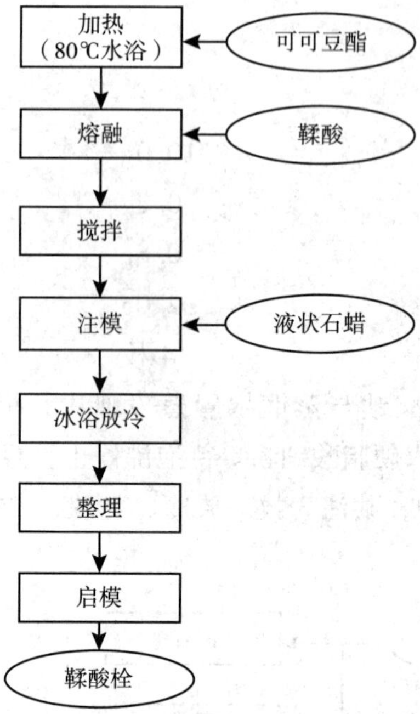

图 7－3　鞣酸栓制备的工艺流程图

（2）根据药物的置换价，计算可可豆脂的用量　已知鞣酸的置换价为 1.6，测得空白栓重量为 x，欲制备 3 枚栓剂，实际投料需按 4 枚用量计算。

$$\text{可可豆脂用量 g} = 4x - \frac{0.2 \times 4}{1.6}$$

（3）栓剂的制备　取计算量的可可豆脂，置蒸发皿内，于 80℃水浴加热至近熔化时加入鞣酸细粉，搅拌均匀，注入已涂过润滑剂的栓模中，冰浴冷却，整理、启模、取出，即得。

3. 用途　肛门栓剂。局部收敛止血，治疗痔疮。

三、醋酸氯己定栓的制备

1. 处方

醋酸氯己定	0.05g
聚山梨酯 80（吐温 80）	0.2g
冰片乙醇溶液（2%）	0.5ml
甘油	9.0g
明胶（细粒）	2.7g
蒸馏水	18.0ml
制成	2 枚

2. 制备工艺　取明胶置烧杯中，加蒸馏水 18.0ml，搅拌，覆盖保鲜膜，浸泡约 30min 使膨胀，加甘油搅匀，80℃水浴加热，搅拌使明胶溶解。另取醋酸氯己定置蒸发皿中，加聚山梨酯 80，搅拌使药物溶解，加冰片乙醇溶液、明胶溶液，80℃水浴加热，搅拌均匀，趁热注入已涂好润滑剂（液状石蜡）的阴道栓模中（共注两枚），冷却，整理、启模，即得。制备工艺流程图见图 7－4。

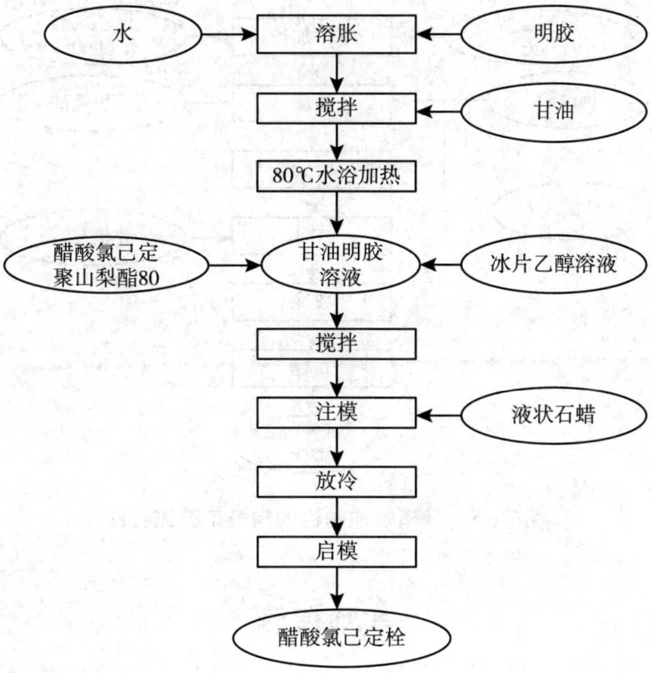

图7-4　醋酸氯己定栓的制备工艺流程图

3. 用途　治疗宫颈糜烂及阴道炎。

四、替硝唑泡腾栓的制备

1. 处方

替硝唑（120 目）	1.0g
聚乙二醇 400	4.6g
聚乙二醇 6000	3.0g
碳酸氢钠	1.12g
枸橼酸	1.04g
制成	4 枚

2. 制备工艺　将柠檬酸、碳酸氢钠干燥，研细，过 20 目筛备用。取聚乙二醇 400 和聚乙二醇 6000 混合，于水浴上加热熔融。在搅拌下加入替硝唑、碳酸氢钠及枸橼酸，混合均匀并趁热倾入模具中，冷却，整理，脱模即得。制备工艺流程图见图 7-5。

3. 用途　治疗滴虫性阴道炎。

五、栓剂质量检查

1. 重量差异　取栓剂 10 粒，精密称定总重量，求得平均粒重后，再分别精密称定每粒的重量；每粒重量与平均粒重比较，超出重量差异的限度不得多于 1 粒，并不得超出限度的 1 倍。限度规定为：1.0g 以下或 1.0g 时为 ±10%，1.0~3.0g 为 ±7.5%，3.0g 以上为 ±5%，栓剂重量差异的限度应符合规定。

2. 融变时限　取栓剂 3 枚，在室温放置 1h 后，参照片剂崩解时限项下规定的装置和方法（可各加一挡板）检查，除另有规定外，脂溶性基质的栓剂应在 30min 内全部融化，或软化变形，水溶性基质的栓剂应在 60min 内全部溶解。

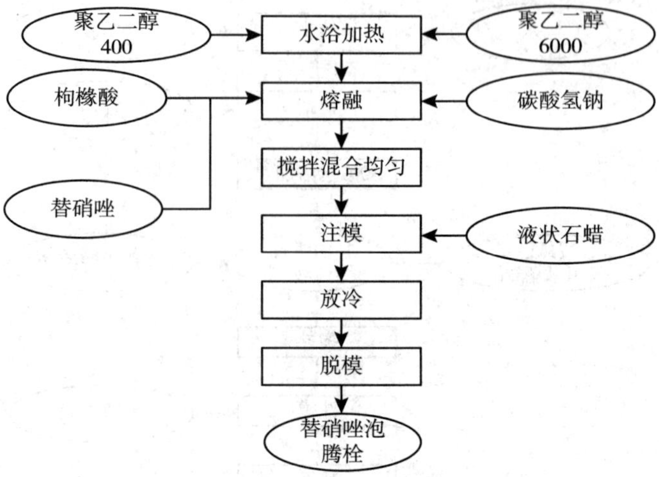

图7－5　替硝唑泡腾栓的制备工艺流程图

实验指导

一、预习要求

1. **掌握**　可可豆脂的主要理化性质，掌握熔融法制备栓剂的方法。置换价的实验方法及其计算。

2. **了解**　甘油明胶基质制备时的注意事项。

二、操作要点和注意事项

1. 制备甘油栓时，水浴要保持沸腾，且蒸发皿底部要接触水面，使硬脂酸细粉（少量分次加入）与碳酸钠充分反应，直至泡沸停止、溶液澄明、皂化反应完全，才能停止加热。化学反应式如下：

$$2C_{17}H_{35}COOH + Na_2CO_3 \longrightarrow 2C_{17}H_{35}COONa + CO_2\uparrow + H_2O$$

产生的二氧化碳须除尽，否则所得的栓剂内含有气泡，影响美观。也有处方用硬脂酸钠直接和甘油加热混合制备，避免了皂化反应过程，提高了栓剂的质量。

2. 甘油栓中含有大量甘油（90%～95%），与皂化产生的钠肥皂，两者均具有轻泻作用。

3. 甘油明胶由甘油、明胶和水三者按一定比例组成，明胶需先用水浸泡溶胀变软，再加热才易溶解。甘油明胶多用于阴道栓的基质，具有弹性，体温条件下不熔融，但能缓缓溶于体液中，释出药物。其溶解速度与明胶、甘油和水三者的比例有关，甘油和水的含量高则易溶解。

4. 制备鞣酸栓时，可可豆脂水浴加热应严格控制温度，勿超过36℃，以防可可豆脂转变晶型，熔点降至23～25℃，不易凝固。鞣酸与可可豆脂搅拌均匀，放冷至近凝固点时，边搅拌边倒入栓模中，栓模应预先冰冷，以便可可豆脂迅速凝固，避免药物沉积于栓模底部。

5. 醋酸氯己定在乙醇中溶解，在水中略溶（1.9∶100），吐温80可以使醋酸氯己定均匀分散于甘油明胶基质中。

6. 为保证栓剂含量准确，在制备脂肪性基质栓剂时应考虑药物的置换价。已知置换价，可按下式计算每枚栓剂所需基质的理论用量。

$$M = E - \frac{D}{f}$$

式中，M 为所需基质量；E 为空白栓剂的质量；D 为每枚栓剂的药量；f 为置换价。

7. 将替硝唑制成阴道泡腾栓，使用后可产生大量泡沫，能增加药物与腔道黏膜的接触，使其渗入到黏膜褶深部，充分发挥疗效。处方中柠檬酸的用量超过理论用量，可使阴道成酸性，有利于杀灭或抑制滴虫与厌氧菌。

三、思考题

1. 甘油栓的制备原理及操作时的注意事项是什么？
2. 甘油栓的作用机制是什么？
3. 结合实验说明计算置换价有何意义？
4. 甘油明胶作为栓剂基质的特点是什么？
5. 替硝唑栓剂柠檬酸为什么用量超过理论用量？
6. 鞣酸栓制备注意事项是什么？

Experiment 7　Preparation of Suppositories

扫码“学一学”

Objectives and Requirements

1. To master the characters and applications of fusion method to prepare suppositories.
2. To be familiar with the calculation of displacement value.
3. To know the characters and applications of the bases of suppositories.

Introduction

A suppository is a solid dosage form that is inserted into the body cavity for local or systemic therapy, consisting of API and other bases. Depending on the location and therapy of the body cavity, the suppository can be prepared with different shape and size, among which vaginal and urethral orifice suppositories are most commonly used. The molds for vaginal and rectal suppositories are displayed in Figure 7 – 1.

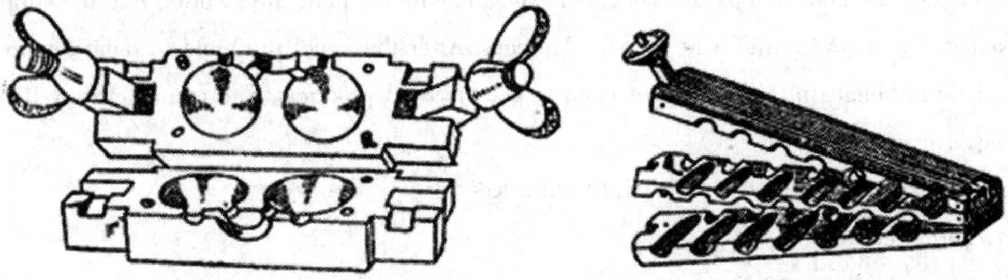

A　　　　B

Figure 7 – 1　The molds for vaginal (A) and rectal suppositories (B)

In general, suppository must satisfy the following requirements: (1) smooth surface and holonomic shape with uniformly mixing the drug and bases; (2) producing local therapeutic effects without irritation for sustaining drug release over time via a process of melting, softening or dissolving and resultant miscibility with body fluids; (3) possessing suitable hardness to prevent the deformation during the process of packing or storage.

Because of the difference in density of drug and bases and thus leading to the changed weight contained in the mold with a fixed volume, the base weight of suppository must be fixed via the displacement value(f). The value is obtained by the weight ratio of drug and cocoa butter with equal volume, such as the f value of tannic acid is 1.6, indicating that 1.6g of the drug has equal volume with 1g of cocoa butter.

The bases commonly used in suppository are classified as lipid - soluble and water - soluble (hydrophilic) matrixes. Fusion method is commonly used to prepare the suppository.

Equipment and Materials

1. Equipment

Mold of vaginal suppository, mold of rectal suppository, evaporating dish, water bath, ice bath, electric hot plate, analytical balance.

2. Materials

Cocoa butter, glycerol, gelatin, stearic acid, sodium carbonate, chlorhexidine acetate, polysorbate 80 (tween 80), tannic acid, acid citric, borneol ethanol solution (2%), distilled water etc.

Experimental Methods

1. Preparation of Glycerol Suppositories

(1) Formulation

Glycerol	10.0g
Sodium carbonate	0.2g
Stearic Acid	0.8g
Distilled water	2.0g
to make	4 suppositories

(2) Manufacturing process

Add distilled water in an evaporating dish, add sodium carbonate and stir to dissolve, add glycerol and mix, heat using a water - bath (100℃), add stearic acid under stirring. Once the bubble boil stopped and the mixture became clear, immediately pour the solution into the suppository mold wetted with liquid paraffin to prepare 3 pieces. After that, cool the mold to room temperature, remove the additional rim and open the mold to get the final products. The manufacturing flow chart is displayed in Figure 7 - 2.

2. Preparation of Tannic Acid Suppositories

(1) Formulation

Tannic acid	0.8g
Cocoa butter	4.0g
To make	3 suppositories

(2) Manufacturing process

Determination of the weight of blank suppository

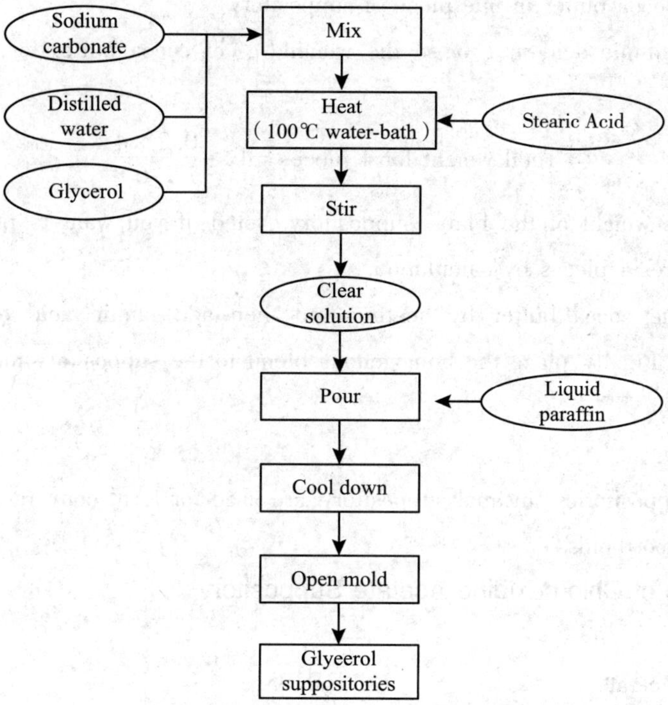

Figure 7 – 2　Manufacturing flow chart of glycerol suppositories

Place cocoa butter(4g) to an evaporating dish, whose bottom is immersed into the water – bath (80℃), and then, take away the disk from the bath as 2/3 of the cocoa butter is melted, and keep the sample under stirring until all butter melt. Place the resulting solution into the suppository mold wetted with a lubricant and cool down to room temperature. Finally, obtain 3 pieces of suppositories and weight accurately. The manufacturing flow chart is displayed in Figure 7 – 3.

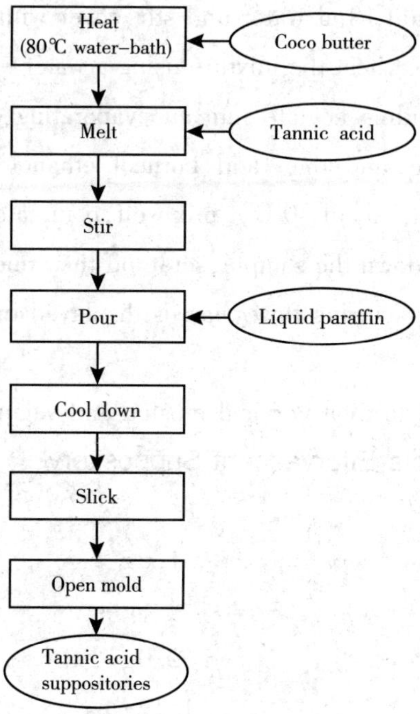

Figure 7 – 3　Manufacturing flow chart of tannic acid suppositories

The weight of cocoa butter in one piece of suppository

The *f* value of tannic acid is 1.6, so the weight (g) of cocoa butter for 3 pieces should be calculated as:

$$\text{Total weight for 4 pieces} = 4x - \frac{0.2 \times 4}{1.6}$$

Where x is the weight of the blank suppository. Noted: if you want to prepare 3 pieces, the actual feeding requires 4 pieces by calculation.

Briefly, melt the cocoa butter by heating and then add tannic acid to the solution with continuous agitation. Finally, place the homogenous blend to the suppository mold and rapidly cool down in an ice-bath.

(3) Application

Tannic acid suppositories, an anal suppository, are used for local convergence to stop bleeding and treatment of hemorrhoids.

3. Preparation of Chlorhexidine Acetate Suppository

(1) Formulation

Chlorhexidine acetate	0.05g
Polysorbate 80	0.2g
Borneol ethanol solution (2%)	0.5ml
Glycerol	9.0g
Gelatin (minute grain)	2.7g
Distilled water	18ml
To make	4 suppositories

(2) Manufacturing process

Add gelatin into a beaker, add 18ml water and stir, cover with a film over 30min to make the gelatin swell, add glycerol and mix, heat the mixture using a water-bath (about 80℃) under stirring to dissolve gelatin. Add chlorhexidine acetate into an evaporating dish, add polysorbate 80 on the drug, stir to make drug dissolve, and then add borneol ethanol solution and gelatin-glycerol solution, heat using a water-bath (about 80℃), mix well, pour into the mold of vaginal suppository wetted with liquid paraffin. Cool down the sample, scrap off the unnecessary parts and open the mold to obtain the products. The manufacturing flow chart is displayed in Figure 7-4.

(3) Application

The present product is used to treat cervical erosion and vaginitis.

4. Preparation of Tinidazole Effervescent Suppository

(1) Formulation

Tinidazole	1.0g
PEG 400	4.6g
PEG 6000	2.0g
Sodium bicarbonate	1.12g
Citric acid	1.04g
To make	4 suppositories

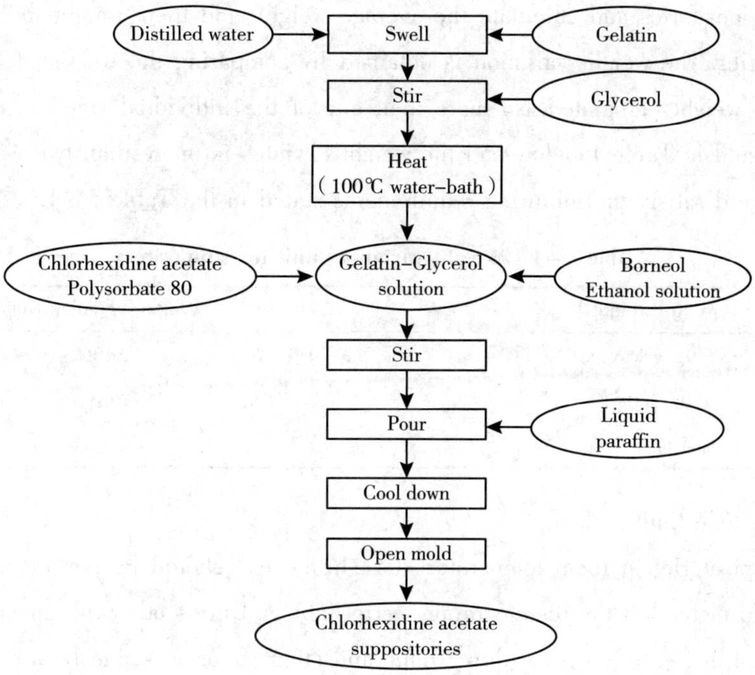

Figure 7 – 4　Manufacturing flow chart of chlorhexidine acetate suppositories

(2) Manufacturing process

Dry sodium bicarbonate and citric acid are pressed through a 120 – screen; meanwhile, mix PEG 400 and PEG 6000 together and melt in water – bath. Subsequently, slowly add tinidazole, sodium bicarbonate and citric acid into the homogenous PEG solution and in sequence place the mixture into the mold of the rectal suppository. The manufacturing flow chart is displayed in Figure 7 – 5.

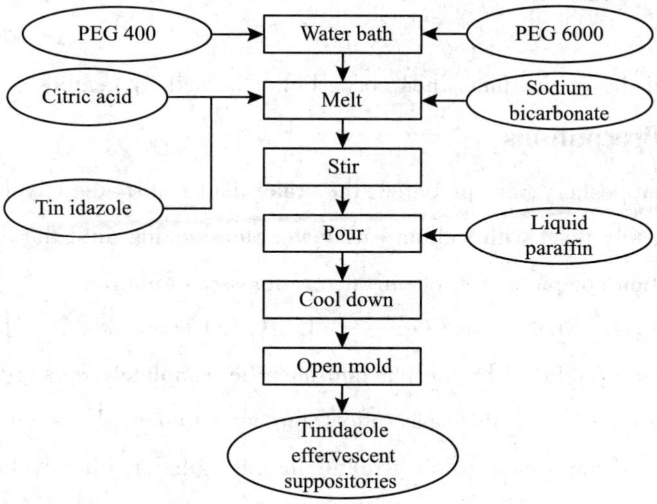

Figure 7 – 5　Manufacturing flow chart of tinidazole effervescent suppository

(3) Application

The present product is used for treatment of infusorium cloudy inflammation.

5. Quality Control of Suppository

(1) Weight variation

The weight variation of suppository can be obtained by sampling 10 suppositories. Weigh accurately 10 suppositories and calculate the average weight, and then, weight individually each of the 10 suppositories. The weight variation is obtained by comparing the weight of each suppository with the average weight calculated. No more than one of the individual weight exceed the weight variation limit listed in Table 1 below and the weight deviates no more than twice of that limit. The suppositories should satisfy the following requirements stated in the Table 7 - 1.

Table 7 - 1 Weight variation limit for suppository

Average weight	Weight variation limit
1.0g or less	±10%
1.0 - 3.0g	±7.5%
Greater than 3.0g	±5%

(2) Melting time limit

Keep 3 suppositories at room temperature for 1h, the test should be performed according with the apparatus and method of the disintegration test of tablets. Unless otherwise specified, fatty - base suppositories must melted or soften within 30min, and other water - soluble base suppositories must dissolve in water within 60min.

Experimental Instructions

Requirements for Preview

1. To preview the physicochemical property of cocoa butter and master the preparation of suppository by the fusion method. To master the experimental method and calculation of displacement value(f).

2. To understand the precautions when cocoa butter is melt by heating.

Procedures and Precautions

1. As glycerol suppository was prepared, the water bath must keep boiling which will allow stearic acid to completely react with sodium carbonate. Stop heating until the mixture becomes clear and saponifying reaction complete. The chemical reaction is as following.

$$2C_{17}H_{35}COOH + Na_2CO_3 \longrightarrow 2C_{17}H_{35}COONa + CO_2\uparrow + H_2O$$

The carbon dioxide produced by the reaction must be completely removed, and otherwise there will be bubbles in suppositories that may affect the appearance. The suppositories can also be prepared by heating sodium stearate and glycerol in the agitation directly that avoid saponifying reaction and improve the quality of the suppositories.

2. The glycerin - suppositories contain plenty of glycerol (about 90% - 95%), which have the same effect of hypocatharsis as soda soap generated by saponifying reaction.

3. The glycerogelatin comprises glycerol, gelatin and distilled water by a certain proportion. The gelatin should be swelling in water to make it soft first so that it can be easily dissolved by heating. It is elastic, does not liquate under body temperature but can dissolve in body fluid gradually and release drug. The dissolving rate can be affected by the preparation of glycerol, gelatin and distilled

water. The bigger the ratio of glycerol or distilled water is, the faster dissolving rate of glycerinated gelatin suppositories.

4. Cocoa butter should be heated in the water bath below 36℃ in the preparation of tannic acid suppository in case that the crystal forms of cocoa butter will transform. The melting point of the new crystal form decreases to 23 – 25℃ so it is difficult to solidify. Stir tannic acid and cocoa butter fully, keep stirring to transfer the mixture to the mold as it cools close to the solidifying point. The mold should keep in ice bath in advance so that the cocoa butter can solidify immediately, avoiding drugs deposit in the bottom of the mold of suppositories.

5. Chlorhexidine acetate is soluble in ethanol, sparingly soluble in water(1.9 : 100), Tween – 80 can help it uniformly disperse in glycerinated gelatin.

6. The displacement value should be considered to ensure accurate content of suppositories in the preparation of fatty bases of suppositories. The amount of bases of each suppository can be calculated by the following equation when the displacement value is known.

$$M = E - \frac{D}{f}$$

Where M is the amount of bases, E is the amount of blank bases, D is dosage of each suppositories, f is the displacement value.

7. Much foam can be produced by the reaction of sodium bicarbonate and acid citric when tinidazole is prepared into effervescent vaginal suppository. It can increase the contact surface of drug and mucous membrane so that the drug can permeate into the deep part of the fold of mucous membrane to play its drug action fully. The dosage of citric acid in the formulation is higher than theoretical dosage that profit for killing or inhibiting infusorians and anaerobe as the vagina is in a tart condition.

Questions

1. What are the principles of preparation and precautions of purpose of the glycerol suppositories?
2. What is the mechanism of action of glycerol suppositories?
3. Why is the displacement value according to the experiment?
4. What are the characteristics of glycerin – gelatin base in suppositories?
5. Why the dosage of citric acid in the formulation is higher than theoretical dosage?
6. What is the important steps in preparation of tannic acid suppositories?

第三部分　片剂的制备

实验8　阿司匹林片剂的设计、制备与肠溶包衣

【目的与要求】

1. **掌握**　片剂的处方设计和处方分析及其基本工艺过程。片剂的肠溶包衣工艺。

2. **熟悉**　单冲压片机的基本构造、使用方法。肠溶包衣材料的组成及其特性。

3. **了解**　包衣机的基本构造、使用方法。

【基本概念与实验原理】

片剂系指药物与适宜的辅料混匀压制而成的圆片状或异形片状的固体制剂，其制法分为直接压片、干法制粒压片和湿法制粒压片。因为粉末直接压片对辅料的要求较高，一般采用把粉末制成疏松的颗粒后，再压片的方法，提高物料的可压性。除对湿、热不稳定的药物外，多数药物采用湿法制粒压片。

片剂设计与制备要点如下：①原料药与辅料应混合均匀。含量小或含有毒剧药物的片剂，可根据药物的性质采用适宜的方法使药物分散均匀。②具有挥发性或遇热分解的药物，在制片过程中应避免受热损失。③具有不适的臭味、刺激性、易潮解或遇光易变质的药物制成片剂后，可包糖衣或薄膜衣。对一些遇胃液易被破坏或需要在肠内释放的药物，制成片剂后应包肠溶衣。④为减少某些药物毒副作用，减少用药频率，避免或减少血浓峰谷现象，提高患者的顺应性并提高药物疗效和安全性，可制成缓、控释制剂。

片剂中加入的辅料，根据其加工功能和附加功能，可分为稀释剂（增加片剂的重量和体积，便于片剂成型和分剂量），崩解剂（使片子在胃内崩解成颗粒），黏合剂（黏合粉末形成颗粒，制湿颗粒/软材），稳定剂（增加药物的稳定性），阻滞剂（用于缓控释片剂），润滑剂（用于压片时，减少摩擦，受力均匀，片子光洁），助流剂（增加颗粒或粉末的流动性）等。

目前，常用的压片机有撞击式单冲压片机和旋转式多冲压片机等。

包衣系指在片剂的外表面均匀地包裹上一定厚度的衣膜，它是制剂工艺中的一种单元操作，也常用于胶囊、颗粒或微丸等其他固体制剂的包衣。

对制剂进行包衣的目的有：控制药物在胃肠道的释放部位；控制药物在胃肠道的释放速度；掩盖苦味或不良气味；防潮、避光、隔离空气以增加药物稳定性；防止药物的配伍变化；改善片剂的外观与光洁度。

包衣类型包括糖衣包衣、薄膜包衣和压制包衣等。生产实践中，前两种最为常用。其中薄膜衣又分为胃溶型、肠溶型和水不溶型三种。但是无论何种包衣，片芯的硬度和脆碎度都应符合要求，以免在包衣过程中破碎或缺损；同时也要求片芯具有适宜的厚度与弧度，

以免片剂相互粘连或衣层在边缘部破裂。

薄膜包衣系指在片剂、颗粒或其他粒子等固体剂型上包裹高分子聚合物薄膜，厚度通常为 20～100μm。薄膜包衣材料通常由成膜材料、增塑剂、释放调节剂、增光剂、抗黏剂、色淀和分散剂等组成。

成膜材料：要求能溶解于适宜的溶剂，成膜性能良好，在胃液或肠液中迅速溶解。常用高分子成膜材料有：①水溶性纤维素衍生物，如羟丙甲纤维素（HPMC），其特点是成膜性能好，膜透明坚韧，但无抗湿性能。羟丙基纤维素（HPC），能溶于水、乙醇中成黏性溶液，可用于包胃溶薄膜衣。甲基纤维素（MC），其低黏度水溶液包薄膜衣时最好与 HPMC 等混合使用。②水不溶性纤维素衍生物，如乙基纤维素（EC）和醋酸纤维素（CA），前者能溶于乙醇，后者能溶于丙酮等有机溶剂，成膜性好，常用作缓、控释包衣材料。③丙烯酸（酯）-甲基丙烯酸（酯）共聚物（国外商品名 Eudragit）。其中Ⅳ号胃溶型丙烯酸树脂（Eudragit E100）以及胃崩型丙烯酸树脂乳胶液（Eudragit E30D）两种可用作胃溶性薄膜包衣。Ⅱ号肠溶丙烯酸树脂（Eudragit L100）、Ⅲ号肠溶丙烯酸树脂（Eudragit S100）、Ⅰ号丙烯酸树脂乳胶液（Eudragit L30D）三种均用于肠溶性薄膜包衣材料。另有不溶型丙烯酸树脂（Eudragit RS 和 Eudragit RL）均可用于制备缓、控释制剂的包衣材料。

增塑剂：增加包衣材料的可塑性，使衣层保持良好的柔韧性，常用水溶性增塑剂有甘油、聚乙二醇、吐温 80、丙二醇等；水不溶性增塑剂有蓖麻油、邻苯二甲酸二乙酯和柠檬酸三乙酯等。

溶剂：常用的溶剂有乙醇、甲醇、丙酮、三氯甲烷及水等，必要时可使用混合溶剂。

其他：如着色剂（如食用色素）、避光剂（如二氧化钛）、润湿剂（如吐温 80）、防黏剂或抗黏附剂（如滑石粉）以及增加表面光泽的二甲硅油等。

肠溶包衣指在片剂、颗粒或胶囊等固体剂型外层包裹可使药物能在规定的时间内在胃中不释放或是几乎不释放，而进入肠道可大部分或全部释放药物的包衣，可防止药物在胃中被破坏以及药物对胃的刺激性等。肠溶衣材料的溶解度随 pH 变化而变化，在胃液（酸性）中不溶，而在肠液（中性、偏碱性）中能迅速崩解或溶解。常用肠溶衣材料主要有以下几种：丙烯酸树脂类（如商品化的 Eudragit L100、Eudragit S100）、邻苯二甲酸醋酸纤维素（CAP）、羟丙甲纤维素邻苯二甲酸酯（HPMCP）、醋酸羟丙甲纤维素琥珀酸酯（HPMCAS）等。但大部分肠溶包衣材料在使用时需要用有机溶剂溶解，易产生爆炸和环境污染问题，近年来随着包衣预混技术的发展，商品化的肠溶包衣水分散体相继问世，如 Eudragit L30D-55 等，有效避免了有机溶剂的使用，应用广泛。

包衣装置可分为锅包衣装置、转动包衣装置和流化包衣装置等。

【仪器与材料】

1. 仪器 电子天平，DP30A 单冲压片机，烘箱，乳钵（中号），尼龙筛网（16 目，18 目），冲头（Φ8mm，Φ11mm），烧杯，磁力搅拌器，搪瓷盘，不锈钢筛网（60 目），恒温干燥箱，包衣机，空气压缩机，喷枪，电吹风。

2. 材料 阿司匹林（粒状结晶），微晶纤维素，交联羧甲基纤维素钠，淀粉，酒石酸，滑石粉，雅克宜（Acryl-EZE93F）肠溶包衣粉，蒸馏水等。

【实验内容】

一、阿司匹林片（100mg 规格）的制备

1. 处方（1000 片用量）

阿司匹林	100g
微晶纤维素	25g
酒石酸	1g
10% 淀粉浆	QS
交联羧甲基纤维素钠	6g
滑石粉	15g

2. 制备工艺 制备工艺流程图如图 8－1 所示。

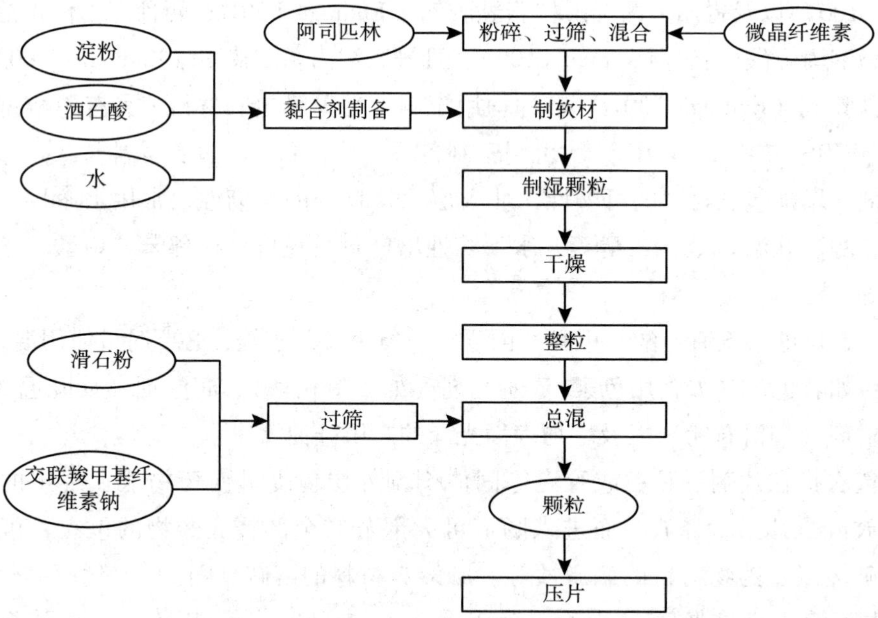

图 8－1 阿司匹林片（100mg 规格）的制备工艺流程图

称取淀粉 5g、酒石酸 1g 分散或溶解于 50ml 的蒸馏水中，加热制备 10% 淀粉浆，放冷备用。

取适量阿司匹林研磨均匀，过 80 目筛，称取处方量阿司匹林、微晶纤维素，混匀，加适量 10% 淀粉浆制成软材，使之手握成团，触之即散。过 16 目尼龙筛制粒，湿颗粒于 60℃烘箱干燥 30min 后，抖动过 18 目筛整粒，将此颗粒与交联羧甲基纤维素钠和滑石粉混匀，使用 Φ8mm 冲头压片。每片含阿司匹林 100mg，硬度控制在 3～4kgf。

3. 用途 本品对血小板聚集有抑制作用，可防止血栓形成，临床用于预防缺血发作，心肌梗死，心房颤动或其他手术后的血栓形成。

二、阿司匹林片（300mg 规格）的制备

1. 处方（1000 片用量）

阿司匹林	300g
淀粉	20g
酒石酸	2g

10%淀粉浆	QS
淀粉（外加）	10g
滑石粉	15g

2. **制备工艺** 制备工艺流程如图 8 -2 所示。

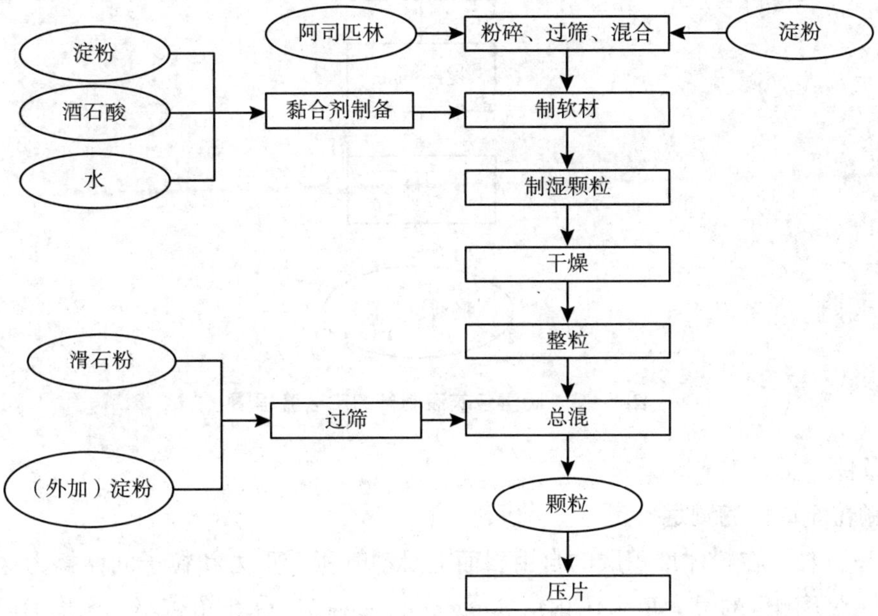

图 8 -2 阿司匹林片（300mg 规格）的制备工艺流程图

称取淀粉 5g、酒石酸 2g 分散或溶解于 50ml 的蒸馏水中，加热制备 10% 淀粉浆，放冷备用。

取适量阿司匹林研磨均匀，过 80 目筛，称取处方量的阿司匹林与淀粉混匀，加适量 10% 淀粉浆制成软材，使之手握成团，触之即散。过 16 目尼龙筛制粒，湿颗粒于 60℃烘箱干燥 30min 后，抖动过 18 目筛整粒，将此颗粒与滑石粉和外加淀粉混匀，使用 Φ 11mm 冲头压片。每片含阿司匹林 300mg，硬度控制在 3 ~4kgf。

3. **用途** 本品用于镇痛、解热、抗炎、抗风湿及关节炎等。

三、阿司匹林肠溶片（100mg 规格）的制备

1. 处方

包衣液处方

雅克宜（Acryl - EZE93F）	15.0g
纯化水	85ml

2. **制备工艺** 肠溶包衣液配制：配制工艺流程见图 8 -3。

取雅克宜 Acryl - EZE93F 肠溶包衣粉，分散于 85ml 纯化水中，搅拌使分散均匀，持续搅拌 30 分钟，过 60 目筛，即得。

肠溶包衣工艺：取片芯 50g，置包衣锅内，片床温度控制在 30 ~35℃，调节包衣锅转速为 30 ~40r/min。将配制好的包衣液用喷枪连续喷雾于转动的药片表面，随时根据片面干湿情况，调控片床温度和喷雾速度，控制包衣溶液的喷雾速度和溶媒挥发速度相平衡，即以片面不太干也不太潮湿为度。一旦发现片面较湿（滚动迟缓），即停止喷雾以防粘连，待药片干燥后再继续喷雾，使肠溶衣增重为 8% ~10%，待达到增重后，停止喷液，将药片于

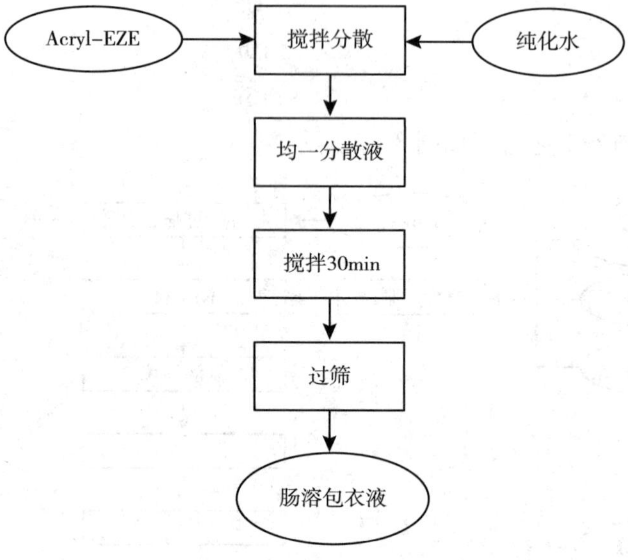

图8-3 肠溶包衣液制备的工艺流程图

30～35℃条件下干燥10min。

四、颗粒流动性的测定

1. 原理 粒子在粉体堆积层的自由斜面上滑动时所受重力和粒子间摩擦力达到平衡而处于静止状态下测得的最大角为休止角（angle of repose）。休止角越小，摩擦力越小，流动性越好，一般认为 $\theta \leqslant 30°$ 时流动性好，$\theta \leqslant 40°$ 时可以满足生产过程中流动性的需求。如图8-4所示，休止角常用的测定方法有注入法、排出法、倾斜角法等。

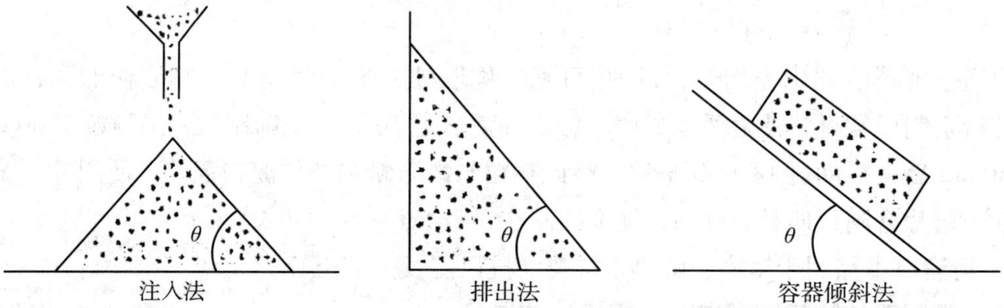

图8-4 休止角测定方法示意图

2. 休止角的测定 将表面皿水平放于实验台上并记录其半径，将玻璃漏斗固定在铁架台上，调节漏斗中心线与表面皿中心在同一垂直线上，使漏斗最低位置与表面皿垂直距离为3.0～6.0cm。将阿司匹林片剂总混颗粒从漏斗轻缓加入，颗粒落入表面皿中心并堆积形成圆锥体，当颗粒从圆锥斜边沿表面皿边缘自由落下时停止加料，并测定圆锥体高度。休止角 θ 用公式计算即得，即 $\tan\theta$ = 高度/半径。

五、单冲压片机的安装与调试

1. 压片机的结构 如图8-5所示，单冲压片机主要部件有冲模、饲料器、出片调节器、片重调节器和压力调节器等。

2. 压片机的安装与调试

（1）首先装好下冲头，旋紧下冲固定螺丝。旋动片重调节器，使下冲在较低的部位。再将模圈装入模板，旋紧模圈固定螺丝，然后仔细地将模板固定在机座上（冲头的周边锋

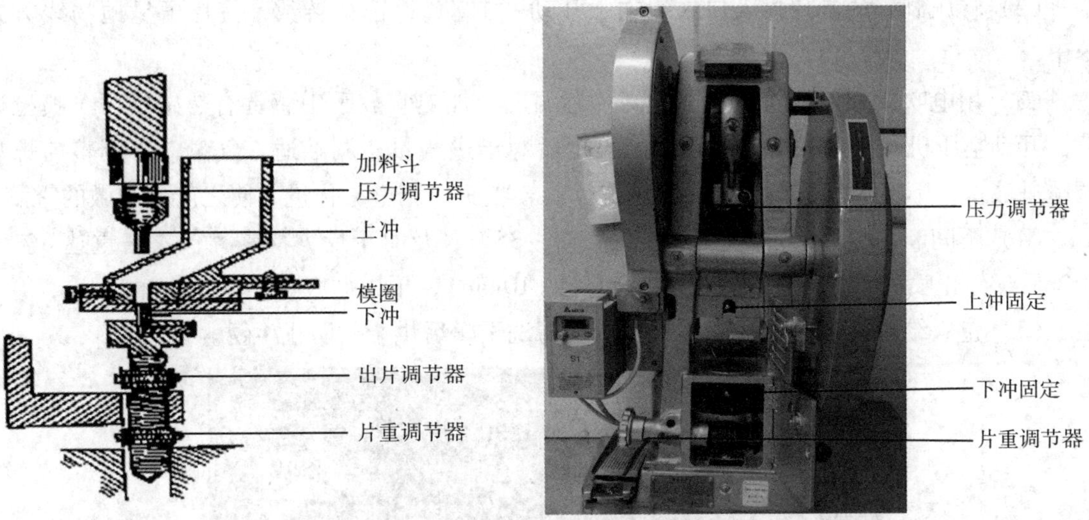

图 8－5　单冲压片机主要构造示意图

利部位容易因碰撞而损坏，故在整个装拆过程中都应小心）。

（2）调节出片调节器，使下冲头上升到恰与模圈相齐平。再装上冲并旋紧上冲固定螺丝，转动压力调节器，使上冲处在压力低的部位，缓缓地用手摇转压片机的转轮使上冲逐渐下降，观察其是否正好在冲模的中心位置。如不在中心位置，应上升上冲头（不得将上冲头强制地冲入模孔，更不应使上下冲头相撞）稍微松动一点模板固定螺丝，移动模板位置直至上冲头恰在模圈模孔的中心位置。旋紧固定螺丝，装好饲料器和加料斗，并加入颗粒。

（3）用手转动转轮，如感到不易转动时，不得用力硬转，应小心倒转少许，然后转动压力调节器使之适当上升减小压力。称其平均片重，调节片重调节器，使压出的片重与应压片重相等，同时调节压力调节器，使压出的片剂有一定的硬度。

（4）在上述一切操作均较顺利后，开动电机进行试压，检查片重和崩解时间，达到要求后方可正式压片。压片机有一定转向，不得反向运转，否则将会损坏机件。单冲压片机压制的片剂硬度不高，切忌为提高硬度而盲目增加压力，在过高压力下，压力调节中心活动螺杆很容易弯曲损坏。若需拆卸时，拆下的次序与安装的次序恰好相反。

3. 冲模的选择　压片机的冲模由上冲、下冲和模圈构成。通常普通的冲头都是圆形的，但有各种不同的凹形弧度。冲头的直径有多种规格，可根据所压药片的重量来选择，见表 8－1。

表 8－1　冲头规格的选择

片重（mg）	50	100	150	200	300	500
冲头直径（mm）	5～6.5	7	8	8.5	10.5	12

4. 压片机的保养　压片完毕，用毛刷刷去药粉，用废纱头揩拭机件，使压片机干燥清洁，最后加好润滑油。下次使用前仍应用手缓缓转动转轮，仔细观察压片机是否有故障，当一切正常后，方可开启使用。

六、包衣操作步骤

1. 操作　包衣装置主要部件有包衣主机、空压机、加热控温装置和喷枪，如图 8－6 所示，包衣操作基本过程如下。

（1）检查包衣主机、喷枪、空压机、加热装置等是否清理干净，有无问题。

（2）将压制好的素片投入包衣锅内，开动“启动”，选择转数，使片子呈抛物线方式落下。

（3）用电吹风加热锅体，适当提高片芯温度，加热宜放手中感觉有热感即可。喷枪试喷：开动空压机，按动喷枪扳机，调准喷枪后螺母进气量，调准适宜气量，再调整前螺母调整进液量，不可太大，以致来不及干燥，旋转喷头可调整雾化量，使之产生细微的雾滴。

（4）不间断边喷液边加热，控制温度30～35℃，及时干燥，待素片包衣增重达8%～10%后，停止喷液后，继续加热一段时间（约10min），干燥彻底。

（5）包衣结束后及时清洗锅体，喷枪，清洗干净后烘干，防止生锈。

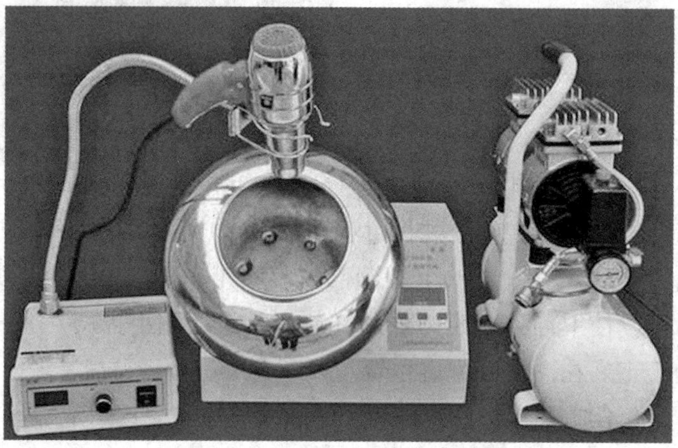

图8－6　包衣装置主要组成部件

2. 保养维护　每次试验完毕必须进行清理，枪头卸下，喷嘴部件清洗，肠溶材料可在碱性条件下溶解，因此可使用浓度3%～5%的NaOH溶液清洗。

七、质量检查

1. 重量差异　照《中国药典》四部通则<0101>“片剂”项下规定，取供试品20片，精密称定总重量，求得平均片重后，再分别精密称定每片的重量，每片重量与平均片重比较（凡无含量测定的片剂或有标示片重的中药片剂，每片重量应与标示片重比较），按表8－2中的规定，超出重量差异限度的不得多于2片，并不得有1片超出限度1倍。

表8－2　片剂的重量差异限度要求

片剂的平均重量（g）	重量差异限度（%）
0.3g以下	±7.5
0.3g或0.3g以上	±5

2. 硬度检查　片剂的硬度与其储运后外形的完整性有关，生产厂家一般均将硬度作为片剂的内控指标之一。硬度的检查法有以下两种。

手工检查法：取一片受试片剂，置中指和食指间，用拇指以适当压力挤压片子，不应立即分裂，否则表示此片剂硬度不足。

片剂硬度测定仪测定：将一片受试片剂径向固定在微调夹头与顶头之间，将“倒”“顺”开关拨至“顺”位置，选择开关拨至“硬度”挡，待药片破碎，读取硬度指示读数表中的读数，共测定3～6片，取其平均值。

3. 崩解时限

（1）测定装置　照《中国药典》四部通则<0921>崩解时限检查法，采用升降式崩解仪。崩解仪的主要结构为一能升降的金属支架与下端镶有筛网的吊篮，并附有挡板。升降的金属支架上下移动距离为55mm ±2mm，往返频率为每分钟30 ~32次。

吊篮：玻璃管6根，管长77.5mm ±2.5mm，内径21.5mm，壁厚2mm；透明塑料板2块，直径90mm，厚6mm，板面有6个孔，孔径26mm；不锈钢板1块（放在上面一块塑料板上），直径90mm，厚1mm，板面有6个孔，孔径22mm；不锈钢丝筛网1张（放在下面一块塑料板下），直径90mm，筛孔内径2.0mm；以及不锈钢轴1根（固定在上面一块塑料板与不锈钢板上），长80mm。

挡板：为一平整光滑的透明塑料块，相对密度1.18 ~1.20，直径20.7mm ±0.15mm，厚9.5mm ±0.15mm；挡板共有5个孔，孔径2mm，中央1个孔，其余4个孔距中心6mm，各孔间距相等；挡板侧边有4个等距离的V形槽，V形槽上端宽9.5mm，深2.55mm，底部开口处的宽与深度均为1.6mm。

（2）检查法　将吊篮通过上端的不锈钢轴悬挂于支架上，浸入1000ml烧杯中，并调节吊篮位置使其下降至低点时筛网距烧杯底部25mm，烧杯内盛有温度为37 ±1℃的水，调节水位高度使吊篮上升至高点时筛网在水面下15mm处，吊篮顶部不可浸没于溶液中。

除另有规定外，取供试品6片，分别置上述吊篮的玻璃管中，启动崩解仪进行检查，各片均应在15分钟内全部崩解。如有1片不能完全崩解，应另取6片复试，均应符合规定。

4. 肠溶包衣增重与包衣质量

包衣增重的计算：包衣增重（%）=（包衣后片剂重量/包衣前片剂重量 -1）×100%。阿司匹林肠溶片的包衣增重应为8% ~10%。

包衣质量检查：检查的项目主要包括外观检查、包衣增重、耐冲击强度、衣层强度、耐湿耐水测试、稳定性检查、耐酸及释放度等。

实验指导

一、预习要求

1. 掌握　影响片剂崩解度的主要因素。

2. 熟悉　制粒压片和粉末直接压片等制备片剂的方法。药用高分子材料学中有关薄膜包衣材料的性质和应用。

3. 了解　单冲压片机的主要构造、装拆和保养过程。肠溶包衣片生产工艺及特点。

二、操作要点和注意事项

1. 压片所用原料一般应先经过粉碎、过筛和混合等操作。阿司匹林除粒状结晶可直接压片外，针状、鳞片状结晶均需粉碎，再与其他成分混合。小剂量药物与辅料混合时，常采用逐级稀释法（等容量递增法）并反复过筛、混合以确保混合均匀。

2. 黏合剂用料要恰当，使软材达到以手握之可成团块、手指轻压时又能散裂而不成粉状为度。再将软材挤压过筛，制成所需大小的颗粒，颗粒应以无长条、块状和过多的细粉为宜。

3. 湿颗粒应根据主药和辅料的性质，以适宜温度尽快干燥。干燥后颗粒往往结团粘连，需过筛整粒，也可加入润滑剂同时整粒并混匀。

4. 阿司匹林在湿、热条件下易水解成水杨酸和醋酸，增加对胃肠黏膜的刺激，严重者可发生溃疡和出血等症状。故在淀粉浆中加入酒石酸，以形成酸性环境，减少阿司匹林的降解。

5. 制备好的淀粉浆，须在完全冷却后使用。为了减少用水量，淀粉浆的浓度可以提高至14% ~17%。在实际生产中，除采用湿颗粒法压片外，亦可采用直接粉末压片，以完全避免湿、热的影响。

6. 硬度测定前，检查指针是否在零位，如不在零位，应使用“倒”挡开关，使指针退回零位。硬度测试完毕，指针应回到零位，以免定力弹簧疲劳、损伤，造成误差。电机在转动的情况下，切勿随意拨动倒顺选择开关，以免烧坏电机。项目选择开关的拨动，应在电机运转的情况下进行。关机后应将项目选择开关置于空挡，倒顺选择开关置于倒挡。

7. 在包衣前，可先将片芯在40℃干燥30min，吹去片剂表面的细粉。在包衣锅内纵向粘贴若干1 ~2cm 宽的长硬纸条或胶布，以增加片子与包衣锅的摩擦，改善滚动性。

8. 包衣喷雾较快时片剂表面若开始潮湿后，在包衣锅内的滚动将减慢，翻滚困难，应立即停止喷雾并开始吹热风干燥。

9. 包衣温度应控制在40℃左右，以避免温度过高易使药物分解；干燥速度过快易使片剂表面产生气泡，衣膜与片芯分离。

三、思考题

1. 对湿热不稳定的药物进行片剂处方设计时应考虑哪些问题？
2. 阿司匹林在压片过程中可能出现哪些质量问题？如何解决？
3. 简述单冲压片机的构造及其工作原理。
4. 简述润滑剂的加入顺序及其作用。
5. 哪些药物制剂需要包肠溶衣？肠溶薄膜包衣材料有哪些？
6. 肠溶包衣中可能出现哪些问题？如何解决？

Experiment 8 Preparation and Enteric Coating of Aspirin Tablets

扫码“学一学”

Objectives and Requirements

1. To master the basic technological course of tablets through the preparation of aspirin tablets. To master the basic technological process of enteric coating for tablets.

2. To be familiar with the basic structure and operation method of single - punch press. To be familiar with the composition and characters of enteric coating materials.

3. To understand the basic structure and operation method of coating machine.

Introduction

Tablets are solid preparations with various shapes, usually round, and obtained by compressing uniform volumes of particles containing one or more active ingredients with suitable excipients. They may vary in size, shape, weight, hardness, thickness, disintegration and dissolution characteristics, and in other aspects. They may be classed, according to the method of manufacture, as compressed tablets or molded tablets. Generally, the methods used for preparing tablets are wet or dry granulation compression and direct compression. Wet granulation compression method has been widely used in tablets production, especially for drugs resistant to wet and heat.

There are some aspects should be considered: (1) APIs and excipients should be mixed uniformly. (2) The APIs tend to degrade with heat or easy to volatilize should free from heat during preparation. (3) For the APIs that have bad flavor or irritation of the gastric mucosa, or tend to degrade when exposed to light, moisture or stomach acid, or those treating intestinal diseases, we should prepare them into tablets and coat the tablets with sugar – film or enteric – coated film. (4) In order to reduce APIs' toxicity or adverse effects, or to decrease the administration frequency, we can prepare sustained – release or controlled – release tablets.

The primary aim of excipients used during preparation of the tablets is to ensure good flow and compressibility properties of the mixture. The choice of excipients is determined by factors such as: (1) the type of product and effect required, (2) the chosen method of manufacture, (3) the influence of excipients on the flow and compressibility properties of the mixture/granulate, (4) the acquirement and assurance of good tableting properties (exclusion of tableting problems such as laminating, capping, punch and the adhesion, etc.). In general, the inclusion of excipients must contribute positively to the quality and effectiveness of the final product. Excipients includes diluents or fillers, binders or adhesives, wetting agents, disintegrants or disintegrating agents, etc.

Now tablet presses are of two basic types, the single – punching press and multi – punch rotary press.

Pharmaceutical film coating, one unit operation in preparation manufacture, a uniform coat applied is to the surface of a solid dosage form including tablet, granules and pellets with certain thickness, with the aims as described below: controlled drug release and modified drug release profiles in specific – site of gastrointestinal tract, taste masking, moisture protection, prevented changes of compatibility between two drugs, enhanced long term stability via providing a physical barrier to environmental storage conditions (light, oxygen or water vapor) as well as facilitated drug product identification and improved esthetic appearance.

The film – coating includes sugar – coating, film – coating and compression – coating, with the two formers being most commonly used; meanwhile, the film – coating is further divided into immediate release coating, enteric release coating and water – insoluble coating. On the other hand, irrespective of the type coating, the tablet cores not only must have certain hardness to resist the breaking or defect but also possess suitable thickness and radian to prevent the sticking and defect within the coating rim.

Film – coating that polymer is used as coating material onto the solid dosages such as tablets, granules, or other particles. The thickness of such a coating is usually between 20 – 100μm. The coating formulations usually contain the following components: film materials, plasticizer release modifier, brightening agent, antiadherent, colorant, solvent, etc.

Film materials: The materials should be soluble in fitting solvent, easy to form film and solute quickly in fluid of stomach or intestines. The macromolecular materials usually include: (1) Water – soluble cellulose derivations, such as HPMC, which is easy to form film and the film is transparent and diligent, but is not resistant to wet; HPC, which can dissolve in water and alcohol forming stick solution, and can be used to coating stomach - soluble film; MC, for its low stickness of water solution, should use with HPMC when used in film - coating. (2) Water - unsolvable cellulose derivations, such as EC and CA, usually used as sustained - release coating materials. (3) Acrylic acid resin (Eudragit), in which Eudragit E100 and Eudragit E30D are used in stomach - soluble film coating; Eudragit L, Eudragit S and Eudragit L30D are used in enteric - coating. Eudragit RS and Eudragit RL are unsolvable and used in controlled release coating.

Plasticizers: The plasticizers are those can increase the plasticity of a coating material, and make the film layer keep the good pliant and tough, including water - soluble, such as glycerin, PEG and propanediol, and water - unsolvable, such as castor oil, Tween 80, diethyl phthalate and triethyl ester citrate.

Solvents: Such as alcohol, methyl alcohol, acetone, chloroform and water etc., if necessary, you can use the mixture of several solvents.

Others: Such as colorants (edible coloring matter, etc.), anti - light agents (Titanium dioxide, etc.), moistening agents (polysorbate 80), weight - adding agents (Talcum powder) and surface - blare - adding agents (dimethyl silicon oil).

Enteric coating refers to the film which coated on the outer layer of a solid dosage form such as a tablet, granule or capsule to prevent the drug released in the stomach for a prescribed period of time, and then released partly or fully in the intestine.

The solubility of the enteric coating material varies with pH, and the material is insoluble in gastric juice (acidic), and rapidly disintegrates or dissolves in intestinal fluid (neutral, alkaline). The commonly used enteric coating materials usually include: acrylic resin (such as Eudragit L100, Eudragit S100), cellulose acetate phthalate (CAP), hypromellose phthalate (HPMCP), hypromellose acetate succinate (HPMCAS) and so on. However, most of the enteric coating materials need to be dissolved by organic solvents, which may cause explosion and environmental pollution problems. In recent years, commercial enteric coating water dispersions have been introduced in the market with the development of premixing technology, such as Eudragit L30D - 55, etc., which effectively avoiding the use of organic solvents.

The coating equipment include pan coating device, rotating coating device, and fluid bed coating device.

Equipment and Materials

1. Equipment

Electronic balance, single - punch press, pestle (medium), oven, nylon sieve (16 and 18 mesh), punch (Φ8mm and Φ11mm shallow concave punch), volumetric flask, watch glass, beakers, magnetic stirrer, stainless steel sieve (80 mesh), coating machines, air compressors, spray guns, hair dryers, etc.

2. Materials

Aspirin acid (in granule crystal), microcrystalline cellulose, croscarmellose sodium, tartaric acid, talcum powder, starch, Acryl - EZE93F enteric coating powder, sodium hydroxide, distilled water, etc.

Experimental Methods

1. Preparation of Aspirin Tablets Ⅰ(100mg strength)

(1) Formulation

Aspirin	100g
Microcrystalline cellulose	25g
Tartaric acid	1g
10% starch paste	QS
Croscarmellose sodium	6g
Talc	15g

(2) Manufacturing process

As shown in Figure 8 – 1, 10% starch paste (about 50ml) is prepared by mixing and then heating some 5g starch and 1g tartaric acid with 50ml water. Aspirin acid is ground to pass the sieve of 80 meshes. Then mix it with microcrystalline cellulose and add 10% starch paste to prepare a damp mass. Wet granules are prepared by screening the damp mass through a stainless – steel sieve or nylon sieve of 16 meshes into pellets or granules. Next dry the wet granules at 60℃ for 30min and force dry granules pass through 16 meshes, then add talcum powder and croscarmellose sodium to dry granules with blending uniformly, and tablet by compression (using Φ8mm shallow concave punch).

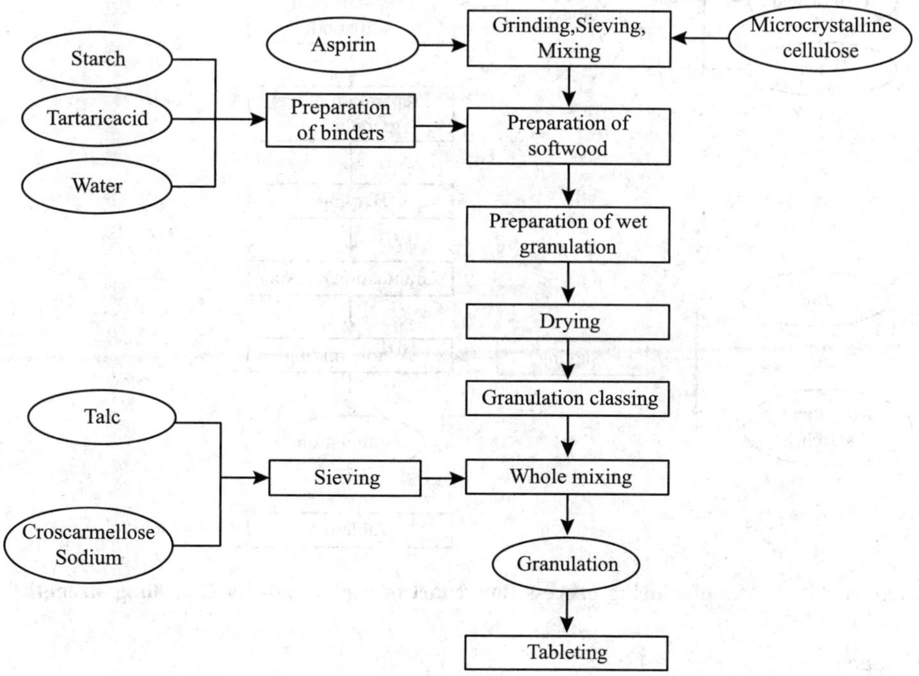

Figure 8 – 1　Manufacturing process flow chart of aspirin tablets Ⅰ(100mg strength)

(3) Usage

This product can prevent the conglomeration of platelets and avoid the formation of thrombus. In clinical, it is used to prevent formations of thrombus after ischemia, cardiac muscle infarct, atrium vibration or other operations.

2. Preparation of Aspirin Tablets Ⅱ(300mg strength)

(1) Formulations

Aspirin	300g
Starch	20g
Tartaric acid	2g
10% starch paste	QS
Starch(Out added)	10g
Talc	15g

(2) Manufacturing process

As shown in Figure 8 - 2, 10% starch paste (about 50ml) is prepared by mixing and then heating 5g starch and 2g tartaric acid with 50ml water. Aspirin acid is ground to pass the sieve of 80 meshes. Then mix it with starch and add 10% starch paste to prepare a damp mass. Wet granules are prepared by screening the damp mass through a stainless - steel sieve or nylon sieve of 16 meshes into pellets or granules. Next dry the wet granules at 60℃ for 30min and force dry granules pass through 16 meshes, then add talcum powder to dry granules with blending uniformly, and tablet by compression(using Φ11mm shallow concave punch).

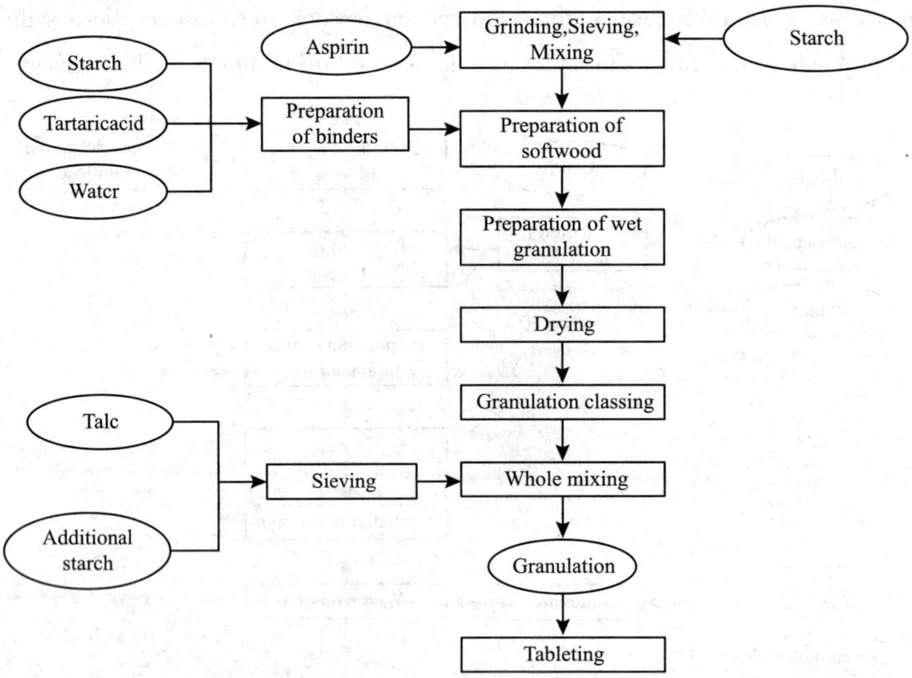

Figure 8 - 2 Manufacturing process flow chart of aspirin tablets Ⅱ (300mg strength)

(3) Usage

This product is used to ease pain, relieve fever, anti - inflammation, anti - rheumatism and treat arthritis.

3. Preparation of Enteric Coated Aspirin Tablets(100mg strength)

(1) Formulation

Acryl - EZE93F	15g
distilled water	85ml

(2) Manufacturing process

As shown in Figure 8 – 3, 15% Acryl – EZE93F enteric coating dispersion is prepared by dispersing 15g Acryl – EZE93F in 85ml water with stirring for 30minutes, and then passing through 60 mesh sieve. Coat the tablet cores using a rotary tablet coating machine. Place 50g of tablet core to the coating pan and preheat the tablet cores for 5min. The coating conditions are listed as follows: a bed temperature of 30 – 35℃, a pan rotation speed of 30 ~ 40 rpm. During the whole process, the spray rate and bed temperature should be adjusted according to the wetness of the tablet surface, aiming to obtain a balance between the spray rate and evaporation rate of solvent and thus avoid sticking. Finally, further dry the coated tablets at 30 – 35℃ for 10min to remove the residual water. The coating weight should be within the range of 8% ~ 10%.

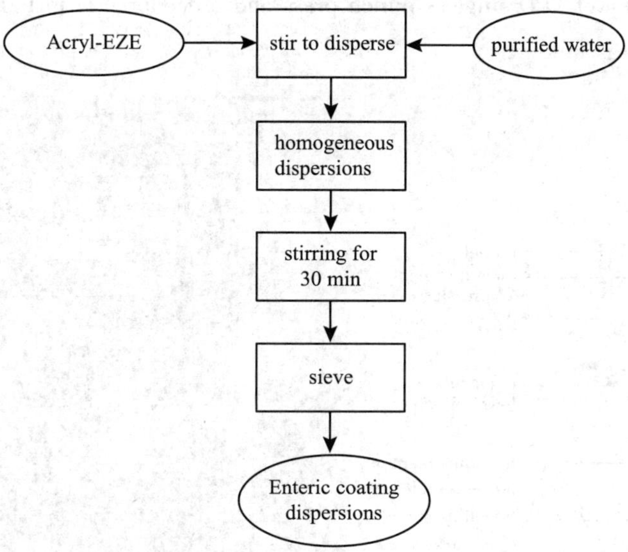

Figure 8 – 3 Manufacturing process flow chart of enteric coating dispersion

4. Determination of Mobility

(1) Principle

Angle of repose is the largest angle at which particles get the balance between gravity and particle friction force and is under stationary state when they slide at the free inclined plane of the powder accumulation. The smaller the angle of repose is, the smaller the friction force will be and the better the flowability will be. We generally think that when $\theta \leqslant 30°$ the flowability is good and when $\theta \leqslant 40°$ that the powder can meet the demand of the productive process. As shown in Figure 8 – 4, the commonly used methods include injection method, discharge method, inclined angle method and so on.

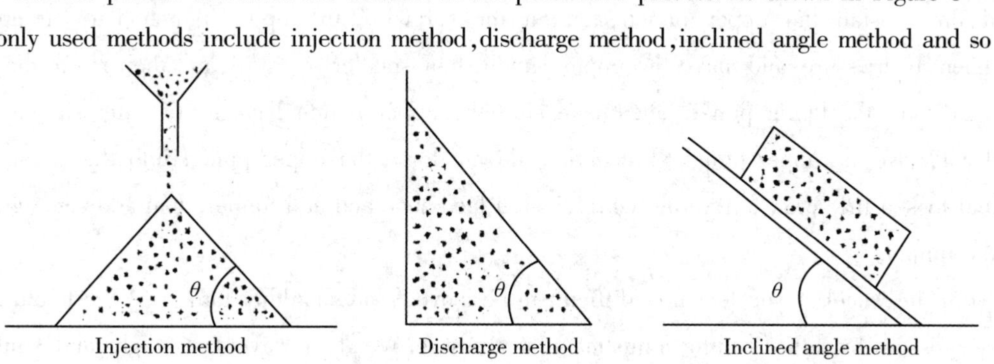

Figure 8 – 4 Illustration of methods for the investigation of angle of repose

(2) Determination of angle of repose

Put watch glass on experiment table horizontally and record it's radius, then connect the glass funnel to iron, let the center line of glass funnel and the center of watch glass are in the same vertical line and the lowest position of glass funnel be 3.0 to 6.0cm to the watch glass. Add aspirin tablets total mixed granules from glass funnel slowly, the granules will heap up on watch glass with the shape of cone, continue to add until the granules free fall along the brim of the cone, and then record the height of the cone. Angle of repose can be worked out by the formula: $\tan\theta$ = height/radius.

5. Installing and Debugging of Single – Punch Press

(1) Structure of single – punch press

The basic structure of TPD single – punch press and procedures of installing and debugging are shown in Figure 8 – 5 as follows.

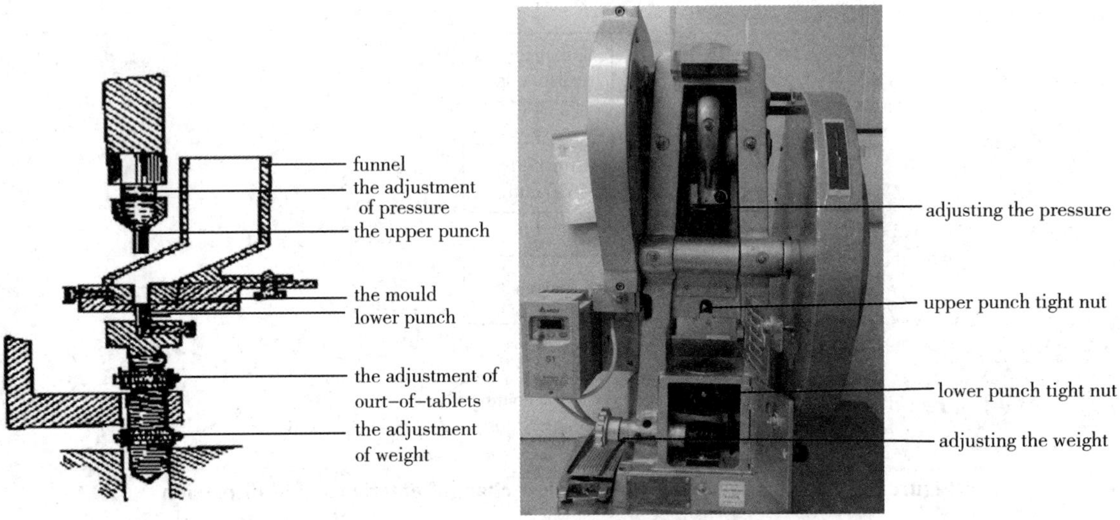

Figure 8 – 5 Illustration of single – punch tablet press

(2) Adjusting and debugging of of single – punch press

Firstly, install the lower punch, tighten the screw of lower punch, rotate the adjustment of weight and make lower punch at the lower part. Then put the die into the mould, tighten the screw of die, and fix the mould (precaution: do not hit and destroy punch).

Adjust the adjustment of out – of – tablets, raise the lower punch to the same level with the mould, then install the upper punch, tighten the screw of the upper punch. Turn around the adjustment of pressure, and make the upper punch show smaller pressure, and then rotate the wheel slowly to lower the upper punch, and make sure the upper punch locates at center station of the die. If not, raise the upper punch (precaution: do not force the upper punch into the canal of the die) and loosen the screw of the die lightly, install feed shoe and add funnel, then add some granules into the funnel.

Turn the wheel. If you feel it is difficult to be moved, you shouldn't force it. You should add or reduce pressure by adjusting the adjustment of pressure. Weigh the average weight and adjust the adjustment of weight to make the compressed tablets fit the requirement of weight, and adjust the adjustment of pressure simultaneously to make the tablets have suitable hardness.

Open power and compress, test weight and disintegration time of the tablets, if the tablets prepared fit the requirement, then compress formally.

(3) Selecting of trimming die

The trimming die of single - punch press is composed of upper punch, lower punch and die. Usually, most punches are round with different foveation radian. As showed in Table 8 - 1, there are many kinds of punches with different diameters, which could be chosen according to the weight of the tablets.

Table 8 - 1 The choosing of the specification of punch

Weight(mg)	50	100	150	200	300	500
Diameter(mm)	5 ~ 6.5	7	8	8.5	10.5	12

(4) Maintenance of tablet press

After the tableting is finished, remove the powder with a brush, and wipe the machine parts to keep the tablet machine dry and clean. Finally add a good lubricant for protection. Before the next use of machine, turn the wheel carefully by hand to make sure whether the tablet machine is in faulty. If everything is normal, start using the tablet machine.

6. Process of Enteric coating

(1) Coating process

The coating device include coating machine, air compressor, heating temperature control device and spray gun, as shown in Figure 8 - 6. The basic process of coating is as follows:

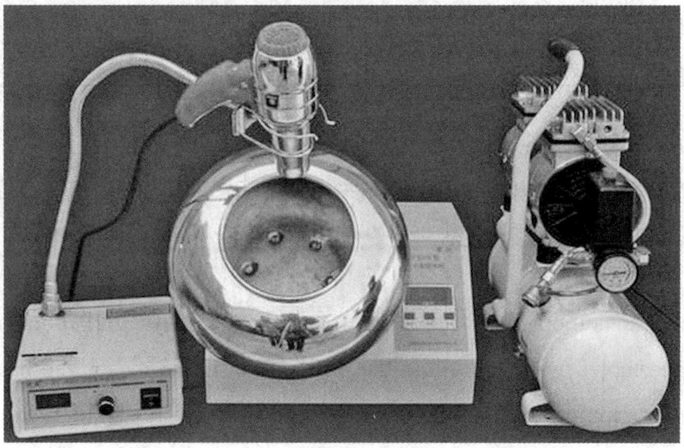

Figure 8 - 6 Illustration of the coating device

①Check the coating main machine, spray gun, air compressor, heating device, etc. and make sure they are normal and clean.

②Put the tablet cores into the coating pan, click the "start" button and set the rotating speed to let the tablets fall in a parabolic manner.

③Use a hair dryer to heat the pan, increase the core temperature appropriately, and heat the tablets to the temperature of feeling hot in hand. Spray gun test: start the air compressor, press the gun trigger and adjust the air intake of the gun, adjust the appropriate gas volume, and then adjust the front nut to spray appropriate liquid volume to make sure the tablets could be dried timely.

④Spray the coating dispersion while heating and control temperature at 30 ~ 35℃. When the coating weight reaches 8% ~ 10%, stop the spray and heat for a period of time (about 10minutes) to dry the tablets completely.

⑤When the coating finished, clean the coating pan and spray gun, and then dried to prevent rust.

(2) Maintenance of coating machine

The machine should be kept clean after each coating test, and the spray nozzle should be removed to clean. As the enteric material can be dissolved under alkaline conditions, it can be cleaned using a concentration of 3% – 5% NaOH solution.

7. Quality Standards

(1) Tablet weight variation

Comply with the requirements of general chapter <0101> of ChP, tablet weight variation test was carried out. Weigh accurately 20 tablets and calculate the average weight, then weigh individually each of the 20 tablets. Compare the weight of each tablet with the labeled tablet (if no labeled weight is stated, compare the weight of each tablet with the average weight calculated). No more than 2 of the individual weights exceed the weight variation limit stated in the Table 8 – 2 above and none doubles the limit. Tablets should comply with the following requirements stated in the table below.

Table 8 – 2 The tablet weight variation limits.

Average weight	Weight variation limit
Less than 0. 3g	±7. 5%
0. 3g or more	±5%

(2) Tablet hardness

The hardness of tablets is concerned with the integrality of tablets after storage and transport. Therefore, hardness is one of the internal control indexes for tablets. The check method of hardness can be divided into two method:

Hand – made check method: Take one piece of the test tablets, and then put it between middle and forefinger. Press the tablet by thumb, while the breakage of tablet means the hardness is not enough.

Tablet hardnessdetermination method: Take one piece of the test tablets, and then fix the tablet between the micro – cartridge and the end radially. Turn the switch to "along", and choose the "hardness" step. Fetch the value of hardness when the tablet is broken. Test 3 – 6 pieces totally, and take the average.

(3) Determination of disintegration

Comply with the requirements of general chapter <0921> of ChP, disintegration test is carried out to determinate the disintegration of aspirin tablets using lift disintegration tester. The disintegration tester is composed of a metal stand that can lift or low, and a basket with an end of mesh, along with apron. The movement distance of metal stand is 55mm ± 2mm, with the frequency of 30 – 32 times per minute.

Hang the basket on the stand through the upper stainless steel shaft, and immerse the basket into a 1000ml beaker. Adjust the basket to guarantee the distance from the sieve to the bottom of beaker is 15mm, when the baskets drop to a low point. Fill the beaker with water of 37 ± 1℃, and adjust the water level so that the basket is below the water surface and the distance is 15cm, when the basket go up to a high point, with the top of the basket not being immersed in the water. If one tablet fails to comply with the requirements of the test, repeat the operation with another 6 tablets. All the tablets should comply with the requirements of the test.

(4) Coating weight and quality

The coating weight (%), within the range from 8% - 10%, was obtained by the following equation: Coating weight (%) = $(W/W_0 - 1) \times 100\%$, where W and W_0 indicate the weight of coated tablets and tablet cores, respectively.

Coating examination: the examination for film - coating process should include the appearance, coating weight (%), impact resistance strength, film intension, water and moisture resistance test, stability, acid resistance and drug release, etc.

Experimental Instructions

Requirements for Preview

1. To preview the main factors those affect the disintegration of tablets.

2. To be familiar with the methods of granulation compression and direct compression. To be familiar with characters and applications of coating materials.

3. To understand the basic structure, installing, dismantling, and maintaining of single - punch press. To understand the procedures and characters of enteric - coating.

Procedures and Precautions

1. All the materials should be crushed, sieved and mixed before tableting. Small dosage of aspirin acid should be milled and forced through stainless steel screen (80 mesh), then mix with excipients, usually we use the method that mass increased as others increased, screen and mix several times to insure uniformly mixed.

2. The dosage of adhesives should be aptitude to make the soft material be conglomeration in hand and when fingers press it slightly, it should disperse but does not turn into powders.

3. The wet granulation should be dried under suitable temperature as soon as possible, according to the properties of active pharmaceutical ingredients and the adjuvant. The dried granulation always be prone to attach with each other, which should be sorted through sieves with lubricants.

4. Aspirin is unstable in wet or heat environment, and when encountering with iron, it can hydrolyze into salicylic acid and acetic acid, the former is irritative to stomach. We can add a few of tartaric acid or citric acid (about 1% dosage of aspirin) to starch solution and mix into granulate.

5. The starch paste should be used when cold. In order to reduce the amount of water, the concentration of starch paste could be improved to 14% - 17%. For practical production, tableting

with dry powder would also be carried out to avoid the influence of wet and heat.

6. Before the test of hardness, please check whether the indicator is fixed at zero. If not, use converse switch to return the indicator to zero. After the test, the indicator should be sent back to zero to avoid the damage of the spring. When the electric machine is rotating, do not turn the switch to make sure the electric machine would not be broken. The operation of switching should be carried out when the electric machine is rotating. Put the switch of proceedings to neutral and the switch of sequence to converse.

7. Dry the tablets at 40℃ for 30minutes before coating, and blow the powders on tablets' surface. Stick lengthways some scrips or adhesive plaster with the wideness of 1 - 2cm on the inner of coating pan to add friction between the tablets and the pans for tablets would roll not well due to the amount of tablets used is small.

8. If spraying is too rapid, when tablets' surfaces grow wet, their rolling in pan will be slower and difficult to overturn, we should stop spraying immediately and blow warm air to dry.

9. The temperature should be controlled at 40℃ to prevent the drugs' decomposition or the formation of air bladder on the surface of tablets; it will make the tablet and coating film separated.

Questions

1. What should be considered in the formulation design of drug unstable in wet and heat environment?

2. What problems would happen in the compression of small dosage drugs, and how to settle them?

3. What's the structure and working principle of the single - punch press?

4. When the lubricants should be added and why?

5. What kind of formulation need to coat with enteric film? Give some examples of enteric coating materials.

6. What problems would happen in enteric coating, and how to settle them?

实验 9　阿司匹林肠溶片释放度的测定

【目的与要求】

1. **掌握**　释放度（溶出度）测定的基本操作和数据处理方法。
2. **了解**　缓释、控释制剂测定释放度的意义。

【基本概念与实验原理】

肠溶片是指在胃液或酸性介质中不崩解，而在肠液或偏中性（pH6.8）介质中能够崩解和释放的一种片剂，它通常是由普通片芯和肠溶包衣构成。由于肠溶制剂在胃内不释放，通常可避免药物对胃的刺激和损伤，同时也可避免部分对酸不稳定的药物在胃部失活。

溶出度系指活性药物从片剂、胶囊剂或颗粒剂等普通制剂在规定条件下溶出的速率和程度，在缓释制剂、控释制剂、肠溶制剂及透皮贴剂等制剂中也称释放度。

与普通口服固体制剂不同，肠溶制剂口服后，在体内胃肠液中，需先经过肠溶包衣在肠液中溶解的过程再经过片芯崩解和药物溶出过程才能被机体吸收。其过程是：肠溶制剂→包衣在肠液中溶解→片芯崩解（或分散）→药物溶出→经生物膜被吸收。

释放度是衡量缓释制剂、肠溶制剂等制剂性能优劣的重要参数，《中国药典》和许多其他国家药典对口服缓释、肠溶制剂的释放度及其测定法都有明确规定。据《中国药典》四部通则 <0931> 溶出度与释放度测定法规定，释放度检查法包括第一法（篮法）、第二法（桨法）、第三法（小杯法）、第四法（桨碟法）和第五法（转筒法）。

以第一法（篮法）为例，溶出装置结构（图 9－1）包括：①转篮。分篮体与篮轴两部分，均为不锈钢或其他惰性材料制成，其形状尺寸如图 9－1 所示。篮体 A 由方孔筛网（丝径为 0.28 ± 0.03mm，网孔为 0.40 ± 0.04mm）制成，呈圆柱形，转篮内径为 20.2 ± 1.0mm，上下两端都有封边。篮轴 B 的直径为 9.75 ± 0.35mm，轴的末端连一圆盘，作为转篮的盖；盖上有一通气孔（孔径为 2.0mm ± 0.5mm）；盖边系两层，上层直径与转篮外径相同，下层直径与转篮内径相同；盖上的 3 弹簧片与中心呈 120° 角。②溶出杯。一般由硬质玻璃或其他惰性材料制成的底部为半球形的 1000ml 杯状容器，内径为 102 ± 4mm（圆柱部分内径最大值和内径最小值之差不得大于 0.5mm），高为 185 ± 25mm；溶出杯配有适宜的盖子，盖上有适当的孔，中心孔为篮轴的位置，其他孔供取样或测量温度用。溶出杯置恒温水浴或其他适当的加热装置中。③篮轴与电动机相连，由速度调节装置控制电动机的转速，使篮轴的转速在各品种项下规定转速的 ± 4% 范围之内。运转时整套装置应保持平稳，均不能产生明显的晃动或振动（包括装置所处的环境）。转篮旋转时，篮轴与溶出杯的垂直轴在任一点的偏离均不得大于 2mm，转篮下缘的摆动幅度不得偏离轴心 1.0mm。④仪器一般配有 6 套以上测定装置。

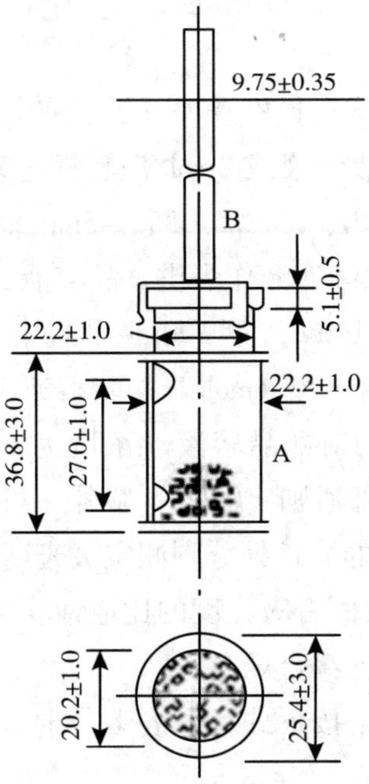

图 9－1　转篮装置（单位：mm）

释放度研究试验主要包括以下内容：释放介质的选择，溶出介质体积的选择，溶出方法的选择，转速的选择，释放度测定方法的验证，释放度均一性试验（批内），重现性试验（批间）等。为了模拟体内环境，溶出试验的温度一般在37℃。这些因素中，溶出介质的选择必须符合漏槽条件（sink condition），即到达溶出终点时，溶液中的药物浓度应远低于其饱和浓度。

在对肠溶制剂进行体外溶出试验时，应充分考虑肠溶制剂在进行制剂设计时的目的，即药物在胃液的酸性条件下不释放而可在肠液的近中性环境下释放。因此肠溶制剂溶出试验的溶出介质的选取应当兼顾模拟胃液的酸性环境和肠液的近中性环境，以期充分反映肠溶制剂口服给药后在胃肠道的释放特点。《中国药典》规定，肠溶片释放度测定试验应分别测定酸中释放度和缓冲液中释放度，其释放介质分别为 pH = 1 的盐酸溶液和 pH = 6.8 的盐酸 - 磷酸钠缓冲液。

【仪器与材料】

1. 仪器 分析天平，溶出试验仪，真空脱气仪，紫外分光光度计，医用注射器（5ml，10ml），量瓶（10ml，100ml），移液管（1ml，2ml，10ml），水系微孔滤膜（0.8μm）等。

2. 材料 阿司匹林肠溶片（规格100mg），盐酸，氢氧化钠，磷酸钠等。

【实验内容】

1. 酸中释放量 取阿司匹林肠溶片6片，按照《中国药典》四部通则 <0931> 溶出度与释放度测定法第一法（篮法）测定，以0.1mol/L的盐酸溶液750ml为溶出介质，设定转速为每分钟100转，取阿司匹林肠溶片6片置于各转篮中央，依法操作，经2h，取溶液5ml，滤过，取续滤液作为供试品溶液，自取样至滤过应在30s内完成，并同时补液5ml。取供试品溶液，按《中国药典》通则 <0401> 要求，以0.1mol/L盐酸溶液为空白，在280nm波长处测定吸光度，并计算酸中释放度，6片中，每片的释放度均不应大于标示量的10%。

2. 缓冲液中释放量 在酸中溶出量检查项下的溶液中继续加入37℃的0.2mol/L磷酸钠溶液250ml，混匀，用2mol/L盐酸溶液或2mol/L氢氧化钠溶液调节溶液的 pH 值至6.8 ± 0.05，继续进行释放试验，在5、10、15、25、35、45min时取溶液5ml，同时补加0.05mol/L磷酸钠缓冲液5ml，滤过样品，取续滤液作为供试品溶液，自取样至滤过应在30s内完成。

另精密称取阿司匹林对照品10mg，置100ml量瓶中，加磷酸钠缓冲液（0.05mol/L）（量取0.2mol/L磷酸钠溶液250ml与0.1mol/L盐酸溶液750ml混合，pH 值为6.8 ± 0.05）适量使溶解，并稀释至刻度，作为对照品溶液（浓度为 C_0）。取上述各时间点的续滤液与对照品溶液，照《中国药典》四部通则 <0401> 紫外 - 可见分光光度法，以磷酸钠缓冲液（0.05mol/L）为空白，在265nm的波长处分别测定吸光度，供试品溶液吸光度记为 A_n（$n = 1 \sim 6$），对照品吸光度记为 A_0，按两者吸光度的比值计算每片的释放量。缓冲液中45min时释放量，限度应为标示量的70%，符合规定。

将上述测定数据填入表9 - 1，按下式计算各取样时间点（$n = 1 \sim 6$）的累积释放百分数 D_n(%)：

$$D_n(\%) = 10 \times \frac{\left(A_n + \frac{10}{1000} \times \sum_{i=1}^{n-1} A_n\right) \times C_0}{A_0} \times 100\%$$

表 9-1　阿司匹林肠溶片释放度测定数据

取样时间	酸中释放 2h	缓冲液中释放					
		5min	10min	15min	25min	35min	45min
吸光度 A_n							
累积释放百分数 D_n（%）							

绘制释放曲线：即 D_n(%)～t 图，以时间（t）为横坐标，D_n(%)为纵坐标作图。

实验指导

一、预习要求

1. **了解**　释放度（溶出度）测定的目的和意义。

2. **了解**　溶出度测定仪器的基本构造和正确使用方法。

3. **了解**　肠溶片剂在不同 pH 环境下的释放性质。

二、操作要点和注意事项

1. 溶出度仪的适用性及性能确认试验除仪器的各项机械性能应符合上述规定外，还应用溶出度标准片对仪器进行性能确认试验，按照标准片的说明书操作，试验结果应符合标准片的规定。

2. 溶出杯内介质的温度是通过外面的水箱控制的。水箱内应加入蒸馏水，不宜用自来水，以免长期使用腐蚀温控零件。

3. 取样位置应固定在转篮上端与溶出介质液面的正中，距杯壁不小于 1cm 处。样品用 0.45μm 微孔滤膜过滤，滤器事先用空气针检漏，过滤时弃去初滤液，取续滤液。

4. 在对溶出液进行吸光度测定时，应注意酸中溶出液和缓冲液溶出液的测定应分别使用两种空白溶出介质作为空白对照样品。

三、思考题

1. 对肠溶制剂进行体外释放度评价的意义是什么？

2. 什么样的药物不适合制成肠溶制剂？

3. 释放度评价时需要研究哪些内容？

4. 简述现行版《中国药典》测定阿司匹林肠溶片释放度的方法。

5. 比较现行版《中国药典》与美国药典测定阿司匹林肠溶片释放度的方法。

6. 简述溶出度仪性能验证的关键点。

扫码“学一学”

Experiment 9　Determination of the Release of Aspirin Enteric Coated Tablets

Objectives and Requirements

1. To master the basic operation and data processing method for the determination of drug release (dissolution) test.

2. To understand the significance of measuring the release rate of sustained release and controlled release preparations.

Introduction

Enteric - coated tablets are tablets that do not disintegrate in gastric juice or acidic medium, but can be disintegrating and released in intestinal juice or neutral(ph6.8) medium. they are usually composed of common core and enteric coating. Because enteric preparation is not released in the stomach, it can usually avoid the stimulation and injury of the drug to the stomach, and also avoid the inactivation of some acid unstable drugs in the stomach.

The dissolution refers to the rate and degree of dissolution of the active drug from the common preparation such as tablet, capsule or granule under the specified conditions, and also the release degree in the sustained - release preparation, the controlled - release preparation, the enteric - coated preparation and the transdermal patch.

Unlike the conventional oral solid preparation, after the enteric preparation is taken orally, the enteric coating in the body needs to be dissolved in the intestinal fluid by the enteric coating, and then the tablet core disintegrates and the drug dissolution process can be absorbed by the body. The process is that the enteric - coated drug - coated tablet is dissolved in the intestinal fluid, and the tablet core disintegrates(or dispersed), and the drug is released and absorbed through the biological membrane.

Release rate is an important parameter to evaluate the performance of sustained release preparation, enteric preparation and other preparations. Chinese Pharmacopoeia and many other pharmacopoeia have clear provisions on oral sustained release, release rate and determination of enteric preparation. According to the general rules of Chinese Pharmacopoeia <0931>, the release rate test methods include the first method(basket method), the second method(paddle method), the third method(small cup method), the fourth method(paddle plate method) and the fifth method (rotating cylinder method).

Taking the first method(basket method) as an example, the structure of the dissolution device includes: (1) the rotating basket is divided into two parts, the basket body and the basket shaft, both of which are made of stainless steel or other lazy materials, and their shape and size are shown in Fig 9 - 1. The basket a is made of square hole screen(wire diameter is 0.28 ±0.03mm, mesh hole is 0.40 ±0.04mm), is cylindrical, the inner diameter of basket is 20.2 ±1.0mm, and the upper and lower ends are sealed. The diameter of the basket b is 9.75 ±0.35mm, and the end of the shaft is connected with a disk as the cover of the basket, and there is a hole on the cover(the aperture is 2.0 ±0.5mm). The diameter of the upper layer is the same as the outer diameter of the basket, and the diameter of the lower layer is the same as that of the basket. The 3 spring plates on the cover are 120 °angle to the center. (2) the dissolution cup is usually made of hard glass or other lazy material at the bottom of the hemispherical 1000ml cup - shaped container with an inner diameter of 102 ± 4mm(the difference between the maximum inner diameter and the minimum inner diameter of the cylindrical part shall not be greater than 0.5mm), and the high 185 ± 25mm; dissolution cup is equipped with a suitable lid, with an appropriate hole on the lid, the position of the central hole as the basket shaft, and other holes for sampling or measuring temperature. The dissolution cup is placed in a constant temperature water bath or other appropriate heating device. (3) the basket shaft is connected to the motor, and the speed of the motor is controlled by the speed regulating device, so that the speed of the basket shaft is within the range of ±4% of the specified speed under each variety. The whole device should be kept stable and cannot produce obvious sloshing or vibration (including the environment in which the device is located). When the basket rotates, the deviation between the basket axis and the vertical axis of the dissolution cup shall not be more than 2mm, and the swing amplitude of the lower edge of the basket shall not deviate from the axial center 1.0mm. (4) the instrument is generally equipped with more than 6 sets of measuring devices.

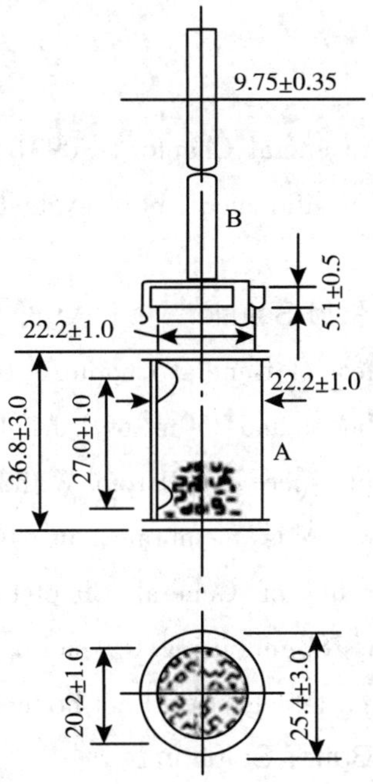

Figure 9 - 1 Rotating basket device (Unit: mm)

The release degree study test mainly includes the following contents: selection of release medium, selection of dissolution medium volume, selection of dissolution method, selection of rotation speed, verification of release method, degree of release uniformity test (in - batch), reproducibility test (lot - to - lot), etc. In order to simulate the in vivo environment, the temperature of the dissolution test is generally at 37℃. In these factors, the selection of the dissolution medium must be in accordance with the sink condition. That means the concentration of the drug in the solution should be much lower than its saturation concentration when the dissolution endpoint is reached.

In the in vitro dissolution test of enteric preparation, the purpose of enteric preparation design should be fully considered, that is, the drug can be released in the near neutral environment of intestinal fluid without release under the acidic condition of gastric juice. Therefore, the selection of dissolution medium in enteric preparation dissolution test should take into account the acidic environment of simulated gastric juice and the near neutral environment of intestinal juice, in order to fully reflect the release characteristics of enteric preparation in gastrointestinal tract after oral administration. According to the 2015 edition of Chinese Pharmacopoeia, the release rate of enteric tablets should be determined by acid release and buffer respectively. The release media were hydrochloric acid solution of pH = 1 and sodium phosphate buffer of pH = 6. 8.

Equipment and Materials

1. Equipment

Analytical balance, dissolution test apparatus, vacuum degassing instrument, ultraviolet spectrophotometer, syringe (5ml, 10ml), volumetric flask (10ml, 100ml), pipette (1ml, 2ml, 10ml), microporous membrane (0. 8μm), etc.

2. Materials

Aspirin enteric - coated tablets (100mg), hydrochloric acid, sodium hydroxide, sodium phosphate, etc.

Experimental Methods

According to drug release test (General Chapter <0931> of ChP, Method 1, the release of aspirin enteric - coated tablets in specific medium is evaluated. Upon dealing with the data by Excel, plot the drug release curve.

1. The Amount Released in Acid Solution

Comply with the drug release test of General Chapter <0931> of ChP, Method 1, using the apparatus of the dissolution test method 1 and 750ml of 0. 1mol/L hydrochloric acid solution as the dissolution medium. Adjust the rotating speed to100 rpm. Withdraw 5ml of the solvent after exactly 2h, filter it using a 0. 8μm microporous membrane, use the successive filtrate as the test solution. Comply with the requirements of General Chapter <0401> of ChP, measure the absorbance of the test solutions at 280nm, using 0. 1mol/L hydrochloric acid solution as the blank. The release rate of each of the 6 tablets should not be more than 10% of the marked amount.

2. The Amount Released in Buffer Solution

Carry out the drug release test of General Chapter <0931> of ChP, Method 1, using the apparatus of the dissolution test. After the test of drug release in acid medium, add 250ml of 37℃ 0. 2mol/L sodium phosphate solution, mix well, adjust the pH to 6. 8 ± 0. 05 with 2mol/L hydrochloric acid solution or 2mol/L sodium hydroxide. Withdraw 5ml of the solvent after exactly 5, 10, 15, 20, 25, 30 and 45min, filter it using a 0. 8μm microporous membrane, use the successive filtrate as the test solution and supply 10ml of 0. 05mol/L sodium phosphate solution.

Accurately weight a quantity of aspirin (10mg), place in 100ml volumetric flask, add 0. 05mol/L sodium phosphate solution (measure 250ml of 0. 2mol/L sodium phosphate solution and 750ml of 0. 1mol/L hydrochloric acid solution, mix well, adjust pH to 6. 8 ± 0. 05) to dissolve and dilute to volume, and mix well, as the reference solution. Comply with the requirements of General Chapter <0401> of ChP, measure the absorbance of the test and reference solutions at 265nm, using 0. 05mol/L sodium phosphate solution as the blank; calculate the amount released in buffer solution per tablet with respect to the absorbance. Not less than 70% of the labelled account is released at 45min.

Calculate the amount released (D_n) in buffer solution with respect to the absorbance, fill the following table (Table 9 - 1), draw the curve of D_n (%) - t, with the time (t) as X - axis and the D_n

(%) as Y - axis.

$$D_n(\%) = 10 \times \frac{\left(A_n + \frac{10}{1000} \times \sum_{i=1}^{n-1} A_n\right) \times C_0}{A_0} \times 100\%$$

Table 9 - 1　data for determination of release of aspirin enteric - coated tablets

Sampling time	Release in acid for 2h	Release in buffer					
		5min	10min	15min	25min	35min	45min
A							
$D_n(\%)$							

Experimental Instructions

Requirements for Preview

1. To understand the purpose and significance of determination of release rate (dissolution rate).

2. To understand the basic structure and correct usage of dissolution measurement instrument.

3. To understand the release characteristics of enteric - coated tablets in different pH environments.

Procedures and Precautions

1. The applicability and performance confirmation test of the dissolution meter in addition to the various mechanical properties of the instrument shall comply with the above regulations, the dissolution standard sheet shall also be used to carry out the performance confirmation test of the instrument according to the specification of the standard sheet, and the test results shall conform to the requirements of the standard sheet.

2. The temperature of the medium in the dissolution cup is controlled by an external tank. Water tank should be added distilled water, should not use tap water, lest long - term corrosion temperature control parts.

3. The sampling position shall be fixed in the middle of the basket and not less than 1cm from the wall of the cup. The sample was filtered with a 0.45μm microporous filter, and the filter was first leak - detected with an air needle, and the primary filtrate was discarded at the time of filtration and the subsequent filtrate was used.

4. When determining the absorbance of the solution, we should pay attention to the determination of the dissolution solution in acid and buffer solution. Two kinds of blank dissolution medium should be used as blank control sample respectively.

Questions

1. What is the significance of evaluating the release of enteric - coated preparations?

2. What kind of drug is not suitable to be prepared as enteric - coated preparations?

3. What should be investigated for release rate evaluation?

4. Describe the method used to evaluate the release rate of aspirin enteric - coated tablet in the

current Chinese Pharmacopeia

5. Compare the release rate evaluation method of aspirin enteric - coated tablet used in the current Chinese Pharmacopeia and USP.

6. Describe the key point in the performance validation of dissolution test apparatus.

实验10 茶碱骨架型缓释片的制备与释放度测定

【目的与要求】

1. **掌握** 骨架型缓释片的制备方法及其释放度检查方法。
2. **熟悉** 骨架型缓释片的设计原理。
3. **了解** 骨架型缓释片的释药机制。

【基本概念与实验原理】

缓释制剂系指口服药物在规定溶剂（水、酸性介质、缓冲液等）中，按要求缓慢地非恒速释放，且每日用药次数与相应普通制剂比较至少减少一次或用药的间隔时间有所延长的制剂。缓释制剂与控释制剂的区别在于，后者能按要求缓慢地恒速或接近恒速释药。缓释制剂按剂型分主要有片剂、颗粒剂、小丸剂、混悬剂、胶囊剂、膜剂、栓剂、植入剂等，其中，片剂又分为骨架片、膜控片、胃内漂浮片、生物黏附片等。骨架型缓释片是目前研究最多、制备工艺相对简单的品种。

骨架片是药物和一种或多种骨架材料以及其他辅料，通过制片工艺而成型的片状固体制剂。使用不同的骨架材料或采用不同的工艺制成的骨架片，可以不同的释药机制延长作用时间、减少服用次数、降低刺激性或不良反应。骨架可呈多孔型或无孔型。多孔型骨架片，药物通过微孔道扩散而释放，服从 Higuchi 方程，个别也可达零级释放；影响释放的主要原因是药物的溶解度、骨架孔隙率、孔径以及孔曲率，一般适于水溶性药物。无孔型骨架片的释药是外层表面的溶蚀 - 分散 - 溶出过程，扩散不是释药的主要途径，这类制剂可通过改变骨架材料用量或采用多种混合骨架材料等来调节释药速率；其释药过程服从一级或近一级动力学过程，少数可调节至零级过程。

适于制备骨架片的药物大多数为固体药物，一般而言，水溶性较大的药物比较合适，溶解度小于0.01mg/ml时问题较多，但可应用固体分散技术，将药物纳入水溶性载体后，再与骨架材料混合制成骨架片。常用的骨架材料有：不溶性骨架材料，如乙基纤维素及其水分散体、聚乙烯、聚丙烯、聚硅氧烷、乙烯 - 醋酸乙烯共聚物和聚甲基丙烯酸甲酯等；生物溶蚀性骨架材料，如硬脂酸、巴西棕榈蜡、单硬脂酸甘油酯和十八烷醇等；亲水凝胶骨架材料，如天然胶（海藻酸钠、琼脂、西黄蓍胶等）、纤维素衍生物（甲基纤维素、羟乙基纤维素、羟丙甲纤维素等）、非纤维素多糖（壳多糖、半乳糖甘露聚糖等）以及乙烯聚合物和丙烯酸树脂（聚乙烯醇和聚羧乙烯等）。骨架片可采用湿法制粒压片、干法制粒压片或者粉末直接压片等工艺制备。

释放度系指药物从缓释制剂、控释制剂、肠溶制剂及透皮贴剂等在规定条件下溶出的速率和程度。检查释放度的制剂不再进行崩解时限的检查。通过释放度的测定，找出其释放规律，从而可选定所需的骨架材料，同时，亦用于控制片剂的质量，确保片剂以适宜的速度释药进而确保其疗效。释放度的测定方法，照溶出度测定法进行，释放介质为人工胃液和人工肠液，有时也可用水或其他介质。一般采用3个时间取样，在规定时间、规定取样点，吸取溶液适量，滤过，进而进行测定并计算释放量。

【仪器与材料】

1. 仪器　乳钵（中号），托盘天平，分析天平，搪瓷盘（31cm×41cm），尼龙筛（18目、16目），不锈钢丝筛（80目、40目），烘箱，单冲压片机，浅凹冲（Φ8mm），片剂硬度测定仪，溶出度试验仪，752型紫外－可见分光光度计，量筒（1000ml，10ml），微孔膜滤器（孔径0.8μm），量瓶（500ml、10ml）等。

2. 材料　无水茶碱，羟丙甲纤维素（HPMC，K15），乙基纤维素水分散体（固含量25%），微晶纤维素（MCC，PH101），一水乳糖，滑石粉，硬脂酸镁，乙醇（90%）等。

【实验内容】

一、茶碱亲水凝胶骨架片的制备

1. 处方　见表10－1。

表10－1　茶碱亲水凝胶骨架片处方

原辅料	每400片用量（g）		
	处方A1	处方A2	处方A3
无水茶碱	40.0	40.0	40.0
HPMC	6.0	8.0	12.0
MCC	2.0	2.0	2.0
一水乳糖	8.0	8.0	8.0
90%乙醇	QS	QS	QS
滑石粉	1.0	1.0	1.0

2. 制备工艺　取无水茶碱、HPMC、MCC及一水乳糖，分别过80目筛。按处方称取上述原辅料，在研钵中混合，过40目筛混合3次，加90%乙醇适量制成适宜软材，过18目尼龙筛制湿颗粒，于50～60℃干燥（约45min），16目筛整粒，加入滑石粉混匀，使用Φ8mm冲压片。每片含无水茶碱100mg，硬度控制在5～7kgf。

二、茶碱不溶性骨架片的制备

1. 处方　见表10－2。

表10－2　茶碱不溶性骨架片处方

原辅料	每400片用量（g）		
	处方B1	处方B2	处方B3
无水茶碱	40.0	40.0	40.0
一水乳糖	50.0	—	25

续表

原辅料	每400片用量（g）		
	处方B1	处方B2	处方B3
微晶纤维素（MCC）	—	50	25
25%乙基纤维素水分散体	40.0	40.0	40.0
滑石粉	1.0	1.0	1.0
硬脂酸镁	0.5	0.5	0.5

2. 制备工艺 取无水茶碱、一水乳糖及MCC，分别过80目筛。按处方称取上述原辅料，在研钵中混合，过40目筛混合3次，加25%乙基纤维素水分散体制成适宜软材，过18目尼龙筛制湿颗粒，于50～60℃干燥（约1h），16目筛整粒，加入滑石粉和硬脂酸镁，混匀，使用Φ9mm冲压片。每片含无水茶碱100mg，硬度控制在5～7kgf。

三、释放度测定

1. 标准曲线的制备 精密称取茶碱对照品约20mg，置500ml量瓶中，加水溶解、定容。精密量取0.5、1.0、2.0、2.5、3.0ml分别置于10ml量瓶中，加水定容，摇匀，制成2.0、4.0、8.0、10.0、12.0μg/ml的溶液。以水为空白对照，在272nm的波长处分别测定吸光度。

2. 释放度测定

取缓释片，照溶出度与释放度测定法(《中国药典》四部通则 <0931 >)，采用第二法（桨法）装置，以水900ml为溶剂，转速为每分钟50转，依法操作，在1、2、3、4、6、12小时分别取溶液3ml，立即经0.8μm微孔滤膜滤过，并及时在操作容器中补充水3ml。分别精密量取续滤液各1ml，分别置于10ml量瓶中，加水至刻度，摇匀，在272nm的波长处分别测定吸光度。

四、实验结果与数据处理

1. 标准曲线

将标准溶液的浓度与吸光度进行最小二乘法线性回归，求得标准曲线。数据记录于表10－3中。

表10－3 标准溶液浓度与相应吸光度

浓度 C（μg/ml）	
吸光度 A	

标准曲线：$C=$

相关系数：$r=$

线性范围：　～　μg/ml

2. 释放度及释放曲线 根据标准曲线，计算各取样时间的药物释放量，并按标示量（100mg）估算各取样时间的累积释放百分率。以累积释放百分率对时间作图，得释放曲线。

3. 释药机制 通常将释放度数据按以下三种数学模型进行拟合，来研究释药机制：

零级方程：
$$M_t/M_\infty = kt \quad (1)$$

一级方程：
$$\ln(1-M_t/M_\infty) = -kt \quad (2)$$

Higuchi 方程：　　　　　　$M_t/M_\infty = kt^{1/2}$　　　　　　（3）

式中，M_t 为在时间 t 的累积释药量；M_∞ 为在时间趋于无穷大时的累积释药量；M_t/M_∞ 为在时间 t 的累积释药百分数；k 为释药速率常数。

表 10－4　释药机理研究数据处理

时间（h）	M_t/M_∞	$\ln(1-M_t/M_\infty)$	$t_{1/2}$
0			
1			
2			
3			
4			
6			
8			
12			

采用最小二乘法分别按以上数学模型进行拟合，求相关系数。相关系数最大且均方差（MSE）最小者为最佳。

实验指导

一、预习要求

1. **复习**　缓控释制剂内容，了解缓控释制剂的类型及其临床意义。溶出度试验的方法、对象及其意义，并参阅《中国药典》四部通则 <0931> 溶出度与释放度测定的有关内容。

2. **了解**　口服缓释制剂的一般制备原理及方法，熟悉常用骨架材料的理化性质及其应用。缓控释制剂与一般口服制剂在质量要求上的异同。

二、操作要点与注意事项

1. 本实验选用亲水凝胶材料 HPMC 制备溶蚀性骨架片。亲水凝胶骨架片的释药过程是骨架溶蚀和药物扩散综合效应的过程，同时，由于药物水溶性的不同，释放机制也不同，水溶性大的药物主要以药物扩散为主，而水溶性较小的药物（如茶碱）则以骨架溶蚀为主。本实验茶碱缓释片中 HPMC 用量增加时，可使片剂遇水后形成凝胶层的速率加快、厚度增加，从而导致水分向片芯渗透速率减小，以致片剂骨架溶蚀减缓、茶碱释放速率减慢；若片中水溶性小分子乳糖用量增加，则在一定程度上可以促使水分渗入片芯，从而使片剂溶蚀加快，进而加快释放速率。因而，茶碱缓释片可通过 HPMC、乳糖用量的改变来调节药物的释放速率，直至达到要求为止。

以 90% 乙醇为润湿剂制软材料时，乙醇用量应适宜，使软材达到手握之可成团，手指轻压时又能散裂而不成粉状为度。制得的颗粒应以无长条、块状和过多细粉为宜。

2. 本实验选用乙基纤维素水分散体作为缓释黏合剂用于制备不溶性骨架片。乙基纤维素水分散体可以提高药物的可压性，药物从不溶性骨架中的释放机制是通过孔道扩散，释放速率受填充剂的影响。乙基纤维素广泛用于膜控包衣材料或作为黏合剂使用，用来制备口服缓释制剂。乙基纤维素的水分散体可用于制备缓释多颗粒系统填充于胶囊或压制成片，也可用于软胶囊的缓释包衣。

3. 骨架型缓释片的硬度对释药速率有较大影响，本实验将硬度控制在 5 ~ 7 kgf 之间为宜。

4. 对所用的溶出度测定仪，应预先检查其是否运转正常，并检查温度、转速的控制等是否精确；桨的位置应按规定高度安装，桨底部距溶出杯底应为 25mm。

5. 样液用微孔滤膜过滤时，应注意滤膜安装是否正确紧密，否则会影响测定数据的正确性。

三、思考题

1. 在茶碱缓释片处方中，HPMC 和 EC 分别起什么作用？MCC、乳糖又各起什么作用？
2. 缓控释制剂释放度标准为何需 3 个控制点？
3. 缓释制剂进行体外释放度检查有何意义？
4. 骨架型缓释片中常用的骨架材料有哪些，各有什么特点？
5. 请设计硝苯地平骨架型缓释片的处方与制备工艺。
6. 请设计盐酸二甲双胍骨架型缓释片的处方与制备工艺。

扫码"学一学"

Experiment 10 Preparation and Drug Release Test of Theophylline Extended – release Matrix Tablets

Objectives and Requirements

1. To master the manufacturing process of extended – release matrix tablets and the procedure of drug release test.

2. To be familiar with design principles of extended – release matrix tablets.

3. To understand the mechanism of drug release from extended – release matrix tablets.

Introduction

Extended – release preparations are preparations which release drugs with non – constant rate generally in rated solvent(water, tart medium, buffer, etc.) and the daily frequency of administration is one time less than the corresponding ordinary preparation at least or the dosing interval is relative longer. The difference between extended – release preparation and controlled – release preparation is that the latter release drug in constant rate or quasi – constant rate. Extended – release preparations are classified as tablets, granules, small pills, suspensions, capsules, pellicles, suppositories and embedded preparations according to dosage form. Among the total, tablets also include matrix tablets, membrane – controlled tablets, gastric floating tablets, biotic adhering tablets, etc. The matrix extended – release tablets are the hottest researching preparation whose preparation process are relatively simple.

Matrix tablets are solid preparations containing one or more matrix materials or other excipients prepared by tabletting techniques. Matrix tablets prepared with different matrix materials or different technology have the different mechanism of drug releasing to extend action time, reduce frequency of administration, irritation and adverse effects. The matrixes include multiporous type or aporate type. For multiporous matrix tablets, drug release by diffusing through the microporous channel whose release rate conforms to Higuchi equation besides few releases with zero order. The main factors that affect the releasing of drugs are the solubility of drugs, the porosity of the matrix and the aperture and curvature of pores. They generally refer to water - soluble drugs. For aporate matrix tablets, drugs release by the corrosion - dispersion - dissolution process of the out surface, diffusion is not the main path of the releasing of drugs. The drug release rate this type of preparation can be regulated by changing the amount of matrix material or using incorporating matrix material. The drug release of first - order or quasi - first - order kinetics, a few can be adjusted to zero - order kinetics.

Drugs which prepared into matrix tablets are most solid drugs. Generally speaking, water - soluble drugs are most suitable for it, if the solubility of drug is less than 0. 01mg/ml, there will be lots of problem, but the drug can be dispersed in water - soluble carrier by solid dispersion technical first, and then prepared into matrix tablets with matrix materials. The commonly used matrix materials are described as follows. Insoluble matrix materials include ethylcellulose (EC) and it aqueous dispersion, polyethylene, polypropylene, polysiloxane, ethylene - vinylacetate copolymer and polymethyl methacrylate (PMM). Biotic erodible matrix materials include stearic acid, carnauba wax, glyceryl monostearate and octadecanol. Hydrophilic gelatinous matrix materials include natural rubber such as sodium polymannuronate, agar, gum tragacanth, etc. , cellulose derivatives such as methylcellulose, hydroxyethylcellulose, hydroxypropyl methylcellulose(HPMC) , etc. , non - cellulose polycose such as chitin, galactomannan, etc. , ethylene polymer and acrylic resin such as polyvinyl alcohol, carbopol, etc. Two basic techniques are used to granulate powders for compression into a tablet: wet granulation and dry granulation. Powders that can be mixed well do not require granulation and can be compressed into tablets through direct compression.

Drug release rate is defined as the rate and degree that medicaments release from extended - release preparations, controlled - release preparations, enteric - coated preparations and transdermal drug delivery systems in the specified condition. It is unnecessary to examine the dissolution rate or disintegration time of the preparation when release rate is determined. The matrix materials can be chosen according to the rule of drug releasing which is obtained by the determination of the release rate. At the same time, it can also be used to control the quality of tablets, so that the tablets can release drug with proper rate to insure the therapeutic effect. The determination of release rate must comply with the requirements of dissolution test, the releasing medium are artificial gastric juice and artificial intestinal juice, water or some other mediums are also used sometimes. Generally sampling at three different time, imbibe solution at certain time in a certain location, filter, determine and calculate the releasing amount.

Equipment and Materials

1. Equipment

Pestle(medium) , counter balance, analytical balance, enamel ware dish(31cm × 41cm) , Nylon sieve(18 and 16 - mesh) , stainless steel sieve(40 and 80 - mesh) , oven, single - punch machine, punch (shallow concave punch, Φ8mm and Φ9mm), hardness tester, dissolution tester, 752 UV - vis spectrometer, measuring cylinder (1000ml, 10ml), membrane filter (0.8μm), measuring flask (500ml, 10ml), etc.

2. Materials

Theophylline anhydrous, hydroxypropyl methylcellulose (HPMC K15), aqueous dispersion of ethylcellulose (Surelease, 25% *W/W*), microcrystalline cellulose (MCC, PH101), lactose, talc, magnesium stearate, ethanol (90%), etc.

Procedures

1. Preparation of Theophylline Hydrophilic Gelatinous Matrix Tablets

(1) Formulations

As shown in Table 10 - 1。

Table 10 - 1 Formulations of theophylline hydrophilic gelatinous matrix tablets

Drug and excipients	400 tablets (g)		
	Formulation A1	Formulation A2	Formulation A3
Theophylline anhydrous	40.0	40.0	40.0
HPMC	6.0	8.0	12.0
MCC	2.0	2.0	2.0
Lactose	8.0	8.0	8.0
Ethanol (90%)	QS	QS	QS
Talc	1.0	1.0	1.0

(2) Manufacturing process

Theophylline, HPMC, MCC, lactose are passed through 80 - mesh sieve respectively. Weigh theophylline and excipients in the formulation and mix uniformly in a mortar, pass through a 40 - mesh sieve for three times, add 90% alcohol solution to prepare damp mass, then pass through a 18 - mesh nylon screen to form wet granules, dry at 50 - 60℃ (about 45min), force dry granules pass through 16 - mesh to create granules of uniform size, then add talc to dry granules, mix uniformly, and compress into tablets using Φ8mm punch. Each tablet contains 100mg of theophylline. The tablet hardness ranges from 5 to 7 kgf.

2. Preparation of Theophylline Insoluble Matrix Tablets

(1) Formulations

As Shown in Table 10 - 2。

Table 10 - 2 Composition of theophylline insoluble matrix tablets

Drug and excipients	400 tablets (g)		
	Formulation B1	Formulation B2	Formulation B3
Theophylline anhydrous	40.0	40.0	40.0
Lactose monohydrate	50.0	—	25
MCC	—	50	25
25% Aqueous EC dispersion	40.0	40.0	40.0
Talc	1.0	1.0	1.0
Magnesium stearate	0.5	0.5	0.5

(2) Manufacturing process

Theophylline, MCC and lactose are passed through 80 – mesh sieve respectively. Weigh theophylline and excipients in the formulation and mix uniformly in a mortar, pass through a 40 – mesh sieve for three times, add 25% aqueous EC dispersion to prepare damp mass, then pass through a 18 – mesh nylon screen to form wet granules, dry at 50 – 60℃ (about 1h), force dry granules pass through 16 – mesh to create granules of uniform size, then add talc and magnesium stearate to dry granules, mix uniformly, and compress into tablets using Φ9mm punch. Each tablet contains 100mg of theophylline. The tablet hardness ranges from 5 to 7 kgf.

3. Drug Release Test

(1) Preparation of the standard curve

Weigh about 20mg of theophylline standard accurately and transfer to a 500ml volumetric flask. Dissolve and dilute to volume with distilled water. Measure accurately 0.5, 1, 2, 2.5, and 3ml of the stock solution into 10ml volumetric flasks and dilute with water to volume separately. Measure the absorbance of each solution at 272nm, using water as the blank.

(2) Drug release test

Carry out the drug release test (general chapter <0931> of ChP 2015, method 2), using 900ml of water as the drug release medium; adjust the rotational speed of the paddle to 50 rpm. Withdraw a sample of 3ml of the solution at exact 1, 2, 3, 4, 6, 8 and 12h respectively, filter through 0.8μm membrane filter and supply 3ml of water accordingly in the vessel immediately. Transfer accurately 1ml of the filtrate solution into 10ml volumetric flasks and dilute with water to volume separately. Measure the absorbance of the resulting solutions at 272nm using an UV – Vis spectrometer.

4. The Experimental Results and Data Processing

(1) The standard curve

Fill the table (Table 10 – 3) and calculate a linear regression equation using the least squares method.

Table 10 – 3 The concentration of the standard solution and the corresponding absorbance.

C(μg/ml)	0					
A	0					

Regression equation: C =

Regression coefficient: r =

Linear range: – μg/ml.

(2) Release rate and release curve

Calculate the drug release amount at each sampling time according to the standard curve, and estimate the accumulated drug release percentage of each sampling time compared with the indicated amount (100mg). The release curve can be obtained by plotting the accumulated drug release percentage versus time.

(3) Mechanism of drug release

To study the mechanism of drug release, the release data can be generally fitted to the following three math models:

Zero - order equation: $M_t/M_\infty = kt$ (1)

First - order equation: $\ln(1 - M_t/M_\infty) = -kt$ (2)

Higuchi's equation: $M_t/M_\infty = kt^{1/2}$ (3)

Where M_t stands for the cumulative release amount at time t, M_∞ is the cumulative release amount while time tends to ∞, M_t/M_∞ is the accumulated drug release percentage at time t, and k is the release rate constant. Fill in Table 10 - 4.

Table 10 - 4 Data processing for the mechanism of drug release.

t(h)	M_t/M_∞	$\ln(1 - M_t/M_\infty)$	$t_{1/2}$
0			
1			
2			
3			
4			
6			
8			
12			

To determine the correlation coefficient for each model using linear least squares fitting technique. The fitted results of the largest regression correlation (r) and the smallest mean square error (MSE) are regarded the best.

Experimental Instructions

Requirements for Preview

1. To preview the chapter concerning controlled and extended release preparations, to understand its type and clinical significance. To preview the method, object and significance of the dissolution test, comply with the requirements of the dissolution test and drug release test in general chapter 0931 of ChP.

2. To understand the general preparation principles and method of oral extended release preparations, to be familiar with the physicochemical property of the commonly used matrix materials. To know the difference and identity of the quality requirements between controlled and extended release preparations and routine preparations.

Procedures and Precautions

1. Hydrophilic gelatinous HPMC is chosen top repare the hydrophilic gelatinous matrix tablets in this experiment. The drug release process of hydrophilic gelatinous matrix tablets is the comprehensive effect of the erosion of the matrix and the diffusion of the drug. The mechanism of release is different if the water - solubility of drug is different, the release of drug with high water -

solubility is controlled by the diffusion of drug, while for drug with low water – solubility (such as theophylline), the erosion of matrix is the rate – limiting step. As the amount of HPMC in matrix tablets of theophylline increase, the rate of gel layer forming when the tablets contact with water is faster, and the thickness of gel layer is thicker, so the rate that water permeate into the centre of tablets is decrease, which lead to the decrease of erosion rate of matrix and release rate of theophylline. If the amount of water – soluble lactose in tablets increased, the water can permeate into the centre of tablets easily to some extent, which makes tablets erode faster and release drug more quickly. So the release rate of drug in theophylline extended release tablets can be adjusted by changing the amount of HPMC and lactose until it complies with the requirements.

When prepare soft material with 90% ethanol, the dosage of adhesives should be aptitude to make the soft material be conglomeration in hand and when fingers press it slightly, it should disperse but does not turn into powders.

2. Aqueousethylcellulose dispersion is chosen as a release retardant binder for the manufacture of insoluble inert matrix tablets in this experiment. The aqueous dispersion of ethylcellulose enhanced the compaction characteristics of drug, and the drug release mechanism from those inert porous matrices was by diffusion. The rate of drug release is influenced by the choice of filler. Ethylcellulose has been widely used as a barrier membrane or binder, to prepare pharmaceutical oral extended – release dosage forms. The aqueous dispersion of ethylcellulose, for example Surelease has been utilized to manufacture extended – release multiparticulates for filling into capsules and single unit tablets or soft – gel capsules through film coating applications.

3. The hardness of extended – release matrix tablets has a direct effect on the drug release. The hardness is controlled at the range of 5 – 7 kgf in this experiment.

4. The apparatus should be checked whether it works properly, temperature control and rotating rate run precisely, the paddle heave smoothly before use. The paddle should be fixed according to the requirements. The distance between the bottom of the beaker and the paddle is 25mm.

5. When filter the sample solution, make sure that the membrane fixed tightly, otherwise it would affect the correctness.

Questions

1. In theophylline extended – release matrix tablets, what actions do HPMC and EC take? And what actions lactose and MCC take?

2. Why three test time points at least are chosen in drug release profile of extended – release preparations?

3. What is the significance of in vitro drug release test for extended – release preparations?

4. What are the commonly used matrix materials in matrix sustained – release tablets and what are their characteristics?

5. Please design the formulation and preparation process of nifedipine sustained release matrix tablets.

6. Please design the formulation and preparation process of metformin hydrochloride sustained release matrix tablets.

第四部分　注射剂的制备

实验 11　维生素 C 的稳定性及其影响因素研究

【目的与要求】

1. **掌握**　影响维生素 C 溶液稳定性的主要因素以及考察药物溶液稳定性的方法。
2. **熟悉**　维生素 C 溶液的有关化学性质以及影响药物氧化速度的因素。
3. **了解**　提高易氧化药物稳定性的基本方法。

【基本概念与实验原理】

药物制剂的基本要求是安全、有效、稳定。如果药物分解变质，不仅会使疗效降低，而且有些药物甚至产生毒副作用，故药物制剂的稳定性对制剂的安全、有效非常重要。而注射剂由于直接进入机体血管，因此对药物的稳定性要求较高。药物的化学不稳定性主要表现在放置过程中发生的降解反应，水解和氧化是其降解的主要途径。

维生素 C（Vitamin C）即抗坏血酸，用于防治坏血病、促进创伤及骨折愈合、预防冠心病等，临床应用十分广泛。维生素 C 外观呈白色或略带黄色的晶体或粉末，具有轻微的酸性，易溶于水，微溶于乙醇，不溶于三氯甲烷、乙醚和苯。维生素 C 的分子结构中，在羰基毗邻的位置上有两个烯醇基，很容易被氧化生成黄色的双酮化合物，再迅速水解、氧化，生成一系列有色的无效杂质。即在有氧条件下，先氧化成去氢维生素 C，然后水解为 2,3－二酮古罗酸糖，再进一步氧化为草酸与 L－丁糖酸。其氧化降解反应过程如图 11－1 所示。

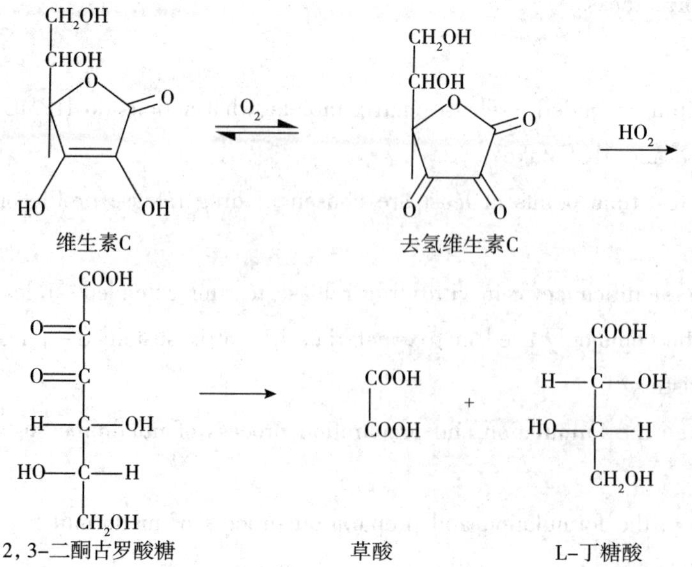

图 11－1　维生素 C 氧化降解反应过程

影响维生素C溶液稳定性的因素主要有空气中的氧气、溶液的pH值、温度及重金属离子等。本实验重点考察下列几个方面：加热时间的影响；溶液pH值的影响，并求出最稳定pH（pH_m）；含氧量的影响，以及通入惰性气体CO_2和加入抗氧剂的抗氧效果；重金属离子的影响以及加入金属离子络合剂的效果。

【仪器与材料】

1. 仪器　紫外-可见分光光度计，pH计，熔封设备，G3垂熔玻璃漏斗，水浴，电炉，烧杯（100ml），量筒（100ml），玻璃棒，玻璃安瓿（2ml），注射器及针头，洗瓶等。

2. 材料　维生素C，碳酸氢钠，亚硫酸氢钠，硫酸铜，依地酸二钠，注射用水，二氧化碳（钢瓶），浓硫酸等。

【实验内容】

1. 加热时间的影响　取注射用水80ml，加入维生素C 12.5g，分次缓缓加入碳酸氢钠5g，随加随搅拌使完全溶解，添加注射用水至100ml，测定并控制pH（5.8～6.2）。用G3垂熔玻璃漏斗滤2～3次使澄明。取10ml样液，作为加热前溶液，其余均灌封于2ml玻璃安瓿中。将安瓿放入沸水中煮沸，间隔一定时间取出6支安瓿，放入冷水中冷却。将6支安瓿内的溶液混合均匀，以蒸馏水为空白，用紫外-可见分光光度计测定420nm波长处各溶液的透光率，按下式计算透光率比并记录于表11-1中。

$$透光率比(\%)=\frac{T_0-T_i}{T_0}\times 100 \quad (1)$$

式中，T_i为加热后各溶液的透光率；T_0为加热前溶液的透光率。

表11-1　加热时间对维生素C稳定性的影响

煮沸时间（min）	透光率（%）	透光率比（%）
0		
15		
30		
60		

2. 溶液pH值的影响　取维生素C 17.5g，加注射用水配成12.5%的溶液140ml，用G3垂熔玻璃漏斗过滤，取样，依法测定波长420nm处的透光率。精密量取20ml该溶液6份，分别置50ml烧杯中，依次加入碳酸氢钠粉末0.2、0.6、0.8、1.0、1.2、1.3g，使溶液的pH值相应为4.0、5.0、5.5、6.0、6.5和7.0（用pH计测定）。用注射器将上述溶液分别灌封于安瓿中，做好标记，同时放入沸水中加热45min，取出冷却。各取6支，将其中溶液混合均匀，以蒸馏水为空白依法测定透光率，按下式计算透光率比并记录于表11-2中。

$$透光率比(\%)=\frac{T_0-T_p}{T_0}\times 100 \quad (2)$$

式中，T_p为不同pH溶液加热后的透光率；T_0为未调整pH值溶液加热前的透光率。

表 11-2 pH 值对维生素 C 稳定性的影响

样品号	pH 值	透光率（%）	透光率比（%）
0	未调整		
1	4.0		
2	5.0		
3	5.5		
4	6.0		
5	6.5		
6	7.0		

3. 含氧量的影响和抗氧剂的作用 分别取出煮沸放冷的注射用水和通 CO_2饱和 3min 的注射用水，按“1”项下方法分别配成 12.5% 的 A、B 两种维生素 C 溶液各 50ml，依法测定其透光率 T_0。然后将 A、B 液各分成两份，每份 20ml，按表 11-3 附加条件操作并将试液灌封于安瓿中，做好标记，于沸水中煮沸 45min，取出放冷。分别混匀各安瓿中的溶液，以蒸馏水为空白，依法测定透光率，按下式计算透光率比并记录于表 11-3 中。

$$透光率比(\%) = \frac{T_0 - T_i}{T_0} \times 100 \qquad (3)$$

式中，T_i为 A 或 B 溶液加热后的透光率；T_0为 A 或 B 溶液加热前的透光率。

表 11-3 含氧量和抗氧剂对维生素 C 稳定性的影响

样品号	附加条件	透光率（%）	透光率比（%）
A	—		
A_1	—		
A_2	加入 0.1g $NaHSO_3$		
B	—		
B_1	—		
B_2	在 CO_2气体中灌封		

4. 重金属离子的影响及金属离子络合剂的作用 按“1”项下方法配制 25% 维生素 C 溶液 80ml，精确量取 12.5ml 置 25ml 量瓶中，共 4 份。按表 11-4 所示加入不同试剂后，用注射用水稀释至刻度，第一份样液立刻测定透光率后和其余样液均灌封于安瓿中，做好标记，放入沸水中煮沸 30min 后取出。各取 6 支安瓿，将安瓿内溶液混匀，以蒸馏水为空白，依法测定透光率，按下式计算透光率比并记录于表 11-4 中。

$$透光率比(\%) = \frac{T_0 - T_i}{T_0} \times 100 \qquad (4)$$

式中，T_i为加热后的透光率；T_0为加热前的透光率。

表 11-4 重金属离子对维生素 C 稳定性的影响

样品号	加入试剂	透光率（%）	透光率比（%）
0	—		
1	0.001mol/L $CuSO_4$2.5ml		
2	0.001mol/L $CuSO_4$5.0ml		
3	0.001mol/L $CuSO_4$2.5ml + 5% EDTA-2Na 1ml		

5. **实验结果** 整理表 11 - 1 ~ 表 11 - 4 数据，并对实验结果进行讨论。

对表 11 - 2 中的数据，以 pH 值为横坐标，透光率比为纵坐标作图，由图中曲线求出最稳定 pH 值（pH_m），曲线中最低 pH 值即为最稳定 pH 值（pH_m）。

实验指导

一、预习要求

1. **掌握** 影响药物稳定性的因素及其稳定化的方法。
2. **熟悉** 维生素 C 的有关化学性质以及影响其氧化的主要因素。
3. **了解** 维生素 C 溶液容易氧化的特点，试设计维生素 C 注射液的处方。

二、操作要点和注意事项

1. 用碳酸氢钠调节溶液 pH 时，要将其分次加入，边加边搅拌，否则易产生大量气泡而使溶液溢出。
2. 灌注时，勿使药液溅到安瓿颈的上端，以防熔封时出现焦头等。
3. 待水浴沸腾时再将样品放入，并开始计算时间。
4. 由于样品较多，编号不要弄错。
5. 测定样品含量时，应将 6 支安瓿中的样液充分混匀（所用烧杯要干燥），以免影响透光率的测定。

三、思考题

1. 影响维生素 C 溶液稳定性的因素有哪些？
2. 何为抗氧剂？注射液中常用的抗氧剂有哪些？
3. 惰性气体驱氧时应注意哪些问题？
4. 通过 pH 值对稳定性的影响，求出维生素 C 注射液最稳定 pH 值。
5. 简述 Cu^{2+} 与 EDTA - 2Na 对维生素 C 溶液稳定性的影响。
6. 针对维生素 C 溶液容易氧化的特点，试设计维生素 C 注射液的处方。

Experiment 11 Studies on the Stability of Vitamin C and its Influence Factors

扫码“学一学”

Objectives and Requirements

1. To grasp the main factors that affect the stability of vitamin C solution and the method to test the stability of the drug solution.

2. To be familiar with the chemical characteristics of vitamin C solution and the influence factors that could affect the drug oxidation speed.

3. To understand the basic method to improve the stability of the oxidative drugs.

Introduction

The basic requirements of pharmaceutical preparations are safe, effective and stable. If the drug is decomposed, it will not only reduce its efficacy, but will also, for some drugs, even produce toxic side effects. Thus, the stability of drug preparation is very important for the safety and effectiveness of the preparation. Since the injection is given directly into the blood circulation in the body, the stability requirement of such drug must be higher. On the other hand, the chemical instability of the drug is mainly manifested in the degradation process. Hydrolysis and oxidation are two main ways of degradation.

Vitamin C is recommended in clinic to prevent and treat scurvy, heal the wound and bone fracture and prevent coronary heart disease. It appears as a white or slightly yellow crystal or powder with a slight acidic taste. It is freely soluble in water; sparingly soluble in alcohol and insoluble in chloroform, ether and benzene. In the molecular structure of vitamin C, there are two enolic groups beside the carbonyl group which are easy to be oxidized to produce a yellow compound, and then rapidly hydrolyzed and oxidized to form a series of colorful impurities. In a nutshell, under aerobic conditions, Vitamin C will firstly be oxidized into dehydroascorbic acid, then hydrolyzed to 2,3 - diketo - L - gulonic acid and finally oxidized to oxalic acid and L - butonic acid. Its oxidation and degradation process are shown as following (Figure 11 - 1).

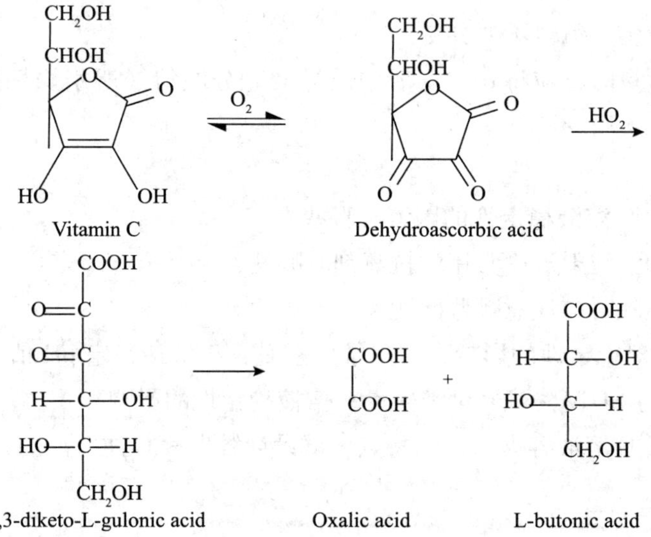

Figure 11 - 1 Oxidation and degradation reaction process of Vitamin C

The main factors that affect the stability of vitamin C solution include oxygen in the air, pH, temperature and heavy metal ions. In this experiment, we will focus on the following aspects: Influence of the heating time, Influence of the pH value of the solution and the most stable pH (pH_m), Influence of the oxygen concentration and the antioxidant effect after adding inert gases (such as CO_2) and antioxidant, Influence of the heavy metal ions and the metal ion complexing agent.

Equipment and Materials

1. Equipment

UV - Vis spectrometer, pH meter, instruments for fill and seal, G_3 sintered glass funnel, water bath, electronic stove, beaker (100ml), Cylinder (100ml), stirring rod, ampoules (2ml), syringes, needles, wash bottles and etc.

2. Materials

Vitamin C, sodium bicarbonate, sodium bisulfite, copper sulphate, natrium edetate, water for injection, carbon dioxide (steel vase), concentrated sulfuric acid and etc.

Experimental Methods

1. Influence of heating time

Add 12.5g of vitamin C into 80ml of water for injection. Then add 5g of sodium bicarbonate slowly into the mixture while stirring to completely dissolve it. Add water for injection to make it a 100ml solution and test the pH value of the mixture (5.8 to 6.2). Filter through a G3 sintered glass funnel 2 – 3 times to make the mixture clear. Take 10ml from the solution and put it aside, the remaining solution will be encapsulated into 2ml ampoules. Put ampoules in the boiling water to boil. At certain time intervals, take 6 ampoules out and put them into cold water to cool down. Mix solutions in the 6 ampoules. Take distilled water as the blank and determine the light transmittance with UV – Vis spectrometer at the wavelength of 420nm. Use the following formula to calculate the transmittance ratio and record in Table 11 – 1.

$$\text{Transmittance ratio}(\%) = \frac{T_0 - T_i}{T_0} \times 100 \tag{1}$$

Where T_i is the light transmittance after heating, T_0 is the light transmittance before heating.

Table 11 – 1　Effect of heating time on the stability of vitamin C

Boiling time (min)	Light transmittance (%)	Transmittance ratio (%)
0		
15		
30		
60		

2. Influence of pH value of solution

Weigh 17.5g of vitamin C and add water for injection to make a 140ml of 12.5% vitamin C solution. Filter through a G3 vertical glass funnel and test the light transmittance of the supernatant by using an UV – vis spectrometer at the wavelength of 420nm. Precisely measure 20ml of the solution and put into six 50ml beakers respectively. Add sodium bicarbonate powder 0.2, 0.6, 0.8, 1.0, 1.2, 1.3g separately into these 6 beakers to make solutions with different pH values of 4.0, 5.0, 5.5, 6.0, 6.5, 7.0 (measured by a pH meter). Use a syringe to inject solutions mentioned above into 2ml ampoules, mark, put these ampoules into boiling water for 45min and cool down. Take 6 ampoules from each branch and mix together separately. Take distilled water as the blank and determine the light transmittance of the mixture. Use the following formula to calculate the transmittance ratio and record in Tablel 11 – 2.

$$\text{Transmittance ratio}(\%) = \frac{T_0 - T_p}{T_0} \times 100 \tag{2}$$

Where T_p is the light transmittance of solutions with different pH values after heating, T_0 is the light transmittance of no adjustment solution before heating.

Table 11 -2 Effect of pH value on the stability of vitamin C

No	pH value	Light transmittance(%)	Transmittance ratio(%)
0	No adjustment		
1	4. 0		
2	5. 0		
3	5. 5		
4	6. 0		
5	6. 5		
6	7. 0		

3. Influence of oxygen concentration and antioxidant

Take one part of water for injection to boil in the boiling water and cool down. Add carbon dioxide into another part of water for injection for 3min. Make 50ml of 12. 5% Vitamin C solutions Aand B(same method under procedure 1)using these two kinds of water respectively. Test their light transmittance. Then separate the solution A and B according to table3 and put into ampoules. Mark and boil the ampoules in the boiling water for 45min. Cool down, mix the solutions in the ampoules separately. Take distilled water as the blank and test their light transmittance. Use the following formula to calculate the transmittance ratio and record in Table 11 -3.

$$\text{Transmittance ratio}(\%) = \frac{T_0 - T_i}{T_0} \times 100 \qquad (3)$$

Where T_i is the A or B solution's light transmittance after heating, T_0 is the A or B solution's light transmittance before heating.

Table 11 -3 Effect of oxygen concentration and antioxidant on the stability of vitamin C

No	Additional condition	Light transmittance(%)	Transmittance ratio(%)
A	—		
A1	—		
A2	Add 0. 1g $NaHSO_3$		
B	—		
B1	—		
B2	Encapsulation in CO_2 gas		

4. Influence of heavy metal ions and metal ion complexing agent

80ml of 25% vitamin C solution was prepared according to the method under procedure 1. Then precisely measure 12. 5ml of the solution 4 times and put into four 25ml volumetric flasks separately. According to table 4, add different reagents into the flasks and dilute to the scale using water for injection. Test the light transmittance of sample 1 immediately and put into ampoules, same as the remaining solutions. Mark and put all the ampoules into boiling water to boil for 30min. Mix solutions in the 6 ampoules taken from each sample. Take distilled water as the blank and test the light transmittance. Use the following formula to calculate the transmittance ratio and record in Table 11 – 4.

$$\text{Transmittance ratio}(\%) = \frac{T_0 - T_i}{T_0} \times 100 \quad (4)$$

Where T_i is light transmittance after heating, T_0 is light transmittance before heating.

Table 11 – 4　Effect of heavy metal ions on the stability of vitamin C

No	Adding reagents	Light transmittance(%)	Transmittance ratio(%)
0	—		
1	0.001mol/L $CuSO_4$ 2.5ml		
2	0.001mol/L $CuSO_4$ 5.0ml		
3	0.001mol/L $CuSO_4$ 2.5ml + 5% EDTA – 2Na 1ml		

5. Experimental results

Sort out the Table 11 – 1 to Table 11 – 4 data, and discuss the experimental results.

Plot light transmittance ratio versus pH values to draw a curve aim at Table 11 – 2 data. Find the most stable pH value(pH_m). The lowest pH value in the curve should be the most stable pH value.

Experimental Instructions

Requirements for Preview

1. Grasp the factors that affect the stability of drugs and its stabilization methods.

2. Understand the chemical properties of vitamin C and analyze the main factors that affect the oxidation process.

3. According to the characteristics of vitamin C solution, try to design an injection formulation of vitamin C.

Procedures and Precautions

1. When using sodium bicarbonate to adjust pH, it should be slowly added into the solution by turns while stirring. Otherwise, it is easy to produce a lot of bubbles and make an overflow of the solution.

2. When pouring vitamin C solutions into ampoules, avoid splashing the solution onto the upper part of the ampoule neck. Otherwise the top of the sealed ampoules might have bubbles or hollows.

3. Start timing and placing ampoules into the water only after the water is boiling.

4. Mark each sample to avoid any confusion.

5. To determine the content of the samples, the vitamin C solutions in 6 ampoules should be fully mixed(keep the beaker dry), so as not to affect the determination of light transmittance.

Questions

1. What are the factors that affect the stability of vitamin C solution?

2. What is an antioxidant ? What antioxidants are commonly used in injection.

3. What problems should be paid attention to when inert gas floods oxygen?

4. How to obtain the most stable pH value of vitamin C injection according to the influence of pH value?

5. Describe the effect of Cu^{2+} and EDTA－2Na on the stability of vitamin C solution.

6. According to the characteristics of vitamin C solution, try to design an injection formulation of vitamin C.

实验12　维生素C注射液处方设计与制备

【目的与要求】

1. **掌握**　溶液型注射剂的制备方法及工艺过程中的操作要点。

2. **熟悉**　注射剂成品质量检查标准和检查方法，了解影响成品质量的因素。提高易氧化药物稳定性的基本方法。

3. **了解**　无菌与灭菌制剂生产工艺中的关键操作。

【基本概念与实验原理】

注射剂系指原料药物或与适宜的辅料制成的供注入体内的溶液、乳状液或混悬液以及供临用前配制或稀释成溶液或混悬液的浓溶液或粉末的无菌制剂。

注射剂的生产车间设施必须符合《药品生产质量管理规范》的要求，注射剂的生产过程包括原辅料和容器的前处理、称量、配制、灌封、灭菌、质量检查、包装等步骤。

注射剂的质量要求：无菌、无热原、澄明度合格、使用安全、无毒性、无刺激性；稳定性合格，即在贮存期内稳定有效。注射剂的pH值应接近血液pH值，一般控制pH在4～9范围内，含量合格；凡大量静脉注射或滴注的输液，应调节渗透压与血浆等渗或接近等渗。

维生素C（Vitamin C）用于防治坏血病，促进创伤及骨折的愈合、预防冠心病等，临床应用十分广泛。维生素C在干燥状态下较稳定，但在潮湿状态或溶液中，其分子结构中的烯二醇结构易氧化，生成黄色双酮化合物，虽仍有药效，但会迅速进一步氧化、断裂、生成一系列有色的无效物质。溶液的pH值、氧、重金属离子和温度对维生素C的氧化均有影响。

针对维生素C溶液易氧化的特点，在注射液处方、工艺设计中应重点考虑怎样延缓药物的氧化分解，通常采取如下措施：除氧，溶液中的氧和安瓿空间的残余氧对药物稳定性影响很大，应设法排除，在配液和灌封过程中通入惰性气体如高纯度的氮气和二氧化碳，可改善易氧化药物的稳定性；加抗氧剂，抗氧剂通常是强还原剂，因其首先氧化从而阻止溶液中药物的氧化，常用于注射剂的抗氧剂有焦亚硫酸钠、亚硫酸氢钠、亚硫酸钠、硫代硫酸钠等；调节溶液pH在最稳定pH范围，药物的降解常受酸、碱催化，选择合适的pH可使降解反应最小化；加金属离子络合剂，金属离子对维生素C的氧化反应有强烈的催化作用，当溶液中仅仅含有0.0002mol/L铜离子时，其氧化速度可以增大10^4倍，故常用依地酸钠或依地酸钙钠络合金属离子，以提高其稳定性。

【仪器与材料】

1. **仪器**　烧杯，量筒，普通天平、G3垂熔预滤器，玻璃安瓿（2ml），熔封设备，水浴，澄明度检查仪。

2. **材料**　维生素 C，碳酸氢钠，依地酸二钠，针用活性炭，二氧化碳，注射用水等。

【实验内容】

1. 处方

维生素 C	52.0g
碳酸氢钠	24.2g
亚硫酸氢钠	2.0g
依地酸二钠	0.5g
注射用水	加至 1000ml

2. **制备工艺**　维生素 C 注射液的制备工艺流程见图 12－1。

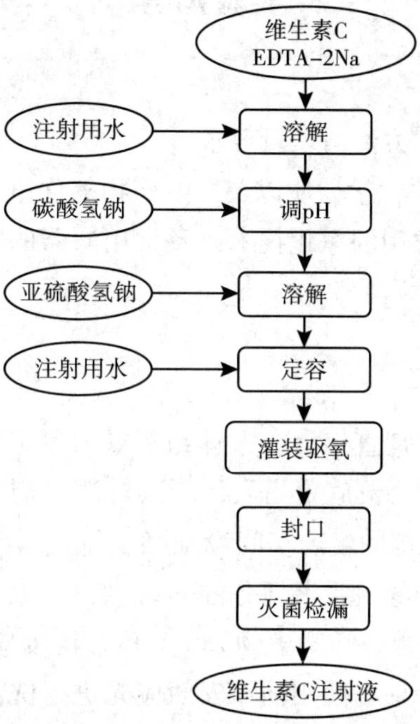

图 12－1　维生素 C 注射液的制备工艺流程图

配液：取处方量 80% 的注射用水，通二氧化碳饱和，加依地酸二钠、维生素 C 使溶解，分次缓缓加入碳酸氢钠，搅拌使溶解，加亚硫酸氢钠溶解，搅拌均匀，检测并调节溶液 pH 至 5.8～6.2，加注射用水至全量。

活性炭吸附：加 0.1% 针用活性炭，室温搅拌 10min。

过滤：先用 G3 垂熔预滤器粗滤，再用 0.22μm 的微孔滤膜精滤。

灌装：取过滤后的药液，灌装于安瓿中，通二氧化碳驱除安瓿上部空间的氧气。

熔封：灌装后立即将安瓿熔融封口。

灭菌：将灌封好的安瓿用 100℃ 沸水浴灭菌 15min。

检漏：灭菌完毕，立即将安瓿放入 1% 亚甲蓝水溶液中，待安瓿冷却，取出，剔除内装溶液变色安瓿。

3. 质量检查

（1）pH 值　应为 5.0～7.0；按《中国药典》四部通则 <0631> pH 值测定法进行；

（2）可见异物　按《中国药典》四部通则 <0904> 可见异物检查法进行；

（3）无菌　按《中国药典》四部通则 <1101> 无菌检查法进行；

（4）含量测定　应为标示量的 90.0% ~110.0%；

（5）其他　按《中国药典》四部通则 <0102> 注射剂项下。

4. 实验结果　将维生素 C 注射液检漏及可见异物检查结果填入表 12－1 中，计算成品率。

表 12－1　维生素注射液质量检查结果

检查总数（支）	检漏（支）	可见异物（支）	成品数（支）	成品率（%）

实验指导

一、预习要求

1. 掌握　注射用水的制备方法与质量要求。

2. 熟悉　维生素 C 的有关化学性质以及影响药物氧化速度的因素。

3. 了解　注射剂生产上常用的净化技术以及常用滤器的特性与使用方法。注射剂成品质量检查的标准与方法。

二、操作要点和注意事项

1. 注射剂制备一般要点

（1）操作环境　由于注射剂直接注入人体组织或血管，吸收快，作用迅速，特别是静脉注射，无吸收过程，常用于抢救危重病人，所以对注射剂的生产原料、生产工艺和质量控制的要求都极其严格。注射剂的生产车间设施必须符合《药品生产质量管理规范》的要求，必须按生产工艺和产品质量的要求划分洁净级别：一般生产区、控制区、洁净区。控制区与洁净区内的空气中尘粒数、活微生物数、温度、湿度应符合有关规定。

（2）安瓿与配制用具的处理　使用前，安瓿应先进行洗涤、干燥（灭菌）等处理，为提高洗涤效果，在洗涤前安瓿内先灌入去离子水（或 0.1% 盐酸溶液），经 100℃蒸煮 30min 的热处理后，再趁热甩水，以滤净的去离子水（或蒸馏水）灌洗数次。大生产时，1 ~2ml 小安瓿须经灌水机和甩水机反复数次操作，洗净的安瓿应立即烘干（灭菌）备用。

调配器具使用前，要用洗涤剂或硫酸清洁液处理洗净。临用前用新鲜注射用水荡洗或灭菌处理，不得引入杂质及热原。

（3）配液方法　有稀配法和浓配法两种，可根据原料药物的纯度加以选用。

（4）药液过滤　有减压过滤、加压过滤以及高位自然滴滤等。过滤用具的种类较多，砂滤棒、压滤机等常用作初滤，再依次经垂熔玻璃滤器和微孔滤膜精滤，使药液澄明并除去微粒。

（5）灌封　灌注药液时尽量不使药液碰到安瓿颈口，以免封口时产生炭化和白点等。灌装后随即封口。手工熔封时，火焰应调节至细而呈蓝色，待玻璃烧红后用镊子夹去顶部并在火焰中断丝。

（6）灭菌与检漏　封口后应及时灭菌，趁热放入亚甲蓝溶液中检漏。

2. 维生素 C 注射液制备要点

（1）维生素 C 显强酸性，加入碳酸氢钠使其部分中和成钠盐，既可调节至维生素 C 较稳定的 pH 值 6.0 左右，又可避免酸性太强，在注射时产生疼痛。加入碳酸氢钠至维生素 C 溶液中时应缓慢，以防溶液溢出，并应充分搅拌以免局部碱性过强。

（2）维生素 C 易氧化变色、含量下降，尤其当金属离子（特别是铜离子）存在时变化更快。故在处方中加入 $NaHSO_3$ 作抗氧剂，EDTA－2Na 作金属离子络合剂，并在药液内和灌封时均通 CO_2 气体，以减少氧化。

（3）活性炭有吸附热原、色素、其他杂质及助滤作用。使用时一般采用加热煮沸后再冷到 45～50℃时过滤除炭，用量为溶液总量的 0.2%，吸附时间以 20～30min 以上较好。因维生素 C 溶液不稳定，故采用 0.1% 用量，室温吸附 10min。

（4）惰性气体的使用：对维生素 C 等易氧化药物的注射液，除加入抗氧剂、金属离子络合剂等外，较有效的方法是在配液和灌封时通入高纯度氮气或二氧化碳等惰性气体。二氧化碳在水中的溶解度大于氮气，采用二氧化碳驱除维生素 C 溶液中的氧，其效果要优于氮气，但应注意二氧化碳可使溶液的 pH 下降，呈酸性。由于氮气的化学性质稳定，故驱除安瓿空间的氧，用氮气效果较好。

惰性气体应先通过洗气装置，除去微量杂质。使用纯度较低的二氧化碳时，可将气体分别通过盛装浓硫酸、1% 硫酸铜、1% 高锰酸钾溶液的洗气瓶处理，以分别除去水分、硫化物、有机物和微生物，最后经注射用水洗气瓶除去可溶性杂质和二氧化硫。若惰性气体纯度较高时，只需通过甘油和注射用水洗涤即可。若是氮气，应依次通过碱式焦性没食子酸溶液和 10% 高锰酸钾溶液（除去氧和有机物质）。

（5）为减少维生素 C 氧化变色，灭菌温度及时间控制在 100℃、15min。

（6）在实验过程中避免使用金属容器或器具。

三、思考题

1. 分析影响注射剂可见异物的因素。
2. 用 $NaHCO_3$ 调节维生素 C 注射液的 pH 值，应注意什么问题？为什么？
3. 影响药物氧化的因素有哪些？如何防止？
4. 何谓注射用水？制备时主要采用哪些方法和设备？
5. 维生素 C 注射液为何采用二氧化碳惰性气体？
6. 根据维生素 C 性质试设计与实验处方不同的注射液处方。

Experiment 12　Formulation Design and Preparation of Vitamin C Injection

扫码“学一学”

Objectives and Requirements

1. To master the key points to prepare vitamin C injection and the related manufacturing process.

2. To be familiar with the standards and methods of quality control of the end injection, to understand the factors influencing on the quality of the products. To be familiar with the means to enhance the stability of easily oxidized drugs.

3. To understand the key points in the manufacturing process of sterile preparation.

Introduction

Injections are sterile products containing medicaments intended for parenteral administration into the body, including solutions, emulsions, suspensions as well as sterile powders or concentrates solutions, which, by the addition of suitable solvents before use, from solutions or suspensions.

The production of injections must follow rigid aseptic procedures. In the preparation of parenteral solutions, the required ingredients are dissolved in water for injection according to GMP. Then the solutions are usually filtered until sparkling clear through a membrane type filter after filtration, are transferred into the final containers as rapidly as possible and with the least possible exposure. The products are then sterilized, preferably autoclaved, and samples of the finished products are tested for sterilization and pyrogens.

The requirements for injections are as following: sterile, no - pyrogen, valid clarity, safe for using, non - toxic, non - irritant, valid stability, pH close to that of human blood (general 4 - 9), qualified content. The osmotic pressure of intravenous injection with a big amount of dose or infusion should be isoosmotic.

Vitamin C is recommended for the prevention and treatment of scurvy, facilitating the wound and bone fracture, preventing coronary heart disease and so on. It is wildly used in clinical treatment. It is reasonably stable in the solid state. In the wet state or solution, it is easily oxidized to dehydroascorbic acid and the latter undergoes further rapid oxidation into the chemical species possessing no vitamin C activity. It is very sensitive to even slight heating, to the light, and to the action of pH and metal ions. In general, the formulation should be mainly designed from the perspectives of the stability of preparation (physical, chemical, and biologic aspects), safety/toxicity and the efficacy in combination with the selected pharmaceutical ingredients.

The formulation need to be primarily plotted to prevent the oxidation of vitamin C, which is found to be oxidized quickly. Several measures have been taken as follows:

1. Depletion of O_2: Oxygen in injections is a serious contributor influencing the stability of injections, one of which is the catalyzing effect of O_2 on the oxidative decomposition of vitamin C. During the preparation and sealing process, the stability is improved by purging the O_2 with an inert gas, such as highly purified N_2 and CO_2. N_2 is chemically inert and stable for its wide application. CO_2 could render the injection acidic.

2. Addition of antioxidants: Antioxidants are usually strong reducing agents, which first oxidized to prevent the oxidation of pharmaceutical active ingredients in solution. The commonly used antioxidants for injections are $Na_2S_2O_7$, $NaHSO_3$, Na_2SO_3, $Na_2S_2O_3$.

3. Adjusting of pH in the range where vitamin C is most stable: As decomposition is often catalyzed by hydrogen, an optional pH can be determined at which the decomposition is retarded to the lowest extent.

4. Addition of EDTA to reduce the influence of heavy metal ions: Heavy metal ions could strongly catalyze the oxidation of some drugs. For instance, the oxidative reaction rate of vitamin C in the solution will be increased by 10000 times when only 0.0002mol/L copper ions are present. Ethylenediamine tetra - acetic acid (EDTA) is used to suppress the catalytic property of the ions by

forming a soluble chelate complex with heavy metal ions in which the ions is held in a non - ionic form.

Equipment and Materials

1. Equipment

Beaker, measuring cylinder, scale, G3 pre filter, glass ampoules (2ml), ampoule melting sealer, water bath, clarity tester, et al.

2. Materials

Vitamin C, sodium bicarbonate, disodium EDTA, activated carbon, carbon dioxide, water for injection, et al.

Experimental Methods

1. Formulation

Vitamin C	52.0g
$NaHCO_3$	24.2g
$NaHSO_3$	2.0g
EDTA - 2Na	0.5g
Water for injection	add to 1000ml

2. Manufacturing process

Manufacturing process flow chart of vitamin C injections was showed in Figure 12 - 1.

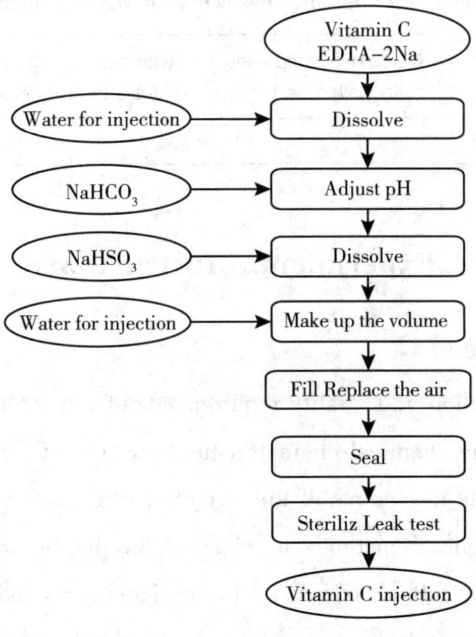

Figure 12 - 1　Manufacturing process flow chart of vitamin C injection

Solution preparing: Add 80% of the total volume water for injection to a suitable beaker and saturated with CO_2. Add EDTA - 2Na and Vitamin C, stir to dissolve. Then add $NaHCO_3$ by turns while stirring, then $NaHSO_3$, mix well. Check and adjust the pH value to 5.8 - 6.2.

Activated carbon adsorbing: Add 0.1% activated carbon, stirring at room temperature for 10min.

Filtrating: Filtrate the solution through a G3 pre filter and then a 0.22μm microfiltration membrane. Add water for injection to the total volume.

Filling: Fill the filtrated solution into glass ampoules, replace the air in ampoules by flushing CO_2.

Sealing: Immediately seal ampoules after filling using an ampoule melting sealer.

Sterilizing: Sterilize the sealed ampoules in a boiling bath for 15min.

Leak – testing: Immediately transfer the hot ampoules into 1% methylene blue dye solution, remove the "blue" ampoules (filled in Table 12 – 1).

3. Quality control of vitamin C injection

(1) pH: The pH value should be controlled between 5.0 to 7.0, carry out the pH test (general chapter <0631> of ChP).

(2) Visible particles: Comply with the requirements and carry out the visible particles test (general chapter <0904> of ChP).

(3) Sterility: Comply with the requirements and carry out the test for sterility (general chapter <1101> of ChP).

(4) Content: The content of vitamin C should be controlled 90.0% to 110.0%.

(5) Other requirements: Complies with the general requirements for injection (general chapter <0102> of ChP).

4. Experimental results

Fill the results in Table 12 – 1 and calculate the qualified rate.

Table 12 – 1 Quality inspection of vitamin injection

Total number of ampoules	Number ofleak ampoules	Number of ampoules with visible particles	Number of ampoules that fulfill the requirements	Qualified rate (%)

Experimental Instructions

Requirements for Preview

1. To master the preparation and quality requirements of water for injection.

2. To be familiar with the chemical characteristics of vitamin C, the factors influencing the rate of the drug's oxidation and the key points of the formulation of oxygen – sensitive drugs.

3. To understand the general methods of cleaning in the preparation of injections and the characteristics and processing methods of general filters. To under stand the standard and methods of quality control of the end injections.

Procedures and Precautions

1. Key points of the preparation of common injections

(1) Conditions for procedures: Injections have a rapid absorption and effect as they are administered into tissue or blood vessel of human body directly, especial for intravenous injections, which are used to rescue seriously ill patients. The production material, manufacturing process and quality control of injection must follow rigid procedures. In the manufacturing plants, the air in which parenteral products are made is maintained bacteria – free through the use of ultraviolet lights, a

filtered air supply, sterile manufacturing equipment, such as masks and sterilized work clothing worn by the personnel in the area. The manufacture plant of injection must comply with good manufacturing practice(GMP). The workshops are divided into following clean grade: general areas, controlled areas, spotless areas. Dust spots, living microorganisms, temperature and humidity must be controlled according with GMP in the controlled areas and spotless areas.

(2) Treatment of ampoules and containers: Ampoules should be tested for their appearance, cleanness, heat resistance, acid resistance, alkali resistance and neutrality before cutting. Fill the ampoules with deionized water or 0.1% HCl solution, and keep at 100℃ for 30min, then wash with deionized water or distilled water for several times. Dry the ampoules immediately.

(3) Preparation method: The preparation method includes dilution method or direct preparation according to the purity of raw material.

(4) Filtration: Filtration method includes filtration under reduced pressure, filtration under pressure and filtration by droplet from the superior position. The procedures are filtration through a press filter, then a funnel sintered glass filter and microfiltration membrane to clarify the solution.

(5) Seal: Don't spatter the liquid on the wall of the ampoule when distribute into ampoules, seal ampoules immediately after filled. Adjust the flame thin and blue, and then seal the ampoules in flame with nipper when the glass exhibits red.

(6) Sterilize the sealed ampoules and check leakage: Sterilize injection immediately after seal, then immerse the ampoules in 1% methylene blue to check leakage.

2. Key points of the preparation of vitamin C injection

(1) Vitamin C solution has strong acidity, so sodium bicarbonate is added to convert the vitamin C to its sodium salts partly, which can create a pH of 6.0 that is benefit for the stability of vitamin C and reduce the irritation. The sodium bicarbonate must be added slowly by complete stirring to prevent inhomogeneous alkalinity of the solution.

(2) Vitamin C solution is easily oxidized and change color, faster especially faced with metal ion. So sodium metabisulfite was added into the formulation as an antioxidant and sodium edetate as a chelating agent. Another effective method is to displace the air in the containers by inert gases such as pure nitrogen and carbon dioxide in the process of filling and sealing.

(3) The activated carbon was widely employed for the absorption of pyrogen, pigment, other impurities and had drainage effect during filtration. The activated carbon was used usually as follows: firstly heat and make the activated carbon added solutions boil, secondly cool down the mixture to 45 – 50℃, and then remove the activated carbon during filtration. The amount of activated carbon added is better to be 0.2% of the total volume of the solution and the absorption time is good to be more than 20 – 30min. In this experiment, as the Vitamin C injection is not stable, we shall use 0.1% activated carbon and absorb for 10min at room temperature.

(4) Inert gases should be passed through a washing instrument so as to get rid of the impurity. Nitrogen should be passed through the alkaline pyrogallic acid solution and 10% potassium permanganate solution by turns so as to get rid of oxygen and organic matter. The pyrogal acid solution was prepared as followed: 160g sodium hydroxide was dissolved 300ml distilled water, and then 10g pyrogallic acid was dissolved in the solution.

Carbon dioxide should be passed through a concentrated sulfuric acid, 1% copper sulfate solution, 1% potassium permanganate solution and water for injection by turns so as to get rid of moisture, sulfide, organic matter and soluble impurity and sulfur dioxide respectively. If the inert gas is relatively pure, they can be passes through the glycerin and water for injection.

(5) In order to decrease the oxidation of vitamin C, the time of sterilization was controlled in 15min at 100℃.

(6) Don't use metal containers and tools.

Questions

1. Analyze the factors that influence the visible foreign body of the injections.
2. $NaHCO_3$ is used to adjust the pH of vitamin C injection, what should be noticed? Why?
3. Describe the factors affecting the oxidation of a drug. How to prevent them?
4. What is water for injection? What are the main methods and instruments in production?
5. Why the inert gas of carbon dioxide is used in the preparation of vitamin C injection?
6. Design formulations of vitamin C injection that is different with this experiment according to its characteristics.

实验 13　维生素 C 注射液稳定性加速实验

【目的与要求】

1. **掌握**　应用恒温加速实验法预测维生素 C 注射液贮存期的方法。
2. **熟悉**　应用化学动力学方法预测注射液稳定性的原理。
3. **了解**　药物制剂稳定性实验方法。

【基本概念与实验原理】

在研究制剂的稳定性以确定其有效期（或贮存期）时，室温留样考察法虽然结果可靠但所需时间较长（一般考察 2～3 年），而加速试验法（如恒温加速试验法等）可以在较短的时间内对有效期或贮存期做出初步的估计。

维生素 C 的氧化降解反应已由实验证明为一级反应。一级反应的速度方程为：

$$-\frac{dC}{dt}=kC \tag{1}$$

式中，$-dC/dt$ 为维生素 C 浓度减少的瞬时速度；C 为维生素 C 在瞬间 t 的浓度；k 为维生素 C 的氧化降解速度常数。

对式（1）积分，C_0为反应开始时（$t=0$）维生素 C 的浓度，则得：

$$\ln C=kt+\ln C_0 \tag{2}$$

由式（2）可知，以 $\ln C$ 对 t 作图呈一直线关系，其斜率为 $-k$，截距为 $\ln C_0$，斜率可求出速度常数 k。

反应速度常数 k 和绝对温度 T 之间的关系，可用 Arrhenius 公式表示：

$$k = A\,e^{\frac{-E_a}{RT}} \tag{3}$$

或

$$\ln k = -\frac{E_a}{RT} + \ln A \tag{4}$$

式中，A 为频率因子；E_a 为活化能；R 为气体常数。

由式（4）可知，以 $\ln k$ 对 $1/T$ 作图呈一条直线，其斜率为 $-E_a/R$，截距为 $\ln A$，由此可求出反应活化能 E_a 和斜率因子 A。将 E_a 和 A 再代回式（4），可求出室温（25℃）或任何温度下的氧化降解速度常数和贮存期（$t_{0.9}$）。

【仪器与材料】

1. 仪器 恒温干燥箱，酸式滴定管（25ml），锥形瓶（50～250ml）等。

2. 材料 维生素 C 注射液（2ml：0.25g），0.1mol/L 碘液，丙酮，稀醋酸，淀粉指示液等。

【实验内容】

一、放样与测定

1. 放样 将同一批号的维生素 C 注射液样品（2ml：0.25g）分别置 4 个不同温度（如 70、80、90 和 100℃）的恒温干燥箱中，间隔一定时间（70℃间隔 24h，80℃间隔 12h，90℃间隔 6h，100℃间隔 3h）取样，每个温度的间隔取样次数均为 5 次。样品取出后，室温冷却后置冰箱保存，供含量测定。

2. 维生素 C 含量测定方法 精密量取各温度维生素 C 注射液样品液 1ml，置 150ml 锥形瓶中，加蒸馏水 15ml 与丙酮 2ml，摇匀，室温放置 5min，加稀醋酸 4ml 与淀粉指示液 1ml，用碘液（0.1mol/L）滴定，至溶液显蓝色并持续 30s 不褪。每 1ml 碘液（0.1mol/L）相当于 8.806mg 的维生素 C（$C_6H_8O_6$），分别测定各样品中的维生素 C 的含量，同时测定未经加热试验的原样品中维生素 C 含量，记录消耗碘液的毫升数。

二、实验数据处理

1. 数据整理 因为含量测定中所用碘液浓度固定，因此只要比较消耗碘液的毫升数即可得维生素 C 各样品的相对浓度百分数。将未经加热的样品（表 13－1 中时间项为 0）所消耗碘液的毫升数（即初始浓度）作为 100% 相对浓度，各加热时间的样品所消耗碘液的毫升数与其相比，得出各自的相对浓度百分数 C（%）。将实验数据填入表 13－1 并计算。

表 13－1 恒温加速试验各时间样品的测定结果

加热温度（℃）	加热时间 t（h）	消耗碘液（ml）				C（%）	ln$C$
		1	2	3	平均		
	0					100	
70	24						
	48						
	72						
	96						
	120						

续表

加热温度（℃）	加热时间 t（h）	消耗碘液（ml）				C（%）	ln$C$
		1	2	3	平均		
80	12						
	24						
	36						
	48						
	60						
90	6						
	12						
	18						
	24						
	30						
100	3						
	6						
	9						
	12						
	15						

2. **求维生素C氧化降解速度常数**　按表13－1，分别将4种加热温度下的ln$C$与加热时间（t，从0开始）进行线性回归计算，得ln$C$～t方程，由斜率求该加热温度下维生素C氧化降解速度常数k（即k_{70}，k_{80}，k_{90}和k_{100}）。计算结果记录于表13－2中。

表13－2　各加热温度下的ln$C$～t方程

加热温度（℃）	70	80	90	100
ln$C$～t方程				
r^2				
k（1/h）				

3. **求维生素C活化能（E_a）和频率因子（A）**　将计算求得的降解速度常数k和对应温度（T）记录在表13－3。根据Arrhenius公式求维生素C氧化降解反应的活化能（E_a）和频率因子（A）。以x'为横坐标，y'为纵坐标，进行回归计算，得ln$k$～$\frac{1}{T}$方程。计算出直线斜率b'，截距a'和相关系数r'，故维生素C氧化降解活化能为：

$$E_a = -b' \times R \tag{5}$$

式中，R为气体常数；频率因子（A）即为直线截距的反对数。

表13－3　不同温度下维生素C注射液的降解速度常数

T（K）	343（273＋70℃）	353（273＋80℃）	363（273＋90℃）	373（273＋100℃）
$\frac{1}{T}\times10^3$，x'	2.915	2.833	2.755	2.681
ln$k$，y'				

4. 求室温时的氧化降解速度常数（k_{25}）　将求得的 E_a、A、R 代入公式（4），计算 k_{25}。

5. 求贮存期 $t_{0.9}$　室温下降解10%所需的时间，即为贮存期 $t_{0.9}$，由下式计算。

$$t_{0.9}=0.1054/k_{25} \tag{6}$$

实验指导

一、预习要求

1. 掌握　研究药物制剂稳定性的目的和意义。

2. 熟悉　维生素C注射液用碘量法测定时的操作要点。实验步骤、要点及数据处理方法。

3. 了解　药物制剂稳定性实验方法。

二、操作要点和注意事项

1. 实验中所用维生素C注射液的批号应全部相同。按规定间隔时间加热、取出后，应立即测定维生素C含量，否则应置低温冰箱保存，以免含量起变化。

2. 测量维生素C含量时，所用碘液的浓度应前后一致（宜用同一瓶的碘液），否则含量难以测准。因各次测定所用的是同一碘液，故碘液的浓度不必精确标定，注射液维生素C含量亦可不必计算，只比较各次消耗的碘液毫升数即可。一般将零时间样品（即未经加热的维生素C注射液）消耗的碘液毫升数作为100%相对浓度，其他各时间消耗的碘液毫升数与其比较，从而得出各时间的 $C_{相}$（%），见表13－1。

3. 经典恒温法常采用4个温度进行加速实验，各温度的加热间隔时间点一般应取5个。间隔时间的确定，应以各次消耗的碘液毫升数有明显差别为宜。

4. 测定维生素C含量时，加丙酮的作用是：因维生素C注射液中加有亚硫酸氢钠等抗氧剂，其还原性比烯二醇基更强，因此要消耗碘；加丙酮后就可避免亚硫酸氢钠和碘的反应发生，因为丙酮能与亚硫酸氢钠起反应。

5. 测定维生素C含量时，加稀醋酸的作用是：维生素C分子中的烯二醇基具有很强的还原性，在空气中极易被氧化。特别在碱性时，氧化反应更易发生。加入适量醋酸保持一定的酸性，以减少维生素C受碘以外其他弱氧化剂的影响。

三、思考题

1. 药物制剂稳定性研究的范围是什么？

2. 留样观察法和加速试验法有何特点？

3. 经典恒温加速试验法的理论依据是什么？

4. 设计实验时应考虑哪些步骤及注意点？

5. 不同剂型的稳定性加速试验有什么异同？

6. 参考数理统计方法等有关内容，试计算加速试验预报的贮存期的可信区间。计算结果说明什么问题，为什么？

扫码“学一学”

Experiment 13 The Accelerated Stability Testing of Vitamin C Injection

Objectives and Requirements

1. To master the method of using constant temperature accelerated test to predict the storage period of vitamin C injection.

2. To be familiar with the principle of applying chemical kinetics method to predict the stability of injection.

3. To understand the experimental method of the stability of drug preparation.

Introduction

Instabilities in modern formulation are often detectable only after considerable storage periods under normal conditions. To assess the stability of a formulated product, it is usual to put the products under nature condition. This result is reliable, but needs long time (generally for 2 – 3 years). The acceleration experiment law (for instance, the constant temperature acceleration test law) can estimate the valid terms tentatively in a shorter time, in turn, will allow unsatisfactory formulations to be eliminated early within a study and will also reduce the commercial process for a successful product.

Oxidation and degradation of vitamin C solution is the first order reaction proved by experiments. The rate of degradation is given by Equation (1):

$$-\frac{\mathrm{d}C}{\mathrm{d}t}=kC \tag{1}$$

Where $-\mathrm{d}C/\mathrm{d}t$ is the instantaneous reducing speed of VC concentration, C is the concentration at the instantaneous time t. k is the rate constant.

Integration of Equ. (1), C_0 is the concentration of vitamin C at the beginning, so:

$$\ln C = kt + \ln C_0 \tag{2}$$

From the equation (2), the line of $\ln C - t$ could be got with a slope of $-$k and an intercept of $\ln C_0$ at $t=0$. The rate constant k may therefore be calculated from the slope.

The effect of temperature on a rate constant k is indicated by the Arrhenius equation:

$$k = A\,e^{\frac{-E_a}{RT}} \tag{3}$$

or

$$\ln k = -\frac{E_a}{RT} + \ln A \tag{4}$$

Where A is constant that is termed the Frequency factor, E_a is the energy of activation, R is gas constant.

It can be seen from Equation (4) that a line will be obtained from a graph of $\ln k$ against $1/T$. The constants E_a and A may be determined from the slope and intercept of this line, which are equal to E_a/R and lnA respectively. Put E_a and A into the formula (4), the rate constant k and shelf – life can be drawn at the room temperature (25℃) or at any temperature.

Equipment and Materials

1. Equipment

Thermostat dryer oven, acid buret (25ml), conical flask (50 – 250ml), etc.

2. Materials

Vitamin C injection(2ml : 0. 25g),0. 1mol/L iodine solution, acetone, dilute acetic acid, starch indicator, etc.

Experimental Methods

1. Preparation and Determination of VC Samples

(1) Preparation of samples

Put the vitamin C injection samples(2ml : 0. 25g) in the thermostat dryer oven of 4 different temperatures(for example:70,80,90 and 100℃) separately. After the certain time(such as 24h at 70℃,12h at 80℃,6h at 90℃,3h at 100℃), take out the samples. Take 5 times' samples at the interval of each temperature. Fast cool samples or put into the refrigerator to keep for determining Vitamin C content of samples respectively.

(2) Determining of VC content

Take 1ml solution from Vitamin C injection accurately, put into the conical flask of 150ml, add 15ml distilled water and 2ml acetone, shaking up evenly. Put it for 5minutes, add 4ml dilute acetic acid and 1ml starch indicator. Titrate it with Iodine solution, until the solution are getting blue, and last 30 seconds fading. Determine Vitamin C content of all samples and unheated samples separately. Write down the volume of Iodine solution assumed. Every 1ml Iodine solution(0. 1mol/L) is equivalent to Vitamin C 8. 806mg($C_6H_8O_6$).

2. Experiment Data Processing

(1) Data processing

Take the Iodine solution milliliters consumed by unheated samples(namely initial concentration) as the relative concentration 100%. Iodine solution milliliters of other samples consumed compare with it, thus get the relative concentration C(%) of every time. Data are recorded in Table 13 - 1 and calculate.

Table 13 - 1　Survey results of constant temperature acceleration experiment

Temperature (℃)	Time (h)	Iodine solution milliliters consumed(ml)				*C*(%)	ln*C*
		1	2	3	average		
	0					100	
70	24						
	48						
	72						
	96						
	120						
80	12						
	24						
	36						
	48						
	60						

续表

Temperature (℃)	Time (h)	Iodine solution milliliters consumed (ml)				C(%)	lnC
		1	2	3	average		
90	6						
	12						
	18						
	24						
	30						
100	3						
	6						
	9						
	12						
	15						

(2) Calculate the oxidization speed constant

According to table 13 - 1, calculate the linear regression between ln$C$ and heating time (T, starting from 0) at four heating temperatures respectively, and obtain the ln$C - t$ equation. Calculate the rate constant k (k_{70}, k_{80}, k_{90} and k_{100}) of oxidation degradation of vitamin C at the heating temperature from the slope. Record the calculation results in Table 13 - 2.

Table 13 - 2 lnC - t equation at different heating temperatures

Temperature (℃)	70	80	90	100
ln$C - t$ equation				
r^2				
k(1/h)				

(3) Calculate E_a and A

Record the calculated degradation rate constant and corresponding temperature (T) in Table 13 - 3. Calculated the activation energy (E_a) and frequency factor (A) of oxidative degradation of vitamin C according to Arrhenius formula. Taking x' as the abscissa and y' as the ordinate, the regression calculation is carried out and the $\ln k - \frac{1}{T}$ equation is obtained. The linear slope b', intercept a' and correlation coefficient r' are calculated, so the activation energy of oxidation degradation of vitamin C is:

$$E_a = -b' \times R \quad (5)$$

Where R is the gas constant, and the frequency factor (A) is the inverse number of the straight intercept.

Table 13 - 3 Degradation rate constants of vitamin C injection at different temperatures

T (K)	343 (273 + 70℃)	353 (273 + 80℃)	363 (273 + 90℃)	373 (273 + 100℃)
$\frac{1}{T} \times 10^3$, x'	2.915	2.833	2.755	2.681
$\ln k$, y'				

(4) Calculate oxidation degradation rate constant at room temperature (k_{25})

To calculate oxidation and degradation speed constant k_{25} under the room temperature, according to the formula (4).

(5) Calculate storage period $t_{0.9}$

Storage period (the necessary time of losing 10% content) under the room temperature, can be calculated from the following formula:

$$t_{0.9} = 0.1054/k_{25} \quad (6)$$

Experimental Instructions

Requirements for Preview

1. To master the purpose and significance of the study on the stability of drug preparation.

2. To be familiar with the operation points of vitamin C injection in the determination of iodine content. To be familiar with the experimental procedures, key points and data processing method.

3. To understand the experimental method of the stability of drug preparation.

Procedures and Precautions

1. The principle of examining the vitamin C is that ethylene glycol in the vitamin C molecule has reducibility, can be oxidized by iodine into 2 ketone bases. The alkaline condition is positive to the reaction.

The vitamin C injection used in the experiment should be the same batch. Heat samples according to the stable time interval. It is necessary to determine the vitamin C content immediately after taking samples out, otherwise put them into the refrigerator to avoid the content changing.

2. At the vitamin C content of examining, the concentration of iodine solution should always be unanimous. Otherwise, the content can't be determined accurately. The concentration of iodine solution needn't be demarcated accurately because the solution used in all experiments are from the same solution The vitamin C content also needn't be calculated, just compare the volume of iodine solution consumed. Iodine solution milliliters consumed by the sample of zero time (namely the vitamin C injection that is not heated) as relative concentration 100% generally. Relative concentration of every time C% is calculated by comparing iodine solution milliliters of other times consumed with zero time.

3. There are 4 temperature points that are often addressed in the acceleration experiment of Classics thermostat law. Generally, there are 5heat interval time points of every temperature. The interval time period should designed to make it sure that there is obvious difference among iodine solution milliliters consumed of different samples.

4. Sodium bisulfate is used as antioxidant in vitamin C injection. It also consume iodine because its reducibility is stronger than ethylene glycol. Therefore acetone is added in the determining of vitamin C to avoid the interference with reaction of acetone and sodium bisulfate.

5. The function of dilute acetic acid in the vitamin C determining is explained as following. The ethylene glycol group in vitamin C molecular has strong reducibility. It is easily oxidized in the

air, especially under the alkaline condition. Moderate dilute acetic acid is added to keep acid condition of the solution to avoid the oxidation between vitamin C and other weak oxidant except for iodine.

Questions

1. What is the range of drug stability study?

2. What are the characteristics of sample - staying observation test and accelerated stability test?

3. What is the theoretical evidence of classics thermostat acceleration law?

4. What are the experimental procedures and precautions?

5. What are the similarities and differences between the stability acceleration tests of different dosage forms?

6. Try to calculate the confidence interval of the storage period predicted by the accelerated test. What does the result suggest?

实验14　注射用维生素C冻干粉针处方设计与制备

【目的与要求】

1. **掌握**　冷冻干燥制品的生产工艺过程和操作要点。
2. **熟悉**　冷冻干燥制品成品质量检查的标准和方法。
3. **了解**　冷冻干燥制品的质量常规检查方法。

【基本概念与实验原理】

注射用无菌粉末又称粉针，系指药物制成的供临用前用适宜的无菌溶液配制成澄清溶液或均匀混悬液的无菌粉末或无菌块状物。无菌粉末的制备方法有溶剂结晶法、喷雾干燥法和冷冻干燥法等，其中采用冷冻干燥工艺制备的注射用无菌粉末称为注射用冻干粉针。

冷冻干燥（freeze - drying）全称真空冷冻干燥（vacuum freeze - drying，简称冻干），是指含水物料先经低温冻结成固体，然后在低温真空状态下，利用水的升华性能使其直接升华而干燥的方法。冷冻干燥工艺适用于热敏感或在水中不稳定的药物。

冻干粉针的工艺过程包括预冻（恒压降温）、升华干燥、解析干燥等过程。此外，药液在冻干前需经配液、过滤、灌装、半加塞、入箱等处理过程。整个冻干过程要严格按无菌操作法进行。共熔点（或共晶点）是预冻温度等冷冻干燥工艺参数的选择依据，系指溶液全部凝结成固体的温度。一般药液的低共熔点在 -10 ~ -20℃之间。

冻干曲线是冻干过程中通过机械和计算机记录产品和隔板温度、冷凝器温度和真空度随时间变化的曲线。冻干曲线中涉及的参数包括预冻温度、预冻时间、预冻速率、冷凝器降温时间、抽真空时间、冻结结束时间、升华干燥阶段的加热时间、箱内真空度控制时间、冻干各阶段产品加热最高允许温度、校正漏空的工作时间、真空报警工作时间、冻干总时间等。

注射用无菌粉末除应符合《中国药典》对注射用原料药物的各项规定外，还应符合下列要求：①粉末无异物，配成溶液后可见异物检查合格；②粉末细度或结晶度应适宜，便于分装；③无菌、无热原。

【仪器与材料】

1. 仪器　天平，烧杯，量筒，玻璃棒，pH 计，定量灌装器，冷冻干燥机，紫外 - 可见分光光度计，电磁炉，G3 垂熔滤器，微孔滤膜过滤器。

2. 材料　维生素 C（注射用规格），无水碳酸钠（注射用规格），甘露醇，二氧化碳，注射用水，针用活性炭（注射用规格），西林瓶，丙酮，碘滴定液（0.1mol/L），稀醋酸（6%，g/g）。

【实验内容】

1. 处方

维生素 C	5.0g
无水碳酸钠	1.25g
甘露醇	5.0g
注射用水	加至 100ml

2. 制备工艺　取注射用水 200ml，通入二氧化碳（20～30min）使其饱和，以除去注射用水中的氧气，备用。取除氧后的注射用水 80ml，加入处方量的维生素 C 使溶解，加入甘露醇溶解。分次缓慢加入无水碳酸钠粉末，不断搅拌至完全溶解，继续搅拌至无气泡产生后，继续缓慢加碳酸钠粉末调节药液 pH 值至 5.0～7.0。加入 0.1g 针用活性炭，室温搅拌 10min。用 G3 垂熔漏斗粗滤除去活性炭，再经 0.22 μm 的微孔滤膜过滤（精滤）。加入二氧化碳饱和的注射用水至 100ml，检测滤液澄明度，合格后灌装于 10ml 西林瓶中，每瓶 3ml，半压塞。将样品置于冷冻干燥机中，－35℃预冻 4h，－35～0℃低温真空干燥 16h，30℃再干燥约 4h。压塞，取出，轧盖即可。工艺流程图如图 14－1。

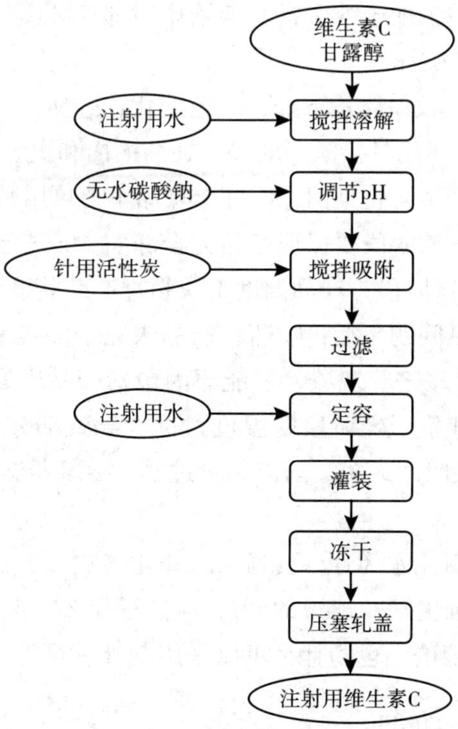

图 14－1　注射用维生素 C 的制备工艺流程图

3. 质量检查 需检查的项目包括外观、澄明度、pH、溶液颜色、含量测定、热原、无菌检查、干燥失重、含量均匀度和装量差异等。

（1）pH 值测定 取本品 0.5g，加新煮沸过的澄明冷水 10ml 溶解后，依法测定（《中国药典》四部通则 <0631> pH 值测定法），pH 值应为 5.0～7.0，符合规定。

（2）含量测定 精密称取本品适量（约相当于维生素 C 0.2g），加水 15ml 与丙酮 2ml，摇匀，放置 5min，加稀醋酸 4ml 与淀粉指示液 1ml，用碘滴定液（0.1mol/L）滴定，至溶液显蓝色并持续 30s 不褪。每 1ml 碘滴定液相当于 8.806mg 的 $C_6H_8O_6$。应为标示量的 90.0%～110.0%。

（3）颜色 取本品，加水稀释成每 1ml 中含维生素 C 50mg 的溶液，照《中国药典》四部通则 <0401> 紫外－可见分光光度法，在 420nm 的波长处测定，吸光度不得超过 0.06。

（4）装量差异 取本品 5 瓶，除去铝盖后，容器外壁用乙醇擦净，干燥，开启时注意避免玻璃屑等异物落入容器中，分别迅速精密称定，倾倒出内容物，容器用水或乙醇洗净，在适宜条件下干燥后，再分别精密称定每一容器的重量，求出每瓶的装量与平均装量，应符合规定。

（5）其他 按《中国药典》四部通则 <0102> 注射剂项下检查，符合要求。

实验指导

一、预习要求

1. 熟悉 冷冻干燥制品的制备工艺和操作要点。

2. 了解 无菌与灭菌制剂生产工艺中的关键操作。药液配制的常用方法。容器的处理方法。冷冻干燥制品封口压盖的方法。

二、操作要点和注意事项

1. 配液时，将无水碳酸钠加于维生素 C 溶液中时速度要慢，同时要不断搅拌，以防局部碱性过强，造成维生素 C 破坏。

2. 维生素 C 容易氧化，致使含量下降，颜色变化，金属离子可加速这一反应过程，因此在制备过程中应避免与金属用具接触。此外，在药液内和灌装时均通 CO_2，以减少氧化。

3. 配制按无菌操作法严格防止染菌，冷冻干燥品不得再用其他方法补充灭菌。

4. 冷冻干燥过程中，预冻阶段要保证产品完全冻实，通常预冻最低温度应比产品的共熔点低 5～10℃；在升华干燥阶段，产品温度不应超过产品共熔点。

5. 冷冻干燥过程中常见问题包括：喷瓶，产品未完全冻实或升温速度过快，可能导致喷瓶；外观有硬壳、萎缩、塌陷等现象，可能原因包括产品干燥不彻底，冻干后成品密封性不好，导致吸潮，或者升华干燥阶段时温度过高，导致部分产品熔化等；含水量偏高，可能原因包括解析干燥阶段时间太短、药液装量过厚、冷凝器温度偏高等。

三、思考题

1. 溶解维生素 C 的注射用水为什么要通入二氧化碳？

2. 用无水碳酸钠调节维生素 C 溶液的 pH，应注意什么？为什么？

3. 配制的维生素 C 溶液的颜色为什么可以采用紫外－可见分光光度计法检查颜色？目的是什么？

4. 冷冻干燥品为什么不能再补充灭菌？

5. 维生素 C 冻干粉针剂中为什么要加入甘露醇?

6. 讨论冷冻干燥制品生产工艺中的关键步骤。

Experiment 14 Formulation Design and Preparation of Vitamin C Lyophilized Powder for Injection

扫码“学一学”

Objectives and Requirements

1. To master the manufacturing process and the key points of preparation of freeze - dried products.
2. To be familiar with the standards and methods of quality control of the freeze - dried products.
3. To understand the routine examination of quality control of the freeze - dried products.

Introduction

Sterile powders for injection are sterile powders or sterile lumps containing medicaments, which form solutions or suspensions by the addition of suitable sterile solvents before use. The preparation methods of sterile powders contain solvent crystallization, spray drying and freeze - drying and so on. Among them, one which made by freeze - drying method is called as lyophilized powder.

Freeze - drying is fully known as vacuum freeze - drying, which works by freezing the materials and then reducing the surrounding pressure to allow the frozen water to directly sublimate from the solid phase to the gas phase. The process of freeze - drying includes freezing (cooling in constant pressure), sublimation drying and secondary drying generally. In addition, the medicine solution should be prepared before lyophilization as followed: solution preparation, filtration, filling, half - filling stopper and putting into the box and so on. The whole preparation process should be strictly followed to the aseptic method. The eutectic melting point is the temperature at which it changes state from a solution to a solid, and is an important reference to set some technical parameters such as freezing temperature in freeze - drying process. The eutectic melting point of the drug solution is usually between -10℃ to -20℃.

The freeze - drying process curve is worked out based on vacuum degree and the temperature of the material and partition combined with freeze - drying duration time. It involves a large number of lyophilization process parameters, including freezing rate, the lowest freezing temperature, freezing time, cooling time of the condenser, vacuuming time, ending time of freezing time, heating time, freeze - drying total time, vacuum alarm working time etc.

Apart from meeting all the requirements of Chinese Pharmacopoeia for the raw materials for injection, the sterile powder for injection should also meet the requirements as follows: No foreign substance, qualified visible foreign substance inspection, suitable powder fineness or degree of crystallinity, easy to dispense; Sterile and no - pyrogen.

Equipment and Materials

1. Equipment

Scale, beaker, measuring cylinder, glass, pH meter, quantitative filling machine freeze - drying machine, UV - Vis spectrophotometer, electric stove, G_3 pre filter, porous membrane filters.

2. Materials

Vitamin C (injection specification), anhydrous sodium carbonate (injection specification), mannitol, carbon dioxide, injection water, activated carbon (injection specification), vials, acetone, iodine solution, diluted acetic acid (6%, g/g).

Experimental Methods

1. Formulation

Vitamin C	5.0g
Anhydrous sodium carbonate	1.25g
Mannitol	5.0g
Water for injection	add to 100ml

2. Manufacturing process

200ml of water for injection is taken and saturated with carbon dioxide (20 - 30min), for the purpose of removing the oxygen. Vitamin C and the mannitol is dissolved in 80ml of water for injection without oxygen, following that anhydrous Na_2CO_3 is dissolved in the above solution by turns while stirring to adjust the pH of the solution to 5.0 - 7.0. Next, 0.1g of activated carbon is added into the solution while stirring for 10min at room temperature to remove the pyrogen. The resulting solution was filtrated through G_3 pre filter, and then 0.22 μm micropore membrane. The water for injection is added to the total amount, and then the clarity of the solution is checked, followed by filling into 10ml vials with each of 3ml solution, and then semi - plugged. The vials are placed in a freeze - drying machine, and then freezing for 4h at - 35℃, followed by vacuum drying for 16h at the temperature between - 35 to 0℃, the secondary drying for another 4h at 30℃, plugged and capped. The scheme of the manufacturing process is shown in Figure 14 - 1.

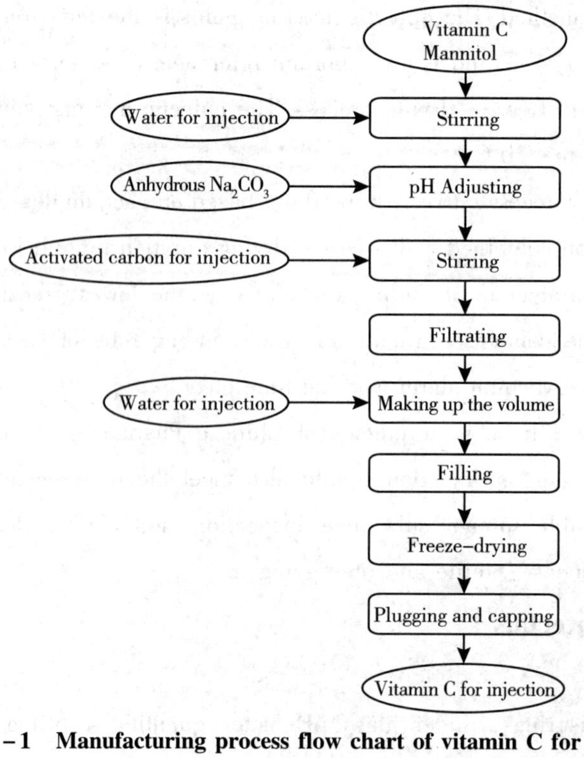

Figure 14 - 1 Manufacturing process flow chart of vitamin C for injection

3. Quality evaluation

The items include appearance, clarity, pH, color, content, pyrogenic, sterility, loss on drying, content uniformity and so on.

(1) pH determination: 0.5mg of vitamin C – loaded lyophilized powder is weighed accurately, and then dissolved with 10ml fresh distilled water. The pH of solution is between 5.0 to 7.0.

(2) Content determination: Contain of vitamin C should be not less than 90.0% and not more than 110.0% of the labeled amount of vitamin C. A certain amount of vitamin C – loaded lyophilized powder (approximately equivalent to the amount of 0.2g vitamin C) is weighed, and then dissolved with 15ml distilled water and 2ml acetone, and stood for 5min after shaking. 4ml of the dilute acetic acid and 1ml of starch indicator are added into the solution, and then titrated with iodine volumetric solution at the concentration of 0.1g/ml until the solution is blue and last for 30s.

(3) Color: A solution of 50mg of vitamin C – loaded lyophilized powder per ml is prepared, and then the absorbance is measured at 420nm. The absorbance should be not greater than 0.06.

(4) Content uniformity: 5 bottles of products is taken, and its aluminum cap is removed, followed that the outer wall of the bottles is wiped with ethanol and dried. It should be paid attention to avoid the glass chip and other foreign matters falling into the container when remove the aluminum cap. Products with inner packing are weighed accurately and then the contents are dumped out. The container is completely washed with water or ethanol and dried under suitable conditions, then weighed accurately. The loading capacity and the average loading capacity are calculated, and should be complied with general chapter <0102> of Chinese Pharmacopoeia.

Other requirements: Comply with general chapter <0102> of Chinese Pharmacopoeia.

Experimental Instructions

Requirements for Preview

1. To understand the basic methods of preparation of the drug solution.

2. To understand the key points in the manufacturing process of aseptic and sterilized products. To be familiar with the key points to prepare lyophilized powder and the manufacturing process. To understand the treatment methods of vessels. To understand the sealing and capping methods of lyophilized powder.

Procedures and Precautions

1. During the preparation of the solution, anhydrous Na_2CO_3 must be added slowly into vitamin C solution by completely stirring to avoid the inhomogeneous alkalinity of the solution.

2. The vitamin C in the solution is easily oxidized followed by the change of the color. The oxidation rate is faster in the presence of metal ion. Therefore, metal container or tool should be inhibited. In addition, the air in the containers should be displaced by inserting gases such as pure nitrogen and carbon dioxide in the process of filling.

3. Aseptic techniques are recommended during the whole preparation process. In general, lyophilized powders are not be sterilized by other sterilization methods.

4. At the first stage of freezing, the solution of the product should be completely frozen, and usually the minimum temperature at the freezing stage should be 5 – 10℃ lower than the eutectic melting point of the product. In addition, the temperature should not exceed the eutectic melting point at the sublimation drying stage.

5. The common problems in the freeze – drying process include as followed: (1) The eruption of products, which may result from the incompletely frozen or too fast heating rate. (2) The appearance of incrustation, atrophy, collapse and other similar phenomena, which may be caused by some reasons as follows: the product is not thoroughly dried, the lyophilized product is not properly sealed which lead to moisture absorption, or the temperature is too high at the secondary drying stage which resulting in the partially melting of the product and so on. (3) High water content, which may result from too much loading capacity, higher temperature in condenser, or shorter time at the secondary drying stage, etc.

Questions

1. Why is carbon dioxide used in the preparation of vitamin C solution?

2. Anhydrous Na_2CO_3 is used to adjust the pH of vitamin C solutions, what should be noticed? Why?

3. Why the UV – Vis spectrophotometer can be used to check the color of vitamin C solution? What is the purpose?

4. Why the freeze – dried product can't be sterilized with other sterilization methods?

5. Why the mannitol is added in the formulation of vitamin C – loaded lyophilized powder?

6. Please discuss the key factors in the manufacturing process of vitamin C – loaded lyophilized powder.

实验 15　静脉注射用脂肪乳的制备

【目的与要求】

1. **掌握**　高速分散 - 高压均质法制备静脉脂肪乳的方法。
2. **熟悉**　静脉注射用脂肪乳的性质及特点。脂肪乳的处方组成。

【基本概念与实验原理】

乳剂是指两种互不相溶的液体混合，其中一种液体以小液滴状态分散在另一种液体中制备成的非均相液体制剂，其对分散相没有明确的液滴尺寸界定，对油相、乳化剂的组成成分以及乳剂的类型也无特别规定，适用范围广泛，可供内服、外用或者注射。与之相区分，亚微乳与纳米乳属于微粒制剂范畴，具体是将药物溶于脂肪油/植物油中，通常经磷脂乳化分散于水相中形成 100 ~ 600nm 粒径的 O/W 型微粒载药分散体系称为亚微乳，粒径在 50 ~ 100nm 之间的称为纳米乳。纳米乳和亚微乳也可经冷冻干燥技术制得固态冻干制剂，称为干乳剂，该类产品经适宜稀释剂水化分散后可得到均匀的亚微乳或纳米乳。

静脉注射用脂肪乳剂属于亚微乳范畴，主要由植物油、乳化剂和其他渗透剂（如甘油等）构成。不含药物的脂肪乳最早用于肠外营养剂，作为必须脂肪酸和能量补充剂已有数十年历史。目前，将脂肪乳作为药物载体制备微粒制剂的研究也日趋广泛，其优点包括：药物被包载于油相或油水界面，避免与水直接接触，可以提高易水解或对水敏感的药物的稳定性；不含或仅含少量有机溶剂，对血管刺激性较小；同时，由于外水相不含或仅含极少量的药物，可有效降低由药物引起的静脉炎发生的概率，增强患者的顺应性；作为微粒给药系统，脂肪乳具有一定的靶向性（尤其是肝脾靶向性），可降低正常组织的药物浓度，降低毒性；由于药物需要从油相扩散并释放入体内，具有一定的缓释作用，因此，注射用脂肪乳剂解决了普通静脉注射制剂所面临的诸多问题。此外，其与其他微粒制剂相比，也具备特有的优势：作为油相的精制植物油和磷脂对人体无毒、安全性好；可使用现有的非胃肠道营养用脂肪乳的生产线进行工业化大生产。

脂肪乳的制备方法主要有高压均质法、超声波法、微射流法等。

【仪器与材料】

1. 仪器　电子天平，高速分散器，ATS 高压均质机，电子恒温水浴锅，激光粒度仪，旋涡混合器，水浴超声，紫外分光光度计，10ml 离心机等。玻璃棒，EP 管托，镊子，刮刀，200μl 移液枪，1ml 移液枪，玻璃滴管，玻璃棒，烧杯（100ml），EP 管（10ml），离心管（10ml），10ml 量筒，称量纸，洗耳球，10ml 量瓶，50ml 量瓶，1ml 移液管。

2. 材料　尼莫地平，注射用大豆油，油酸，甘油，1.5% 依地酸二钠（EDTA－2Na）溶液，卵磷脂，注射用水，氢氧化钠等。

【实验内容】

一、空白脂肪乳

1. 处方

卵磷脂	0.3g
注射用大豆油	2ml
注射用水	30ml

2. 制备工艺　取 0.3g 卵磷脂，置 10ml EP 管中，加入 2ml 注射用大豆油，超声使卵磷脂溶解，制得油相。将油相加入 30ml 水中，在 10000r/min 的条件下高速分散 0.5min，在 600bar 条件下高压均质并循环 20 次，过 0.22μm 滤膜除菌，即得。

空白脂肪乳的制备工艺流程图见图 15－1。

二、尼莫地平脂肪乳

1. 处方

尼莫地平	0.1g
卵磷脂	0.6g
注射用大豆油	4ml
油酸	0.02ml
甘油	1.4ml
1.5% EDTA－2Na 溶液	0.02ml
注射用水（pH 8.5）	54ml

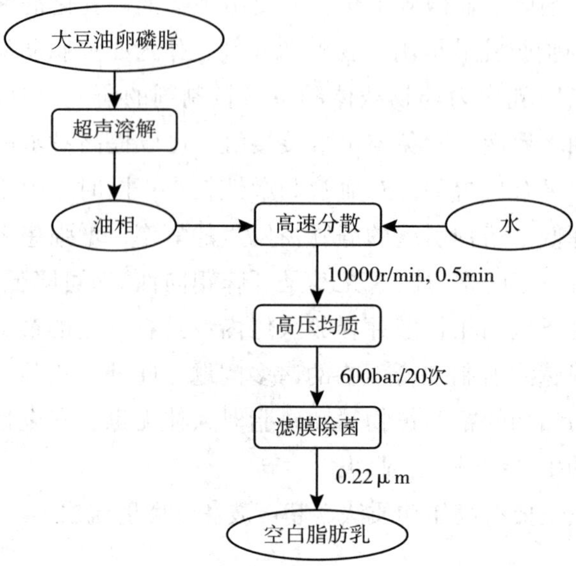

图 15-1　空白脂肪乳的制备工艺流程图

2. **制备**　取处方量注射用大豆油和尼莫地平，置 10ml EP 管中，加入卵磷脂和油酸，超声的同时玻璃棒搅拌溶解，制得油相。取甘油、1.5% EDTA-2Na 溶液和 54ml 注射用水（pH 8.5），置 50ml 烧杯中，混匀，制得水相。将油相加入水相，在 10000r/min 的条件下高速分散 0.5min，最后在 600bar 条件下高压均质并循环 20 次，过 0.22μm 滤膜除菌，即得。

尼莫地平脂肪乳的制备工艺流程图见图 15-2。

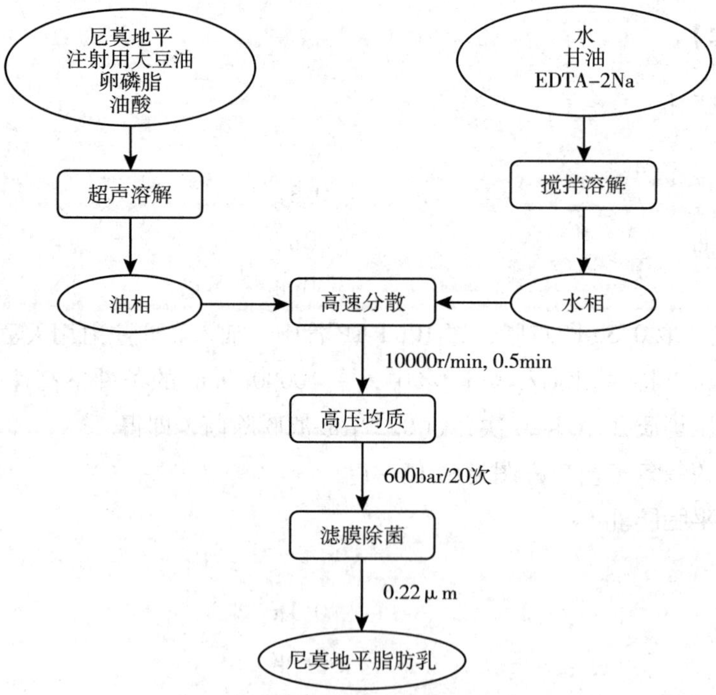

图 15-2　尼莫地平脂肪乳的制备工艺流程图

三、质量控制

1. **外观**　脂肪乳剂应呈乳白色，表面无油滴、静止时不分层，振摇后不挂壁。

2. **粒径与电位**　取脂肪乳 0.5ml，加蒸馏水稀释 10 倍，采用激光粒度仪测定。

3. **包封率**　取适量脂肪乳，3000r/min 离心 15min，取上清液，使用无水乙醇稀释 500 倍，涡旋混合 5min，采用紫外分光光度计于 236nm 处测定吸光度，并根据尼莫地平标准曲线计算纳米乳的药物浓度 C，根据公式计算包封率。尼莫地平标准曲线绘制：制备 200μg/ml 的尼莫地平贮备液，使用 1ml 移液管移取贮备液，制备 2μg/ml、4μg/ml、8μg/ml、12μg/ml、16μg/ml 的尼莫地平无水乙醇稀释液。基线校正后，以无水乙醇为空白对照，在 236nm 记录各尼莫地平标准品稀释液的吸光度。以吸光度 A 对浓度 C_i 作图，进行线性回归分析。

$$包封率 = \frac{CVX}{M} \times 100\% \tag{1}$$

式中，C 表示测得稀释后的脂肪乳药物浓度；X 表示稀释倍数；V 表示脂肪乳体积；M 表示初始药物投料质量。

实验指导

一、预习要求

1. **掌握**　高速分散 - 高压均质法制备静脉脂肪乳的方法。

2. **熟悉**　制备静脉注射用脂肪乳的基本原理。

3. **了解**　脂肪乳的构成。

二、操作要点及注意事项

1. 磷脂存在相转化温度，在相转化温度附近制备成的脂肪乳粒径较小且比较稳定。此外，温度越高，磷脂氧化速度越快。因此，应控制制备的温度。

2. 高速分散剪切搅拌速度和时间会影响初乳的状态，从而影响最终乳化的效果，影响粒径的大小及分布；因此应保证有足够大的剪切力，确保初乳的形成（油水不分层）。

3. 因为高速分散和匀浆过程中不可避免会接触金属器具，所以必须使用金属离子螯合剂以减缓氧化。

4. 由于脂肪乳易发生酸败，需要提供偏碱的环境以维持脂肪乳稳定性。

5. 应用激光粒度仪测定粒径时要注意稀释至一定的倍数，浓度太高容易影响测定数据的准确性。

6. 粒径是脂肪乳的重要质量指标之一，通常上市或已报道的脂肪乳粒径一般粒径分布均匀且小于 1000nm。测定方法可以采用电镜法与激光粒度测定仪。

7. 脂肪乳剂的物理稳定性除通过粒径变化考察外，还可以通过其他方法考察其稳定性，如离心分光光度法。

三、思考题

1. 制备脂肪乳的关键是什么？应如何进行操作？

2. 制备脂肪乳的常用方法有哪些？

3. 脂肪乳的一般处方组成有哪些？

4. 静脉注射用脂肪乳作为药物载体与其他微粒给药系统相比具有何优势？

5. 静脉注射用脂肪乳在药物制剂中有何意义？

6. 普通乳剂、亚微乳和纳米乳有什么区别？

扫码“学一学”

Experiment 15 Preparation of Intravenous Lipid - emulsions

Objectives and Requirements

1. To master the preparation of intravenous lipid - emulsions via mechanical mixing and high - pressure homogenization.

2. To be familiar with the formulation of lipid - emulsions. To be familiar with the properties and applications of intravenous lipid - emulsions.

Introduction

Emulsion refers to a heterogeneous liquid preparation prepared by mixing two mutually incompatible liquids, wherein one liquid is dispersed in the other liquid in the form of small droplets. Emulsion has no clear droplet size definition for the dispersed phase. There are also no special regulations on the composition of the emulsifier and oil phase, as well as the type of the emulsion. Emulsion is widely used through parenteral, oral, and injective administration. In contrast, submicron emulsions and nanoemulsions are in the category of microparticles. Specifically, the drug in submicron emulsions is dissolved in fatty oil or plant oil, emulsified by a phospholipid, and then dispersed in an aqueous phase to form an O/W type dispersed microparticle delivery system with a particle size of 100 - 600nm. If the particle size locates between 50 to 100nm, the system is denominated as nanoemulsions. Nanoemulsions and submicron emulsions can also be obtained by freeze - drying techniques to obtain solid lyophilized preparations, which are called dry emulsions. These products can be hydrated and dispersed by a suitable diluent to achieve a uniform submicron emulsion or nanoemulsion.

Intravenous lipid - emulsion is a submicron O/W emulsion system, consisting of plant oil, emulsifiers and penetrating agents (such as glycerin). Drug - free lipid - emulsion was first used as parenteral nutrients and has been used as essential fatty acids and energy supplements for decades. At present, the research on the microparticle preparations by using lipid - emulsion as a drug carrier is becoming more and more extensive. The drug in general is loaded in the oil phase or oil - water interface of emulsions, avoiding the contact of drug with aqueous conditions, thus the stability of water - sensitive or easily hydrolyzed drug can be improved. The lipid - emulsions with little organic solvent have no vascular irritation. Moreover, because little drug is exposed in the outer aqueous phase, the corresponding phlebitis can be efficiently reduced. Furthermore, lipid - emulsions possess certain targeting ability, especially to live and spleen, thus reducing drug concentrations in normal tissues and the corresponding side effects. Finally, as a result of the drug diffusion behavior across the oil drops, the sustained drug release characteristic is achieved in lipid - emulsions. Taken together, the lipid - emulsions can address the problems that the conventional intravenous formulation cannot. In addition, it has unique advantages compared with other microparticle preparations. For example, refined plant oils and phospholipids used in lipid - emulsion as oil phases are non - toxic and safe to human body. Meanwhile, the associated industrial production can be performed using existing production lines of lipid - emulsion for parenteral nutrition supplement.

Intravenouslipid – emulsion can be prepared by methods including high – pressure homogenization, ultrasonic, and microjet technologies.

Equipment and Materials

1. Equipment

Electronic balance, high speed disperser, ATS high pressure homogenizer, electronic constant temperature water bath, laser particle size analyzer, vortex mixer, water bath ultrasonic, UV spectrophotometer, 10ml centrifuge, etc. Glass rod, EP tube holder, tweezers, spatula, 200μl pipette, 1ml pipette, glass dropper, glass rod, beaker(100ml), EP tube(10ml), centrifuge tube(10ml), 10ml measuring cylinder, weighing paper, ear washing, 10ml volumetric flask, 50ml volumetric flask, 1ml pipette.

2. Materials

Nimodipine, injection grade soybean oil, egg phospholipid, oleic acid, glycerol, EDTA, water for injection, sodium hydroxide.

Experimental Methods

1. Preparation of Blank Lipid – Emulsion

(1) Formulation

Egg phospholipid	0.3g
Soybean oil	2ml
Water for injection	30ml

(2) Manufacturing process

The blank lipid – emulsion is prepared using a two – step procedure. First, a coarse emulsion is prepared by homogenizing oil phase containing egg phospholipid with the aqueous phase using a high – speed Ultra – Turrax blender operating at 10000r/min for 0.5min. Afterwards, the emulsions are further homogenized for 20 cycles at 600bar using a high – pressure homogenizer and sterilized with a 0.22μm filter.

The manufacturing flow chart of blank lipid – emulsion is shown in Figure 15 – 1.

2. Preparation of Nimodipine Lipid – Emulsion

(1) Formulation

Nimodipine	0.1g
Egg phospholipid	0.6g
Soybean oil	4ml
Oleic acid	0.02ml
Glycerol	1.4ml
EDTA	0.02ml
Water for injection(pH 8.5)	54ml

(2) Manufacturing process

Prepare oil phase by dissolving the egg phospholipid, oleic oil and drug in soybean oil by ultrasonication with glass – stick mixing. Add the oil phase to aqueous phase containing 54ml water,

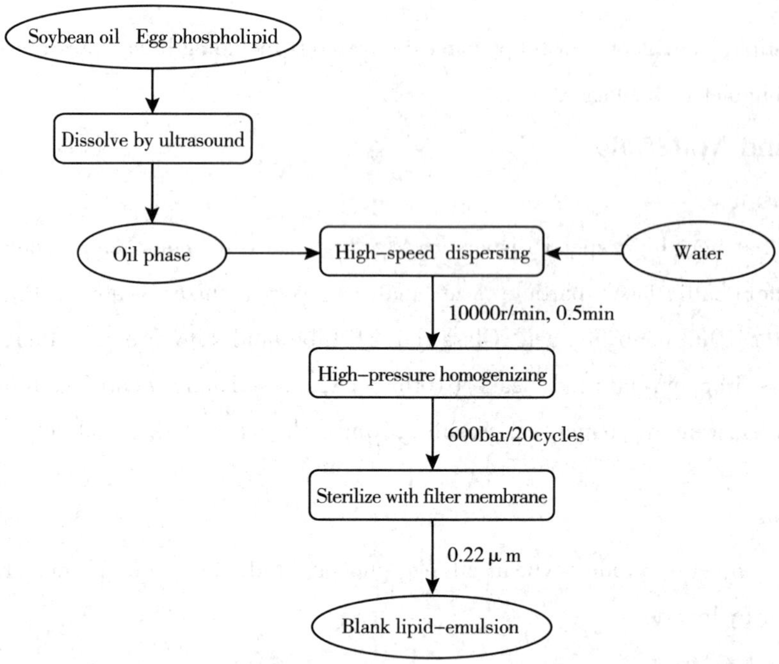

Figure 15 – 1 Manufacturing flow chart of blank lipid – emulsion

glycerol, and EDTA, followed by mixing the two phases homogeneously with high – speed Ultra – Turrax blender operating at 10,000r/min for 0. 5min and in subsequence homogenizing for 20 cycles at 600bar, and finally sterilize with a 0. 22μm filter

The manufacturing flow chart of nimodipine lipid – emulsion is shown in Figure 15 – 2.

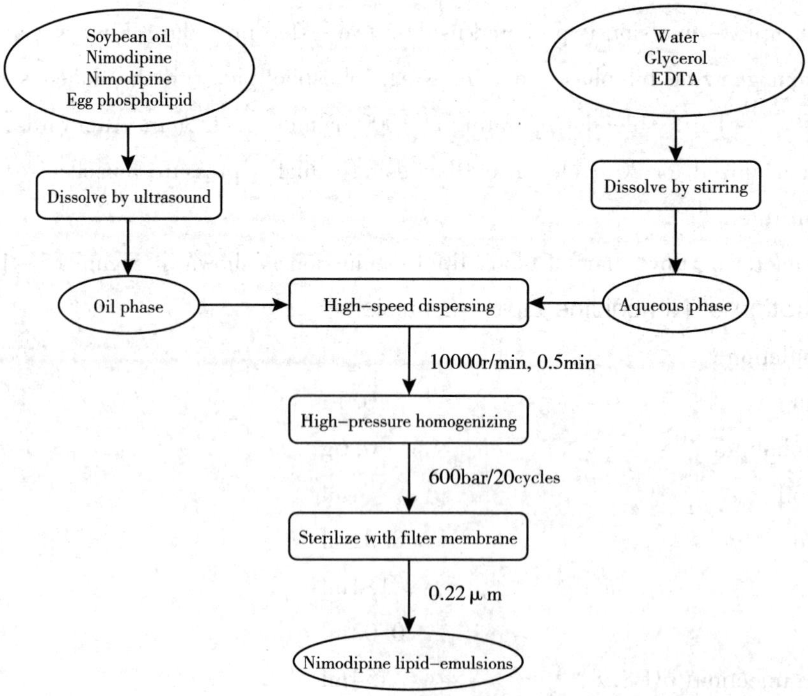

Figure 15 – 2 Manufacturing flow chart ofnimodipine lipid – emulsion

3. Quality Control

Appearance: The lipid – emulsions should be milk white and uniform without oil drops, stratification in static state and wall built – up upon being shaken.

Particle size and size distribution: Withdraw 0. 5ml of lipid – emulsion suspensions and dilute by 10 – fold with water, determine the particle size by a laser particle size analyzer.

Encapsulation efficiency: Pipette an adequate volume of nimodipine lipid – emulsion for centrifuge (3000r/min, 15min) and collect the supernatant, then dilute it for 500 times with ethanol by vortex. Finally, measure the absorbance of the obtained solution at 236nm using the UV spectrophotometer, and then calculate the drug concentration (C) according to the equation (1). Thus, the encapsulation efficiency can be calculated. To obtain the nimodipine standard curve, a series of solutions with different nimodipine concentration are needed to be prepared. Prepare 200μg/ml nimodipine stock solution, and prepare ethanol diluted solutions at the concentration of 2μg/ml, 4μg/ml, 8μg/ml, 12μg/ml, 16μg/ml using a 1ml pipetting tube. After correction of the baseline, the absorbance of each nimodipine solution was recorded at 236nm. Linear regression analysis was performed by plotting the absorbance A against the concentration C_i.

$$\text{Encapsulation efficiency (EE, \%)} = \frac{CVX}{M} \times 100\% \tag{1}$$

C: the detected concentration of the obtained lipid – emulsion product, X: dilution factor, V: the volume of the obtained lipid – emulsion product; M: the feeding amount of drug.

Experiment Instructions

Requirements for Preview

1. To master the preparation of intravenous lipid – emulsions by high – speed dispersion – high – pressure homogenization procedures.
2. To be familiar with the preparation methods of intravenous lipid – emulsions.
3. To be familiar with the formulation of lipid – emulsions.

Procedures and Precautions

1. To obtain lipid – emulsions with small size and better stability, the temperature for preparation of emulsions should be controlled near the phase inversion temperature of phospholipid. Moreover, the higher the temperature is, the faster the oxidation of phospholipid is. Therefore, the temperature control in the preparation should be focused on.
2. The quality of coarse emulsions, size and size distribution, are affected by the blend speed and time; thus, the shearing force from high – speed blend should be high enough to ensure the formation of the coarse emulsions, which oil and aqueous phases are mixed homogeneously.
3. Because metal tools are inevitably contacted during high – speed dispersion and homogenization, metal ion chelators must be used to reduce the oxidation of the oil phase.
4. Since lipid emulsion is prone to rancidity, it is necessary to provide a basic environment to maintain the stability of lipid emulsions.

5. The samples for size determination using a laser particle size analyzer should be diluted; otherwise, the accuracy of the determination might be reduced.

6. Generally, the size of marked or reported lipid – emulsions products is less than 1000nm with uniform size distribution. The size can be determined by electron microscopy and particle size analyzer.

7. The stability of lipid – emulsions can be tested through the change of particle size or other methods like centrifugal spectrophotometry.

Questions

1. What are the key points in the formation of intravenous lipid – emulsions? How to operate it?

2. What are the common methods for preparing lipid emulsions?

3. What are the general formulations of lipid emulsions?

4. What advantages over other particulate drug delivery systems do intravenous lipid – emulsions have?

5. What is the importance of intravenous lipid – emulsions in pharmaceutical dosage forms?

6. What is the difference between emulsion, submicron emulsion and nanoemulsion?

第五部分　新型制剂/载体的制备

实验16　固体分散体的制备与鉴定

【目的与要求】

1. **掌握**　固体分散体中共沉淀物及熔融法的制备方法。
2. **熟悉**　固体分散体提高溶出速率的原理和应用。
3. **了解**　聚乙烯吡咯烷酮及聚乙二醇的基本性质。

【基本概念与实验原理】

固体分散体是利用一种新技术将难溶性药物高度分散于固体载体材料而形成的。其原本应用于增加难溶性药物的溶出，可提高药物的生物利用度。近年来，人们应用水不溶性材料、肠溶性材料等为载体制备固体分散体，且利用固体分散技术制备缓控释制剂的研究进入新的发展阶段。按释药性能可将固体分散体分为三类：速释型、缓控释型、肠溶型。按药物分散状态可分为：低共熔混合物、固体溶液、玻璃溶液或混悬液、共沉淀物，其中药物分别以微晶态、分子态、玻璃态、无定形态分散在载体中。

固体分散体的制备方法有熔融法、溶剂法、熔融－溶剂法等。熔融法是将药物与载体混匀，加热至熔融，将熔融物在剧烈搅拌下迅速冷却成固体。溶剂法又称共沉淀法。将药物与载体共同溶解于有机溶剂中，蒸去溶剂后，得到药物分散在载体中形成的共沉淀物。溶剂－熔融法是将药物用少量有机溶剂溶解后加入熔融的载体混合，搅拌均匀，冷却固化后得到固体分散体。制备的固体分散体可采用显微镜、热分析、X射线衍射、红外光谱、核磁共振等方法加以鉴别。药物形成固体分散体后，溶解度和溶出速率会改变。因此可通过测定溶出度或溶出速率以评价固体分散体的质量。

本试验主要介绍速释型固体分散体。一般认为该类型固体分散体之所以能显著增加难溶性药物溶出度是基于药物的高度分散状态以及载体材料对药物溶出的促进作用。常用的载体材料有：聚乙二醇、聚维酮、泊洛沙姆、有机酸类、糖类与醇类等。

【仪器与材料】

1. **仪器**　分析天平，水浴，电炉，刮刀，尼龙筛（60和80目），乳钵，烧杯，752型紫外－可见分光光度计，磁力恒温搅拌器，电子调温加热套，恒温水浴锅，冰箱，智能溶出度测定仪，圆底烧瓶，真空干燥器，粉碎机等。

2. **材料**　磺胺噻唑（sulfathiazole，ST），聚维酮K30（PVP K30），95%乙醇，蒸馏水，浓盐酸，联苯双酯对照品，联苯双酯原料药，聚乙二醇6000（PEG6000），*N*,*N*－二甲基甲酰胺，蒸馏水，其他试剂均为分析纯。

【实验内容】

一、ST－PVP 共沉淀物的制备及溶出度测定

1. 处方

原辅料	处方 A1	处方 A2
ST	1.0g	3.0g
PVPK30	3.0g	1.0g

2. 制备工艺 ST－PVP 共沉淀物的制备：取处方量的 ST 置蒸发皿中，加适量 95% 乙醇使 ST 溶解（必要时可加热）；将处方量的 PVP K30 加入，搅拌使溶解；在沸水浴上蒸发乙醇近干，取下蒸发皿，置 50℃真空干燥 2～3h。取出凝固物，研磨，过 60 目筛，即得。

ST－PVP 物理混合物的制备：按药物、载体比例为 1∶3 和 3∶1 置研钵中，混合研磨，过 60 目筛，即得。

3. 溶出度测定 溶出介质的配制：取浓盐酸 9ml，加蒸馏水适量使成 1000ml，即得 0.1mol/L 盐酸溶液。

试验样品：相当于 ST 50mg 的原料、各比例共沉淀物和物理混合物。

溶出度测定：取上述样品，照溶出度与释放度测定法（《中国药典》四部通则 <0931> 第二法），以 0.1mol/L 盐酸溶液 500ml 为溶出介质，转速为 50r/min，依法操作，分别在 1、3、5、12 和 25min 时，取溶液 5ml 滤过，并同时补入溶出介质 5ml（37℃保温）。精密吸取续滤液 1ml，置 10ml 量瓶中，加 0.1mol/L 盐酸溶液稀释至刻度，摇匀。照紫外－可见分光光度法（《中国药典》四部通则 <0401>），在 282nm 波长处测定吸光度（A_t）。另取各组样品分别置于溶出杯中参照上述操作 25min 后，将溶出液全部转移至烧杯中，100℃加热搅拌 5min，放冷至 37℃，按前述方法取样及稀释，测定其 100% 溶出的吸光度（A_∞）。

4. 实验结果与数据处理 将上述测定值记入表 16－1。

表 16－1 ST、ST－PVP 共沉淀物及物理混合物的溶出度（以吸光度表示）

样品	吸光度（A）					
	1min	3min	5min	10min	25min	∞
ST						
ST－PVP（1∶3）共沉淀物						
ST－PVP（3∶1）共沉淀物						
ST－PVP（1∶3）物理混合物						
ST－PVP（3∶1）物理混合物						

按下式计算各时间点的累计溶出百分率 D_t（%）：

$$D_1(\%) = A_1/A_\infty \times 100\%$$

$$D_3(\%) = (A_3/A_\infty + 5/500 \times A_1/A_\infty) \times 100\%$$

$$D_5(\%) = [A_5/A_\infty + 5/500 \times (A_1 + A_3)/A_\infty] \times 100\%$$

$$D_{12}(\%)=[A_{12}/A_{\infty}+5/500\times(A_1+A_3+A_5)/A_{\infty}]\times100\%$$

$$D_{25}(\%)=[A_{25}/A_{\infty}+5/500\times(A_1+A_3+A_5+A_{12})/A_{\infty}]\times100\%$$

以时间（t）为横坐标，累计溶出百分率（D_t）为纵坐标作图，比较各样品的溶出程度和溶出速率。

二、联苯双酯－PEG6000固体分散体的制备及溶出度的测定

1. 处方

原辅料	处方 B1	处方 B2	处方 B3	处方 B4	处方 B5
联苯双酯（mg）	100	100	100	100	100
PEG6000（mg）	100	300	500	700	1000

2. 制备工艺

（1）联苯双酯－PEG6000固体分散体的制备

非溶剂熔融法：按照质量比为1∶1、1∶3、1∶5、1∶7、1∶10的比例分别精确称量联苯双酯及PEG6000。将联苯双酯置于圆底烧瓶中，于恒温电磁搅拌电热套上加热至熔融，熔融温度156～159℃，其次将处方量的PEG6000于70℃水浴加热至熔融；将后者加入圆底烧瓶，电磁搅拌至完全混匀；最后将熔融物倾倒在冰浴的不锈钢板上涂成薄片，置冰箱中存放12h，用药匙将凝结的固体分散体刮出，置真空干燥器中，待脆化后用粉碎机进行粉碎，过80目筛，密封保存。

溶剂熔融法：按照质量比为1∶1、1∶3、1∶5、1∶7、1∶10的比例分别精确称量联苯双酯及PEG6000。将联苯双酯置于圆底烧瓶并溶于N,N－二甲基甲酰胺中，于恒温电磁搅拌电热套上加热至熔融形成N,N－二甲基甲酰胺－联苯双酯饱和溶液，熔融温度156～159℃，其次将处方量的PEG6000于70℃水浴加热至熔融；加入适量的N,N－二甲基甲酰胺－联苯双酯饱和溶液混匀；最后将熔融物倾倒在冰浴的不锈钢板上涂成薄片，置冰箱中存放12h，用药匙将凝结的固体分散体刮出，置真空干燥器中，待脆化后用粉碎机进行粉碎，过80目筛，密封保存。

（2）联苯双酯－PEG6000物理混合物的制备　按照质量比为1∶1、1∶3、1∶5、1∶7、1∶10的比例分别精确称量联苯双酯及PEG6000，于研钵里充分研磨为联苯双酯－PEG6000物理混合物，过80目筛，密封保存。

3. 溶出度测定

溶出介质的配制：取浓盐酸9ml，加蒸馏水适量使成1000ml，即得0.1mol/L盐酸溶液。

试验样品：50mg的联苯双酯、联苯双酯－PEG6000固体分散体及物理混合物。

溶出度的测定：取上述样品，照溶出度与释放度测定法（《中国药典》四部通则<0931>第二法），以0.1mol/L盐酸溶液900ml为溶出介质，转速为50r/min，依法操作，分别于1、5、10、20、40、60min注射器取样5ml，并同时补入溶出介质5ml（37℃保温）。精密量取滤液1ml置25ml量瓶中，加溶出介质定容、摇匀，照紫外－可见分光光度法（《中国药典》四部通则<0401>），于278nm测定吸光度（A_t）。另取各组样品分别置于溶出杯中参照上述操作60min后，将溶出液全部转移至烧杯中100℃加热搅拌5min，放冷至37℃，按前述方法取样及稀释，测定其100%溶出的吸光度（A_{∞}）。

4. 试验结果与数据处理　将上述测定值记入表16－2。

表 16-2 联苯双酯、联苯双酯-PEG6000 固体分散体及物理混合物的溶出度（以吸光度表示）

样品	吸光度（A）						
	1min	5min	10min	20min	40min	60min	∝
联苯双酯							
处方 B1 固体分散体							
处方 B1 物理混合物							
处方 B2 固体分散体							
处方 B2 物理混合物							
处方 B3 固体分散体							
处方 B3 物理混合物							
处方 B4 固体分散体							
处方 B4 物理混合物							
处方 B5 固体分散体							
处方 B5 物理混合物							

按下式计算各时间点的累计溶出百分率 D_t（%）：

$$D_1(\%) = A_1/A_\infty \times 100\%$$

$$D_5(\%) = (A_5/A_\infty + 5/900 \times A_1/A_\infty) \times 100\%$$

$$D_{10}(\%) = [A_{10}/A_\infty + 5/900 \times (A_1 + A_5)/A_\infty] \times 100\%$$

$$D_{20}(\%) = [A_{20}/A_\infty + 5/900 \times (A_1 + A_5 + A_{10})/A_\infty] \times 100\%$$

$$D_{40}(\%) = [A_{40}/A_\infty + 5/900 \times (A_1 + A_5 + A_{10} + A_{20})/A_\infty] \times 100\%$$

$$D_{60}(\%) = [A_{60}/A_\infty + 5/900 \times (A_1 + A_5 + A_{10} + A_{20} + A_{40})/A_\infty] \times 100\%$$

以时间（t）为横坐标，累计溶出百分率（D_t）为纵坐标作图，比较各样品的溶出程度和溶出速率。

实验指导

一、预习要求

1. **掌握** 固体分散体的分类和制备方法。
2. **熟悉** 固体分散体溶出度测定操作规程及注意事项。
3. **了解** 聚乙烯吡咯烷酮的基本性质。

二、操作要点及注意事项

1. 共沉淀物中药物的分散性质不仅与所选择的载体有关，也与使用的载体量有关。实验一中选择的 1∶3 比例量，更有利于 ST 以微晶状态分散。不同药物所使用的载体种类及载体用量各不相同，应根据试验筛选确定。

2. 在制备共沉淀物时，所加乙醇以能溶解 ST 和 PVP 为限，过量乙醇不利于共沉淀物的快速结晶和分散。

3. 乙醇的蒸发在沸水浴中进行，并加以搅拌，可使乙醇快速挥发，有利于药物和载体的快速析出，保证药物的高度分散。

4. 乙醇蒸发得到的凝固物应真空干燥，挥尽液体，但真空干燥的温度不宜超过 50℃，以免共沉淀物受热熔融而改变药物分散性质。

5. 液态药物和剂量小于50mg的固态药物或原料药与辅料熔点相差较大一般采用溶剂熔融法制备固体分散体。

6. 恒温电磁搅拌电热套、恒温水浴锅将原料药和辅料熔融搅拌至透明状液体、无可见颗粒即可。*N*,*N*－二甲基甲酰胺在156～159℃条件下易挥发，故该操作应在通风橱进行。

7. 熔融法制备固体分散体的关键在于骤冷，必须将搅拌均匀的样品立刻倾倒在冰浴环境中的不锈钢板上并铺成薄片。

8. 为了比较相等粒径范围的主药、固体分散体、物理混合物等的溶出速率，应注意研磨时的平行操作。

三、思考题

1. 通过比较不同样品的溶出试验结果，可得出哪些结论？

2. 试述本实验中固体分散制备选用共沉淀法和熔融法的原因。

3. 制备固体分散体时如何选择载体？

4. 分别计算不同比例磺胺噻唑固体分散体及其物理混合物，联苯双酯固体分散体及其物理混合物的溶出速率常数。

5. 试举例说明除固体分散体外，哪些方法还可以增加难溶性药物的溶解度和溶出速率。

6. 本实验中还有哪些方面需要改进，你是否可以设计其他的相关实验？

Experiment 16 Preparation and Identification of Solid Dispersions

扫码“学一学”

Objectives and Requirements

1. To master the methods of preparing the solid dispersions.

2. To be familiar with the principles of increased dissolution rate of solid dispersion and its uses.

3. To understand the properties of PVP and PEG.

Introduction

Solid dispersions refer to the dispersion of one or more active ingredients in an inert carrier or matrix at solid state by some methods. Although most solid dispersion system initially focused on producing increased dissolution rates, recent attempts have been aimed at achieving other goals such as sustained release of drugs by the dispersion of the drug in water－insoluble polymeric carriers, and altered solid－state properties. Solid dispersions have been classified mainly into the following four major categories, such as simple eutectic mixtures, solid solution, glass solutions or suspensions, amorphous precipitations, and the drugs have been dispersed in carriers with microcrystalline, molecular level, a glassy state and amorphous form respectively.

Generally, there are only two methods of preparing solid dispersion, including fusion and solvent process. However, a third method of fusion－solvent may also be reported. In the fusion method of preparation, carrier is heated to a temperature just above its melting point and the drug is incorporated into the bases. The mixture is fast cooled with constant stirring to homogeneously disperse the drug throughout the bases. In the solvent method of preparation, the carriers and the active ingredients are dissolved in a suitable organic solvent; and the solvent is evaporated at an elevated temperature or under vacuum. As the solvent is removed, super saturation occurs followed by simultaneous precipitation of the constituents resulting in a solid residue, named coprecipitate. In the fusion - solvent method, carriers are melted and the drugs are incorporated in the form of a solution. A number of methods have been used to characterize solid dispersions including microscopy detection, thermal methods of analysis, X - ray diffraction, spectroscopic methods, especially I. R, and nuclear magnetic resonance (NMR). Dissolution rate determination is also an important tool to evaluate the solid dispersion.

This experiment discusses solid dispersion of poorly water - soluble drugs using water - soluble polymers. The increased dissolution rate of poorly water - soluble drugs can be attributed to the highly dispersion of drugs and the promotion effect of carriers on the dissolution.

Equipment and Materials

1. Equipment

Analytical balance, electric stove, water - bath, scraper, mortar, sieve (60 and 80 mesh), beaker, dissolution test instrument, constant temperature water bath, vacuum dryer, UV spectrophotometer, magnetic constant temperature agitator, electronic temperature control heating jacket, refrigerator, round bottom flask and grinder.

2. Materials

Sulfathiazole (ST), polyvinylpyrrolidone (PVP), ethanol (95%, *V/V*), distilled water, hydrochloric acid, bifendatatum control article (99.8%), bifendatatum (99.0%), *N*, *N* - Dimethylformamide, PEG6000, ultrapure water and other reagents (AR).

Experimental Methods

1. Preparation and dissolution of ST - PVP solid dispersions

(1) Formulations

Materials	A1	A2
ST	1.0g	3.0g
PVP K30	3.0g	1.0g

(2) Manufacturing process

Preparation of ST - PVP solid dispersions: ST - PVP solid dispersions were prepared using the solvent method by fast evaporation from a 95% ethanol solution followed by drying at 50℃ for 2 - 3hours. The samples were ground and sieved through 60 - mesh.

Preparation of ST - PVP physical mixtures: ST - PVP physical mixtures were mixed and grounded, then the samples were sieved through 60 - mesh.

(3) Dissolution rate determination

According to dissolution test (general chapter <0931> of ChP, method 2), 500ml hydrochloric acid solution (9→1000) is prepared as dissolution solvent, and then rotational speed of the paddle was adjusted to 50 rpm. Withdraw 5ml of the solution after 1,3,5,12 and 25min and filter it; and supplement 5ml of dissolution solvent. Discard the initial filtrate, and measure accurately 1ml of the successive filtrate to a 10ml volumetric flask. Then, dilute with the same solvent to volume and mix well. Measure the absorbance (A_t) of the resulting solution at 282nm (general chapter <0401> of ChP). Samples in the dissolution cup after 25min was transferred and heated at 100℃ for 5min, then the solution was cooled to 37℃ again, and the same procedure including sampling and diluting were made. Measure the absorbance (A_∞) of the solution at 282nm as the 100% dissolution.

(4) The experimental results and data analysis

Table 16 – 1　Absorbance of ST – PVP coprecipitates and physical mixtures in different sampling time

Samples	Absorbance (A)					
	1min	3min	5min	12min	25min	∞
ST						
ST – PVP (1 : 3) coprecipitate						
ST – PVP (3 : 1) coprecipitate						
ST – PVP (1 : 3) physical mixture						
ST – PVP (3 : 1) physical mixture						

Calculate the accumulated drug release percentage D_t (%) from each sample according the following equation:

$$D_1(\%) = A_1/A_\infty \times 100\%$$

$$D_3(\%) = (A_3/A_\infty + 5/500 \times A_1/A_\infty) \times 100\%$$

$$D_5(\%) = [A_5/A_\infty + 5/500 \times (A_1 + A_3)/A_\infty] \times 100\%$$

$$D_{12}(\%) = [A_{12}/A_\infty + 5/500 \times (A_1 + A_3 + A_5)/A_\infty] \times 100\%$$

$$D_{25}(\%) = [A_{25}/A_\infty + 5/500 \times (A_1 + A_3 + A_5 + A_{12})/A_\infty] \times 100\%$$

Draw the curve of $D_t(\%) \sim t$, and compare the dissolution degree and rate of each sample.

2. Preparation and dissolution of bifendatatum – PEG6000 solid dispersions

(1) Formulations

Materials	B1	B2	B3	B4	B5
Bifendatatum (mg)	100	100	100	100	100
PEG6000 (mg)	100	300	500	700	1000

(2) Manufacturing process

Non – solvent melting method: According to the mass ratio of 1 : 1, 1 : 3, 1 : 5, 1 : 7, 1 : 10, accurately weigh an appropriate amount of bifendatatum and PEG 6000, respectively. Bifendatatum is set in round bottom flask and placed in a constant temperature – controlled electromagnetic stirring electric to melt, and the melting temperature was 156 – 159℃. The corresponding amount of PEG6000 in 70℃ water bath is heated to melt; and then, the latter is added in a round bottom flask and completely mixed with bifendatatum. Pour the melts on stainless steel plate into thin slices in an ice bath, and store in refrigerator for 12h. Then coagulated solid dispersion is scraped by medicine spoon, set in a vacuum dryer to be pulverized through grinder after embrittlement, and sealed over 80 – mesh sieve.

Solvent melting method: According to the mass ratio of 1 : 1, 1 : 3, 1 : 5, 1 : 7, 1 : 10, accurately weigh appropriate amount of bifendatatum and PEG6000. Bifendatatum is placed in a round bottom flask, and dissolved in N, N – dimethylformamide, then arranged in an isothermal electromagnetic stirring electric to melt into saturated N, N – dimethylformamide – bifendatatum solution. The melting temperature is 156 – 159℃. The corresponding amount of PEG6000 in 70℃ water bath is heated to melt; an appropriate amount of saturated N, N – dimethylformamide – bifendatatum solution is added and mixed. Pour the melts on stainless steel plate into thin slices in an ice bath, and store in refrigerator for 12h. Then coagulated solid dispersion is scraped by medicine spoon, set in vacuum dryer to be pulverized through grinder after embrittlement, and sealed over 80 – mesh sieve.

Preparation of bifendatatum – PEG6000 physical mixtures: In accordance with the quality ratio of 1 : 1, 1 : 3, 1 : 5, 1 : 7, 1 : 10, appropriate bifendatatum and PEG6000 are accurately weighed and grinded completely in mortar, then sealed over 80 mesh sieve.

(3) Dissolution rate determination

According to dissolution test (general chapter <0931> of ChP, method 2), 900ml hydrochloric acid solution (9→1000) is prepared as dissolution solvent, and then rotational speed of the paddle is adjusted to 50 rpm. Dissolution Tester water bath temperature is adjusted (37 ± 0.5) ℃. Accurately weighed 900ml dissolution medium is poured into the analyzer dissolution vessel, preheating and maintaining (37 ± 0.5) ℃. The impeller speed is adjusted to 50r/min. Test samples (bifendatatum, bifendatatum – PEG6000 solid dispersions and physical mixtures with 50mg API contained) are placed into dissolution cup. Withdraw 5ml of the solution after 1, 5, 10, 20, 40 and 60min and filter it; supplement 5ml of dissolution solvent. Discard the initial filtrate, measure accurately 1ml of the successive filtrate to a 25ml volumetric flask, dilute with the same solvent to volume and mix well. Measure the absorbance (A_t) of the resulting solution at 278nm (general chapter 0401 of ChP). Samples in the dissolution cup after 60min are transferred and heated at 100℃ for 5min, then the solution is cooled to 37℃ again; the same procedure including sampling and diluting are made. Measure the absorbance (A_∞) of solution at 278nm as the 100% dissolution.

(4) The experimental results and data analysis

Table 16 – 2 Absorbance of bifendatatum, bifendatatum – PEG6000 SD and physical mixtures in different sampling time

Samples	Absorbance (*A*)						
	1min	5min	10min	20min	40min	60min	∞
Bifendatatum							
Formulation B1 SD							
Formulation B1 physical mixtures							
Formulation B2 SD							
Formulation B2 physical mixtures							

续表

Samples	Absorbance(A)						
	1min	5min	10min	20min	40min	60min	∞
Formulation B3 SD							
Formulation B3 physical mixtures							
Formulation B4 SD							
Formulation B4 physical mixtures							
Formulation B5 SD							
Formulation B5 physical mixtures							

Calculate theaccumulated drug release percentage $D_t(\%)$ from each sample according the following equation:

$$D_1(\%) = A_1/A_\infty \times 100\%$$

$$D_5(\%) = (A_5/A_\infty + 5/900 \times A_1/A_\infty) \times 100\%$$

$$D_{10}(\%) = [A_{10}/A_\infty + 5/900 \times (A_1 + A_5)/A_\infty] \times 100\%$$

$$D_{20}(\%) = [A_{20}/A_\infty + 5/900 \times (A_1 + A_5 + A_{10})/A_\infty] \times 100\%$$

$$D_{40}(\%) = [A_{40}/A_\infty + 5/900 \times (A_1 + A_5 + A_{10} + A_{20})/A_\infty] \times 100\%$$

$$D_{60}(\%) = [A_{60}/A_\infty + 5/900 \times (A_1 + A_5 + A_{10} + A_{20} + A_{40})/A_\infty] \times 100\%$$

Draw the curve of $D_t(\%) \sim t$, and compare the dissolution degree and rate of each sample.

Experiment Instructions

Requirements for Preview

1. To master the classification and preparation methods of solid dispersions.
2. To be familiar with dissolution test procedures and precautions.
3. To understand the properties of PVP and PEG.

Procedures and Precautions

1. Factors that influence the dispersion state of drugs include the physical properties and ratio of the carriers. In this experiment, ratio of 1 : 3 is more advantageous to formation of microcrystalline of ST in the carrier.

2. The volume of ethanol should be reduced to a minimum to just dissolve the drug and carrier in order to obtain the quick evaporation of the solvent and highly dispersion of drugs.

3. The temperature of the vacuum - dry should not go beyond 50℃ to prevent the melt of the coprecipitates and the change of dispersion state of drugs.

4. When APIs are liquid drug, or solid drug whose dose is less than 50mg, or the melting point between drug and excipients are largely different and solvent/fusion method is commonly used in molten solid dispersions.

5. APIs and excipients are melted and stirred through magnetic stirring electric and water bath to become transparent liquid without visible particles. N,N - dimethylformamide is easy to volatilize

at 156 - 159℃, so the operation should be carried out in a fume hood.

6. The key for solid dispersion preparations using fusion method is quencher, and the sample was immediately poured onto a stainless steel plate in an ice bath environment and paved sheet.

7. Parallel operation in grinding and sieving should be followed in order to compare the dissolution rate of coprecipitates and physical mixtures in the same size.

Questions

1. What conclusions can be made from these experiment results?

2. Explain the reasons of choosing the solvent or fusion method for solid dispersion preparation?

3. How to select suitable carriers in the preparation of solid dispersion?

4. Calculate the dissolution rate constant of each sample.

5. Are there other methods to increase the solubility and dissolution rate of poorly water - soluble drug?

6. Which aspects of this experiment need to be improved, and can you design any other related experiments?

实验 17　包合物的制备与鉴定

【目的与要求】

1. **掌握**　饱和水溶液法制备包合物的工艺。
2. **熟悉**　β - 环糊精（β - CD）的性质与应用。
3. **了解**　包合物的鉴别方法。

【基本概念与实验原理】

包合物是由客分子和主分子两种组分加合而成，主分子具有较大的空穴结构，足以将客分子容纳在内形成分子胶囊。

药物制成包合物后，具有如下优点：增加药物的溶解度和溶出速度；提高药物的稳定性，使液体药物粉末化；改善药物的吸收和生物利用度；降低药物的刺激性与毒副作用；掩盖药物的不良嗅味；调节释药速率。

目前应用最多的主分子是环糊精及其衍生物。环糊精是一类由 6 ~ 12 个葡萄糖分子通过 α - 1，4 - 糖苷键连接而成的环状低聚糖化合物，为中空圆筒状结构。常见的环糊精有 α、β、γ 三种，分别由 6、7、8 个葡萄糖分子构成，其中以 β - 环糊精（β - CD）应用最为广泛。β - CD 空洞大小合适，在三种环糊精中，水中溶解度最小，易从水中析出结晶。其溶解度随温度升高而增大。其筒状结构内部显疏水性，开口处显亲水性。动物实验证明其口服毒性很低。以上这些性质为 β - CD 包合物的制备和应用提供了有利条件。同时，客分子的大小、极性、解离状态等均能影响环糊精包合物的形成及稳定。

CD 包合物制备方法很多，有饱和水溶液法、研磨法、冷冻干燥法、喷雾干燥法、中和法、密封加热法等，其中以饱和水溶液法最为常用。

包合物的验证主要是鉴别药物是否已被环糊精包入空穴以及包合的方式，可采用显微镜、相溶解度、X射线衍射、红外光谱、核磁共振、差热分析、薄层色谱等一系列方法加以验证。

本实验中客分子为薄荷油，主要成分为薄荷脑、薄荷酮等，具有发汗、抗菌、解痉等作用，但容易挥发，制成环糊精包合物后可延缓和减少其挥发，同时可使液态油转换成固态，便于配方，且兼具缓释作用。

【仪器与材料】

1. 仪器　磨塞锥形瓶（100ml），量筒（10ml、5ml），干燥器，水浴锅，电炉，分析天平，差示扫描热分析仪和X射线衍射仪等。

2. 材料　β-环糊精（β-CD），吡罗昔康，薄荷油，无水乙醇，95%乙醇。

【实验内容】

一、薄荷油包合物

1. 处方

β-CD	4.0g
薄荷油	1.0ml
蒸馏水	50ml

2. 制备工艺　称取β-CD 4.0g，置100ml带塞锥形瓶中，加蒸馏水50ml，加热溶解，降温至50℃。加入薄荷油1.0ml，恒温搅拌2.5h，冷却至室温，有白色沉淀析出，待沉淀完全后过滤。用无水乙醇5ml洗涤沉淀3次，至表面近无油渍。将包合物置低温真空干燥器中干燥，称重，计算收率。

二、吡罗昔康包合物

1. 处方

β-CD	4.0g
吡罗昔康	0.6g
无水乙醇	1ml
蒸馏水	10ml

2. 制备工艺　称取4.0g β-CD，置研钵中，加10ml水，研磨分散均匀。另取0.6g吡罗昔康溶于1.0ml无水乙醇中。将吡罗昔康乙醇溶液加入β-CD分散液中，充分研磨至糊状，低温干燥后用无水乙醇5ml洗涤3次。将包合物置低温真空干燥器中干燥，称重，计算收率。

三、包合物鉴别与质量评价

1. 包合物的鉴别　一般需要通过几种不同方法验证包合物的形成。

差热分析法（DSC）：测定药物分子、β-CD、包合物与物理混合物的热分析曲线，根据曲线上的吸热峰的变化判断包合物的形成。以空白坩埚为参比，升温扫描，扫描速度为10K/min，扫描范围20~250℃，气氛为氮气（流速100ml/min）。

X射线衍射法（PXRD）：测定药物分子、β-CD、包合物与物理混合物的PXRD曲线，根据衍射峰的位置或强度的变化判断包合物是否形成。测定条件：铜靶，kα线，管压40kV，管流60mA，后置式石墨单色器，扫描范围（2θ）：2.5°~50°，扫描速度0.3°/min，扫描步长0.02°。

2. **载药** 称取包合物（约1.0g），置圆底烧瓶中，加入乙醚5ml振荡10min，过滤；取滤液蒸干后，加入适量有机溶剂（如甲醇）溶解残渣后，测定药物含量。按以下公式计算载药情况：

$$药物含量(\%)=\frac{包合物中药物量(g)}{包合物量(g)}\times 100\%$$

$$药物包封率(\%)=\frac{包合物中药物量(g)}{药物投药总量(g)}\times 100\%$$

$$包合物收率(\%)=\frac{包合物量(g)}{\beta-CD(g)+药物量(g)}\times 100\%$$

实验指导

一、预习要求

1. **预习** 包合物形成的原理与作用，了解环糊精的种类、性质及特点。

2. **掌握** 环糊精包合物的常用制备方法及鉴别方法。

3. **了解** 药物的性质与包合物应用的关系。

二、操作要点及注意事项

1. 本实验采用饱和水溶液法制备包合物，主分子β-CD在25℃时水中溶解度为1.85%，但在50℃时溶解度可增加至4.0%。故在实验过程中，应控制好温度，包合过程结束后，通过降低温度使包合物从水中析出。

2. 包封率取决于环糊精种类、药物与环糊精的配比量以及包合时间，应按照实验内容的要求进行操作。

3. DSC与PXRD检测的特征峰一般会随着β-CD与客分子的比例变化而变化，而当客分子被完全包合时，客分子的特征峰消失。

三、思考题

1. 环糊精的结构特征是什么？药用环糊精有哪些？

2. 制备β-CD包合物的关键是什么？应如何进行操作？

3. 哪类药物适合制备成环糊精包合物？

4. 本实验采用饱和水溶液法与研磨法制备β-CD包合物，还有哪些方法可以制备包合物？各有何优缺点？

5. 鉴别包合物的方法主要包含哪些？各自有什么特点？

6. 包合物在药物制剂中有何意义？

Experiment 17 Preparation of Inclusion Complexes

Objectives and Requirements

1. To master the preparation methods of cyclodextrin inclusion complexes.

2. To be familiar with the properties and applications of β - CD.

3. To understand the identification methods of inclusion complexes.

Introduction

Inclusion complexes, also named molecule capsules, consisted of host and guest molecules, being prepared by incorporating the latter into the inner hydrophobic cavity of the former.

Inclusion complexesfor drugs have various advantages, including increasing the stability of drug, masking the unpleasant taste, enhancing bioavailability of poorly soluble drugs, reducing side effects, modifying drug release profile.

Cyclodextrins (CDs), cyclicα - 1,4 - linked D - glucose oligomers, are most commonly used host molecules and classified as α, β and γ - CDs that possess six, seven and eight D - glucopyranose units, respectively. The shape of the inner hydrophobic cavity of CDs is like a truncated cone. Hydroxyl groups are located at the rims of the cavity resulting in somewhat hydrophilic properties outside of the CD molecule. Among the three CDs, β - CDs are the most commonly used in pharmaceutics due to its cavity with suitable size for drug inclusion, lowest water - solubility and the increase in solubility as the temperature rise, which enables the inclusion complexes to be deposited in cold water and thus facilitate the inclusion preparation, as well as lowest oral toxicity. Indeed, the size, polarity and dissociated state of guest molecule also affect the formation and stability of cyclodextrin inclusion complexes.

The cyclodextrin inclusion compounds can be prepared by various methods, such as, coprecipitate, kneading, freeze - dried, spray - dried, neutralization and heating methods.

The cyclodextrin inclusion compounds are characterized by microscopical studies, phase - solubility behavior, X - ray diffraction, H - NMR, IR, UV spectra, thermal analysis, and thin layer chromatography (TLC).

Herein, peppermint oil is used as guest molecule for preparation of inclusion complexes. The oil consisted of menthol and menthone, having various therapeutic effects like sweating, antimicrobial, antispasmodic. The oil is a volatile compound and the formation of inclusion complexes can thus prevent the evaporation; meanwhile, the oil can be transformed into solid form by inclusion, therefore facilitating the manufacturing.

Equipment and Materials

1. Equipment

Coned flask, graduated cylinder, developing chamber, volatile oil extractor, desiccator, thin layer plate, water bath, electric stove, analytical balance, differential scanning calorimeter (DSC) and PXRD diffractometer, etc.

2. Materials

β - CD, peppermint oil, piroxicam, ethanol, silica gel G, ethyl acetate, petroleum ether.

Experimental Methods

1. Preparation of Peppermint Oil Inclusion Complexes

(1) Formulation

β - CD 4.0g

Peppermint oil	1.0ml
Distilled water	50ml

(2) Manufacturing process

Dissolve β - CD in 50ml distilled water by heating, following by cooling down to 50℃, add drop - wise the oil to the β - CD solution and stir at 50℃ for 2.5h; after that, cool down the mixture to room temperature to deposit the sample. Subsequently, filter the obtained solution and wash the deposition for 3 times with 5ml ethanol to remove the residue oil and dried in desiccators.

2. Preparation of Piroxicam Inclusion Complexes

(1) Formulation

β - CD	4.0g
Piroxicam	0.6ml
Ethanol	1ml
Distilled water	10ml

(2) Manufacturing process

Place β - CD to 10ml distilled water and the mixture and blended uniformly by grinding. Subsequently, add the piroxicam in ethanol to the β - CD dispersion, following by grinding to obtain a paste sample. Dry the sample at low temperature, follow by washing for 3 times with 5ml ethanol and finally dry the sample in a drier.

3. Characterization ofInclusion Complexes

(1) Identification of inclusion complexes

The formation ofinclusion complexes should be confirmed by more than one method.

DSC: The samples including the pure drug, β - CD, physical mixture of pure drug and β - CD and β - CD complexes are subjected to DSC determinations. Heat the samples from 25 to 300℃ at a heating rate of 10K/min. Calibrate the instrument using indium. All of the DSC determinations are conducted in a nitrogen atmosphere at a flow rate of 100ml/min. The absence of characteristic peaks of the drug indicates the formation of β - CD complexes.

PXRD: PXRD of the samples are evaluated by diffractometer over the 2.5 - 50° 2θ range at a scan rate of 3°/min, where the tube anode is Cu with Kα = 0.154nm monochromatized with a graphite crystal. Collect the diffraction pattern at 40 kV of tube voltage and 60 mA of tube current in step scan mode (step size 0.02°, counting time1 s/step).

(2) Drug loading

To extract the drug from the inclusion complexes, place a fixed amount of the sample (1g) and 5ml of ether to a round bottom, following by shaking for 10min and filtrating. Then, dry the filtrated solution by distillation and dissolve the residual with organic solvent like methanol to determine the drug content. The drug loading of the inclusion complex is calculated by the following equations:

$$\text{Content of inclusion complexes}(\%) = \frac{\text{drug weight in inclusion complexes(g)}}{\text{weight of inclusion complexes(g)}} \times 100\%$$

$$\text{Encapsulation efficiency}(\%) = \frac{\text{drug weight in inclusion complexes(g)}}{\text{weight of inclusion complexes(g)}} \times 100\%$$

$$\text{Yield}(\%) = \frac{\text{weight of inclusion complexes(g)}}{\text{weight of }\beta - \text{CD(g)} + \text{weight of drug(g)}} \times 100\%$$

Experiment Instructions

Requirements for Preview

1. To preview the categories, properties and uses of β－CD.

2. To be familiar with the preparation procedure, investigation and evaluation of inclusion complexes.

3. To know the relationship of drug's properties and inclusion complex preparation and uses.

Procedures and Precautions

1. The water－solubility of β－CD is 1.85% at 25℃ and 4.0% at 50℃. Thus the temperature should be controlled carefully in procedure. The deposit of inclusion complex can be obtained by falling the temperature.

2. Drug loading and encapsulation efficiency depend on the type of β－CD, the ratio of β－CD and drug, operating time.

3. The characteristic peaks of the drugs in PXRD diffractograms and DSC thermograms would be alternated for the change in the ratio of β－CD and guest molecules; however, the characteristic peaks would disappear as the guest molecules are completely encapsulated in the complexes.

Questions

1. What is structure of CD? what types of CD are used in pharmaceutical science?

2. What are the key points in the formation of cyclodextrin inclusion complexes? How to operate it?

3. What kinds of drug are suitable to be prepared into cyclodextrin inclusion complexes?

4. Besides the saturated aqueous solution and grinding methods, are there other methods can be used to prepare the inclusion complexes? Describe the advantages and disadvantages of these methods.

5. What methods are used to characterize complexes? what are their properties?

6. What is the importance of inclusion complexes in pharmaceutical dosage forms?

实验18 微球和微囊的制备

【目的与要求】

1. **掌握** 制备微球和微囊的基本原理和方法。
2. **熟悉** 影响微囊成型的因素。
3. **了解** 制备微球和微囊常用的高分子材料。

【基本概念与实验原理】

微球是将药物溶解或分散在适宜的载体辅料中形成的微小球状实体，粒径范围可为1～250μm（也有的定义为1～1000μm）。粒径在10～100nm范围的称为纳米球（nanospheres）或纳米粒（nanoparticles），属于胶体范畴；0.1～1μm的可称为亚微球（sub－microspheres）。

微球的制备方法常见的有：物理法，如喷雾干燥法；物理化学法，如乳化－加热法、乳化－交联法以及乳化－溶剂挥发法；化学法，如聚合法和交联法等。喷雾干燥法是将药物分散在合适的高分子材料溶液中，以喷雾法将此混合物喷入热气流中使液滴干燥固化得到微球。乳化－加热法是利用蛋白遇热变性的性质制备微球。乳化－交联法是利用高分子材料中活性基团可以和相应的化合物发生反应的特点，交联制得微球。乳化－溶剂挥发法则是采用适宜的高分子溶于有机溶剂中，在水相中乳化并逐渐挥发掉溶剂而制得微球。聚合法是将单体化合物分散到一定的介质中使其发生加聚或缩聚反应形成微球。

制备微球的高分子材料主要包括：天然高分子材料，如明胶、海藻酸钠、淀粉、血清蛋白、壳聚糖等）；半合成类高分子材料，如纤维素类衍生物；合成类高分子材料，如聚乳酸、聚羟基乙酸等。明胶为非特异性蛋白，价廉易得，可与醛类物质进行氨醛缩合反应而交联化，交联后的明胶机械强度好，化学性质稳定，遇水不溶胀，微球载药量较大，且可缓慢释药，是较好制备微球或微囊的材料之一。海藻酸钠是从海带、马尾藻等海洋植物中提取得到的白色或淡黄色线性天然多糖，无毒、无刺激，且具有独特的理化性质和良好的生物相容性，广泛应用于食品、印染、水污染处理、生物医药等领域。海藻酸钠主要由α－L－甘露糖醛酸（M单元）与β－D－古洛糖醛酸（G单元）依靠β－1,4－糖苷键连接，并由不同比例的GM、MM和GG片段组成的共聚物。海藻酸钠的GG片段可与二价以上的金属离子（如钙离子）络合交联，生成具有水、酸不溶性的“蛋盒结构”的海藻酸钙凝胶，可作为酶固定化、蛋白多肽类药物口服给药以及缓控释给药的载体，也可以利用海藻酸钠的这个性质采用交联法制备海藻酸钠微球。

微型胶囊（简称微囊）系利用高分子材料（通称囊材）、将固体药物或液体药物（通称囊心物）包裹成直径为1～250μm的微小胶囊。药物微囊化后，具有缓释作用，可提高药物的稳定性，掩盖药物的不良气味和口味，降低药物对胃肠道的刺激性，减少复方药物的配伍禁忌，改善药物的流动性与可压性，使液态药物可固体化。根据临床需要，可将微囊制成散剂、胶囊剂、片剂、注射剂、软膏等。

微囊的制备方法很多，可归纳为物理化学法、化学法以及物理机械法三大类。可根据药物和囊材的性质与微囊的粒径、释放性能等要求进行选择。本实验采用单、复凝聚法制备胶囊，工艺简单，可用于多种类药物的微囊化。复凝聚法的原理是利用一些高亲水性胶体带有电荷的性质，当两种或两种以上带相反电荷的胶体液混合时，因电荷中和而产生凝聚。例如：阿拉伯胶液带负电，而A型明胶在等电点（pH 7～9）以上也带负电荷，故两者混合并不发生凝聚现象；若用醋酸调节胶液pH至A型明胶等电点以下（约pH 3.8～4.0）时，明胶电荷全部转为正电荷，即与带负电荷的阿拉伯胶相互凝聚。当溶液中存在药物时，就包在药物粒子周围形成微囊，此时囊膜较松软，当降低温度使达到胶凝点以下时，则逐渐胶凝、硬化，再加入甲醛使囊膜变性固化而得微囊成品。单凝聚法制备微囊的原理是利用凝聚剂（强亲水性电解质或非电解质）与高分子囊材溶液的水合膜中水分子结合，致使囊材的溶解度降低，在搅拌条件下自体系中凝聚成囊而析出，这种凝聚是可逆的，一旦解除促凝聚条件，就可发生解凝聚现象，需根据囊材性质进行固化。

【仪器与材料】

1. 仪器 电动搅拌器，烧杯（500、250及50ml），循环水真空泵，抽滤瓶，布氏滤器，注射器（6号针头），水浴，电炉，显微镜，研钵，普通天平等。

2. 材料　液状石蜡，明胶A型，明胶B型（等电点pH 4.8~5.2），油酸山梨坦（司盘80），甲醛，石油醚，2%氯化钙溶液，海藻酸钠，磺胺二甲嘧啶，10%醋酸溶液，60%硫酸钠溶液等。

【实验内容】

一、微球的制备

（一）明胶微球

1. 处方

液状石蜡	50ml
明胶	1g
油酸山梨坦（司盘80）	0.5g
蒸馏水	5ml

2. 制备工艺

乳化：量取50ml液状石蜡置烧杯中，加入适量司盘80（1%，*W/V*），预热至60℃，将螺旋形搅拌桨置于烧杯中央液面下2/3高处，调节转速约400r/min。另取明胶1g，置于5ml蒸馏水中，溶胀，60℃溶解配制成20%（*W/V*）明胶溶液，在搅拌下缓缓加入液状石蜡中，继续搅拌15min使充分乳化。

洗涤：将上述乳液在搅拌下迅速冷却至5℃，抽滤，置于通风橱中，从滤器上用适量石油醚分3次洗去微球表面的液状石蜡，抽干，转移至平皿上，加少量丙酮分散后在红外灯下40℃挥去丙酮。

固化：取干燥的微球置盛有40%甲醛溶液的密闭容器中，35℃保持6h后取出，挥去残留甲醛即得明胶微球。

粒径：显微镜下观察其粒子形态并测定其粒径。

（二）海藻酸钠微球

1. 处方

海藻酸钠	1g
蒸馏水	50ml
2%氯化钙溶液	100ml

2. 制备工艺

海藻酸钠溶液的配制：称取1g海藻酸钠，加50ml水溶解，放置溶胀12h，即得。

钙化：用注射器将海藻酸钠溶液逐滴滴入不断搅拌（转速为80r/min）的$CaCl_2$（2%，*W/V*）溶液中，针头距液面8cm，钙化2h。

干燥：胶凝完毕后，用去离子水冲洗3次，抽滤后置干燥箱中干燥12h，即得海藻酸钠空白微球。

粒径：显微镜下观察其微球形态并测定其粒径。

二、微囊的制备

（一）磺胺二甲嘧啶微囊

1. 处方

磺胺二甲嘧啶	1.2g

明胶 1g

阿拉伯胶 1g

10%醋酸 适量

37%甲醛溶液 1.6ml

2. **制备工艺**

胶液的配制：分别称取处方量的阿拉伯胶和明胶，加蒸馏水分别制成3%浓度的胶液，明胶液用20%氢氧化钠溶液调节pH值至7~8，备用。

混悬：称取磺胺二甲嘧啶细粉1.2g，置研钵研细，加入阿拉伯胶液与明胶液，边加边研，将混合胶液转移至烧杯中，置45℃水浴中，搅拌，混匀。取样置显微镜下观察。

凝聚及固化：将药物与囊材混悬液撤离水浴加热并在不断搅拌下，滴加10%醋酸，调节混悬液pH值至3.8~4.1，即产生凝聚，用显微镜观察凝聚成囊的情况。凝聚后继续搅拌5min，加入37℃蒸馏水80ml稀释，移去热水浴，使微囊混悬液的温度降至25℃后，移置冰浴中，等温度降至10℃以下后，加入37%甲醛溶液1.6ml，固化0.5~1h，然后加20%氢氧化钠溶液调节pH值至9.0左右。通过光学显微镜观察微囊形态学特征、粒径和粒径分布。

干燥：将湿囊过滤，用蒸馏水洗涤至无甲醛味，抽干，置70℃以下干燥，即得。

3. **实验记录** 将实验过程中的各处方用量及溶液pH值填入表18-1中。

表18-1 SM_2微囊制备记录

处方组成	实验值	pH值
阿拉伯胶溶液浓度（%）		—
明胶溶液溶液浓度（%）		
调节明胶溶液pH值的20%氢氧化钠溶液量		
SM_2用量		—
稀释加水总量		—
调节pH值的10%醋酸量		
固化用甲醛溶液量		—
固化后调节pH值的20%氢氧化钠溶液量		

（二）液状石蜡微囊的制备

1. **处方**

液状石蜡 2g

明胶 2g

10%醋酸溶液 适量

60%硫酸钠溶液 适量

37%甲醛溶液 3ml

蒸馏水 适量

2. **制备工艺**

明胶溶液的配制：称取明胶2g，加蒸馏水10ml使溶胀、溶解，50℃保温。

液状石蜡乳的制备：称取处方量液状石蜡，加明胶溶液，于研钵中研磨成初乳，加蒸馏水至60ml，混匀，用10%醋酸溶液调节pH值至4（3.5~3.8）。

微囊的制备：将上述乳剂转移至烧杯中，置于50℃恒温水浴内，量取一定体积的60%硫酸钠溶液，在搅拌下滴入乳剂中，至显微镜下观察，以成囊为度，由所用硫酸钠体积计算体系中硫酸钠的浓度。另配制成硫酸钠稀释液，浓度为体系中浓度加1.5%，体积为成囊溶液3倍以上，稀释液温度为15℃，倾入搅拌的体系中，使微囊分散，静置待微囊沉降，倾去上清液，用硫酸钠稀释液洗2~3次。再将微囊混悬于硫酸钠稀释液300ml中，加甲醛溶液，搅拌15min，用20%氢氧化钠溶液调节pH值至8~9，继续搅拌1h，静置待微囊沉降完全。通过光学显微镜观察微囊形态学特征、粒径和粒径分布。倾去上清液，用蒸馏水洗至无甲醛气味（或用Schiff试剂调至不显色），抽干，即得。

实验指导

一、预习要求

1. **复习** 微球、微囊的一般制备方法，掌握单、复凝聚法制备微囊的原理和操作注意点。
2. **熟悉** 明胶和海藻酸钠的性质，影响微囊粒子大小的因素。
3. **了解** 微球和微囊的临床应用与特点。

二、操作要点和注意事项

1. 微球的制备

（1）海藻酸钠和明胶均为黏性较大的高分子化合物，配制溶液时需充分溶胀。

（2）明胶微球采用乳化交联法，先制备W/O型乳液，故选择司盘80为乳化剂，用量为油相的1%（*W/V*）左右。乳化剂用量太少，形成的乳液不稳定，在加热时易粘连。

（3）乳化搅拌时间不宜过长，否则分散液滴碰撞机会增加、液滴粘连而增大粒径。搅拌速度增加有利于减小微球粒径，但以不产生大量泡沫和漩涡为度。

（4）适当降低明胶溶液浓度、升高温度、加快搅拌速度和提高司盘80的加入量均可减小微球的粒径，在实验条件下，微球粒径范围为2~10μm。

（5）甲醛和明胶会产生胺醛缩合反应使明胶分子相互交联，达到固化目的。交联反应在pH 8~9容易进行，所以预先将明胶溶液调节至偏碱性有利于反应完全，完全交联固化时间约在12h以上。

（6）采用化学交联法制备海藻酸钠微球，将预先配制好的海藻酸钠溶液注入氯化钙时需注意以下几点：液滴要逐滴滴入，且滴速控制在每2~3秒1滴；针头距液面的高度在8~15cm，以保证所得的微球较为圆整，太高所得微球呈扁平状，太低则容易拖尾。

（7）海藻酸钠的浓度与黏度有关，黏度较大时可采用较低的浓度，黏度较小时则采用较高的浓度。但其浓度一般在1%~3%，浓度太低不易成型；浓度太高则不易滴制，同时所得的微球易拖尾。

（8）为能直观的观察微球的制备，本实验采用6号针头，并采用滴制法。6号针头的直径为0.5mm，海藻酸钠在水中的吸水率可高达500倍左右，因此在钙溶液中肉眼可见0.5~1mm的微球，干燥后微球可收缩为约0.5mm。如需获得更小粒径的海藻酸钠微球，则可采用更小直径的针头或其他方法进行制备。

2. 微囊的制备

（1）根据生产方法的不同，明胶有A型和B型之分，A型明胶的等电点为pH 7~9，B

型明胶的等电点为 pH 4. 8 ~5. 2。

（2）操作过程所用的水均应为蒸馏水或去离子水，以免干扰凝聚。

（3）用复凝聚法制备时，须注意：磺胺二甲嘧啶细粉置研钵中，需研磨充分并过 80 目筛，以利于囊材包埋。10% 醋酸溶液调 pH 值时，应逐渐滴入，特别是当接近 pH4 时更应小心，并随时取样在显微镜下观察微囊的形成。当降温接近凝固点时，微囊容易粘连，故应不断搅拌并用适量水稀释。

（4）用单凝聚法制备时，须注意：液状石蜡乳的乳化剂为明胶，乳化力不强，亦可将液状石蜡与明胶溶液 60ml，用乳匀器或组织捣碎器乳化 1 ~2min，即制得均匀乳剂。

60% 硫酸钠溶液（硫酸钠是含 10 分子结晶水的晶体），由于其浓度较高，温度低时，易析出晶体，故应配制后加盖放置于 50℃ 保温备用。

凝聚成囊后，在不停搅拌条件下，立即计算硫酸钠稀释液的浓度。若硫酸钠凝聚剂用去 21ml，乳剂中蒸馏水为 60ml，体系中硫酸钠的浓度为（60% ×21ml/81ml），应再增加 1. 5%，即 17. 1% 硫酸钠溶液为稀释液，用量为体系的 3 倍多（300ml），液温 15℃，可保持成囊时的囊形。若稀释液的浓度过高或过低时，可使囊黏结成团或溶解。

成囊后加入稀释液稀释后，再用稀释液反复洗时，只需要倾去上清液，无需过滤，目的是除去未凝聚完全的明胶，以免加入固化剂时明胶交联形成胶状物。固化后的微囊可过滤抽干，然后加入辅料制成颗粒，或可混悬于蒸馏水中放置，备用。

（5）甲醛可使囊膜的明胶变性固化。甲醛用量的多少能影响明胶的变性程度，亦可影响药物的释放速度。

（6）用 5% 氢氧化钠溶液调节 pH 值至 7 ~8 时，可增强甲醛与明胶的交联作用，使凝胶的网状结构孔隙缩小而提高热稳定性。

（7）微囊大小的测定：可用光学显微镜目测微囊的粒径大小及粒径分布。具体操作方法：取少许湿微囊，加蒸馏水分散，盖上盖玻片（注意除尽气泡），用有刻度标尺（刻度已校正其每格的 μm 数）的接目镜的显微镜测量 600 个微囊，按不同大小计数。亦可将视野内的微囊进行显微照相后再测量和计数。

三、思考题

1. 哪些材料可以用乳化法制备微球？
2. 影响微球粒径的主要因素有哪些？控制微球粒径对临床应用有何意义？
3. 分别绘制复凝聚性和单凝聚法制成的微囊形态图，并解释成囊机理。
4. 试分析影响微囊粒径的因素。
5. 试分析影响微囊释药速度的因素。
6. 试述微球和微囊在定义和制备上的异同。

扫码"学一学"

Experiment 18　Preparation of Microspheres

Objectives and Requirement

1. To master the basic principle and method of preparing microsphere and microcapsules.

2. To be familiar with the factors that influence microcapsules' forming.

3. To understand the common materials of microsphere and microcapsule formation

Introduction

Microspheres refer to the small spherical particles with diameters in the micrometer range typically 1μm to 250μm (sometimes defined as 1μm ~ 1mm), manufacturing from drug dissolved or dispersed into suitable materials. It often called nanospheres or nanoparticles when its particle size is less than 10 ~ 100nm; while it called sub – microspheres if it ranges from 0.1 to 1μm.

The reusually have three kinds of methodology for microsphere formation including physical method of spray drying, physical – chemical method of emulsion – heating, emulsion – crosslinking and emulsion – solvent evaporation, and chemical method of polymerization and crosslinking. Spray drying method is suitable for industrialized production, which sprays the mixture of the drug and polymer solution into a stream of dry droplet, and then solidifies it to form microspheres. The fundamental theory of emulsion – heating (or crosslinking) method is to add drug and polymers together, emulsifying and heating (or crosslinking). The emulsion solvent evaporation (or solvent extraction) technique, also called the oil – in – water (O/W) emulsion, is a common method for forming drug encapsulated polymeric microspheres. The polymer is dissolved in an organic solvent as an "oil" solution along with the drug to be encapsulated and added to an aqueous solution containing a stabilizer. The organic solvent is then removed by evaporation and the drug encapsulated microspheres are recovered. The methodologies for microcapsule preparation are induced into three types, such as physicochemical method, chemical method and physicochemical method. How to choose suitable methods is depending on the properties of drug, coating material, particle diameter of microcapsules and release profiles etc. This simple coacervation and complex coacervation was applied to prepare microcapsules, respectively; the technologies are simple and suitable to microencapsulate of many drugs.

Polymers of microsphere formation include naturally polymer such as gelatin, sodium alginate, starch, albumin and chitosan, semi – synthetic polymer of cellulose derivatives and synthetic polymer such as PEG, PLA and PLGA. Gelatin is a common naturally polymer with cheap, stable and high drug loading properties to form microspheres. Gelatin will react to form a reticular polymer with aldehydes. The formed cross – linked polymer has good mechanical strength and stable chemical properties, which can swell and sustained release in the water. Sodium alginate (SA) is a white or light yellow anionic natural polysaccharide extracted from brown algae. SA has been used in the fields of food, textile and dyeing, water treatment and biomedical industry, due to its unique properties and good biocompatibility. SA is a linear copolymer with homopolymeric blocks of (1 – 4) – linked β – D – mannuronate (M) and α – L – guluronate (G) residues, respectively, covalently linked together in different sequences or blocks. The monomers can appear in homopolymeric blocks of consecutive G – residues (G – blocks), consecutive M – residues (M – blocks) or alternating M and G – residues (MG – blocks). Alginate gelation takes place when divalent cations (usually Ca^{2+}), interact ionically with blocks of GG blocks, resulting in formation of three – dimensional network which is usually described by "egg – box" model. This gelation of calcium alginate is insoluble in water and acid and can be applied in the enzymatic immobilization, oral delivery system of proteins and peptides, and carries of control released system. Here SA will be used as the materials of microspheres by the method of crosslinking.

Microcapsules are mini capsules of solid drugs or liquid drugs (usually called core material) with diameters of 1 – 250μm, encapsulated by high polymer material (usually called coating material). After micro – encapsulated, drug can display sustained – release, enhance stability, cover unfavorable flavor and taste, reduce irritation to the gastrointestinal tract, decrease matching taboo of multiple medicine, improve fluidity and compressibility, and make liquid drug into solid. According to clinical demanding, microcapsules can be prepared into powders, capsules, tablets, injections and ointments etc.

The principle of complex coacervation is based on the property that some highly hydrophilic colloids have electric charges. When two or more colloid liquids which have opposite electric charges are mixed, they will agglomerate because of neutralization of electric charges. For example, acacia liquid takes negative charges, as well as gelatin "A" liquid takes. When pH is above isoelectric point (pH 7 – 9), so no condensation take place after mixed; while gelatin "A" liquid is adjusted to under isoelectric point (about pH 3.8 – 4.0), charges of gelatin are completely changed into positive charges, *i. e.*, gelatin condense with acacia after mixed. If there are drugs in the solution, condensing surround these drug particles form microcapsules. At this time, membrane of microcapsule is fairly soft; when lowering the temperature to below the condensing point, they will coacervate and solidificate gradually, so we should add methyl aldehyde to make the membrane dissolute and solidificate and get microcapsule products. The principle of simple coacervation is as follows: conglomerater combine water molecule in hydrated film of high polymer solution, that decrease the solubility of high polymer coating material, they condense surrounding drugs, then microcapsules appear from this system during stirring. This kind of coacervation is reversible, once removing the condition; uncoacervation phenomenon will take place, so microcapsules need to be consolificated based on the properties of coating material.

Equipment and Materials

1. Equipment

Electrical stirrer, baker (500, 250 and 50ml), Circulating water vacuum pump, filter flask, colander, syringe needle (No. 6), water bath, stove, microscope, pestle, scales etc.

2. Materials

Liquid paraffin, gelatin A, gelatin B, sorbitan oleate (span 80), formaldehyde, sodium alginate (SA), 2% calcium chloride solution, sulfadimerazin, 10% acetic acid solution, and 60% sodium sulfate solution etc.

Experimental Methods

Ⅰ. Preparation of Microspheres

1. Preparation of Gelatin Microspheres

(1) Formulation

Liquid paraffin	50ml

Gelatin	1g
Sorbitan oleate(span 80),	0.5g
Distilled water	5ml

(2) Manufacturing process

Emulsification: Liquid paraffin (50ml) was measured and put into the beaker; span 8 (1%, *W/V*) was added. The mixture was heated at 60℃ and stirred at 400 rpm using a paddle stirrer under the beaker of 2/3height. While 1g gelatin was swelled and dissolved into 5ml distilled water to form the 20% (*W/V*) solution at 60℃ and this gelatin solution was then added into above liquid paraffin to emulsify sufficiently for 15min.

Washing: The emulsion solution was quickly cooled to 5℃ using ice water, and then filtrated by millipore filter. The formed microspheres were washed by petroleum ether for three times to remove the liquid paraffin of the microspheres' surface in airing chamber. Filtered microspheres were transferred into a plate and dispersed with a little acetone in airing chamber. Acetone then evaporated under the lamp at 40℃.

Crosslinking: Above microsphere was put in the airtight chamber with 40% formaldehyde to crosslink for 6h at 35℃ water bath. The gelatin microsphere was obtained by evaporation of formaldehyde.

Particle size: The particle size was measured by a microscope.

2. Preparation of Alginate Microspheres

(1) Formulation

Sodium alginate	1g
Distilled water	50ml
2% calcium chloride solution	100ml

(2) Manufacturing process

Preparation of SA solution: Sodium alginate weighted 1g was dissolved in the distilled water of 50ml to form the solution of 2%.

Crosslinking: Solution of SA was dropped into 100ml of 2% calcium chloride solution to form the microspheres by injection syringe with the stirred speed of 80 rpm. The height of needle was 8cm and the reaction time of crosslinking was at least for 2hours.

Drying: The formed microspheres was filtered and washed 3 times with distilled water, then dried at the oven of 60℃ for 12hours.

Particle size: The particle size was measured by a microscope.

Ⅱ. Preparation of Microcapsules

1. Sulfadimerazine microcapsules

(1) Formulation

Sulfadimerazine	1.2g
Gelatin	1g
Acacia	1g
10% acetic acid solution	QS
37% methyl aldehyde solution	1.6ml

(2) Manufacturing process

Preparation of colloid solution: weigh gelatin and acacia separately according to the formulation, add distilled water to form 3% colloid solution, adjust pH of gelatin solution to 7 – 8 with sodium hydroxide, reserve.

Suspending: weigh 1. 2g sulfadimerazine powder and ground to pass the sieve of 80 meshes; add acetic solution and gelatin solution. At the same time, grind them, and transfer the mixed colloid solution into a beaker; place it in 45℃ cleansing bath, and stir, suspend to form uniform solution. Observe the sample under the microscope.

Coacervate and solidificate: Suspension of drug and coating materials is removed from the water bath. Drop 10% acetic acid for adjusting suspension to pH 3. 8 – 4. 1 during continuing stirring, and then coacervate, observe microencapsulating state by microscope. Continually stirring for 5min after coacervated, add 80ml 37℃ distilled water to dilute, and remove warm cleansing bath tub. Then decrease the temperature of microcapsules suspension to 25℃, and put them into an ice bath tub. When the temperature is below 10℃, add 1. 6ml 37% methyl aldehyde solution, and solidification for 0. 5 – 1hour, then add 20% sodium hydroxide solution to adjust pH to 9. 0 or so. The morphology, particle size and size distribution of microcapsules are characterized by microscope.

Dry: filter the wet microcapsules, wash them with distilled water until no methyl aldehyde flavor, depressure and filter until dry, add proper quantity starch to granulate, dry below 70℃ to get products.

(3) The experimental records

Fill the amount of formulation components into the table 18 – 1.

Table 18 – 1 Preparation records of sulfadimerazine microcapsules

Formulation components	Experimental value	pH value
Concentration of acacia solution (%)		—
Concentration of gelatin solution (%)		
Amount of 20% sodium hydroxide solution		
Amount of sulfadimerazine		—
Amount of diluted water		—
Amount of 10% acetic acid solution		
Amount of methyl aldehyde solution		—
Amount of 20% sodium hydroxide solution after solidification		

2. Chrismaline microcapsules

(1) Formulation

Chrismaline	2g
Gelatin	2g
10% acetic acid solution	QS
60% sodium sulfate solution	QS
37% methyl aldehyde solution	3ml

Distilled water QS

(2) Manufacturing process

Preparation of gelatin solution: Weigh 2g gelatin, add 10ml distilled water to swell; and dissolve, keep the temperature at 50℃.

Preparation of chrismaline emulsion: Weigh chrismaline according to formulation, add gelatin solution, and mill to form emulsions in pestle. Add distilled water to 60ml, mingle until uniform, and adjust to pH3.8 with 10% acetic acid solution.

Preparation of microcapsules: Move the emulsion into beaker, and put it in 50℃ homeothermic cleansing bath. Measure certain volume 60% sodium sulfate solution, and drop the emulsion during stirring. Observe microencapsulating phenomenon by microscope, and calculate sodium sulfate concentration in this system through used volume of sodium sulfate at once. Prepare sodium sulfate diluted solution, and its concentration should be 1.5% higher than the system's concentration, while its volume is more than 3 times of microencapsulating solution, and the temperature of diluted solution is 15℃. Pour it into the stirring microencapsulating solution and disperse microcapsules; statically wait until microcapsules precipitate settle, and discard the above solution for washing it 2 - 3 times with sodium sulfate diluted solution. Then, suspend microcapsules in 300ml sodium sulfate diluted solution, and add methyl aldehyde solution; stir for 15min, and adjust to pH 8 - 9 with 20% sodium hydroxide solution. continually stirring for 1 hour, statically wait until microcapsules precipitate settle completely. The morphology, particle size and size distribution of chrismaline microcapsules are characterized by microscope. Discard the above solution, and filter microcapsules; wash with distilled water until no methyl aldehyde flavor (or until no color with Schiff reagent). Depressure and filter until dry, then obtain the products.

Experiment Instructions

Requirements for Preview

1. To preview the common preparations of microspheres and microcapsules; to master the basic principle and methods of simple coacervation and complex coacervation.

2. To be familiar with properties of gelatin and sodium alginate. To be familiar with the influencing considerations on microcapsules particle size.

3. To understand the application and characteristics of microspheres and microcapsules.

Procedures and Precautions

1. Preparation of Alginate Microspheres

(1) Sodium alginate and gelatin both need to be swelled sufficiently to prepare their solution during to their viscous property.

(2) The emulsion - crosslinking method was used to prepare the gelatin microspheres. 1% Span 80 was used as an emulsifier. Lower this percentage, the emulsion will not stable and microspheres will easy to adhere with each other.

(3) The stirring time in emulsification should not too long so as to increase the drop - side of

emulsion. The faster the stirring rate is used, the smaller will the particle sizes of microspheres be. But it should avoid producing bubbles and vortex during stirring.

(4) Particle size of our microspheres ranges from 2 to 10 μm. Reduction in the concentration of gelatin, temperature and stirring rate, increasing the amount of span - 80 can decrease the particle size of microsphere.

(5) Cross links reaction of gelatin and formaldehyde was carried out at pH 8 to 9. And the crosslinking reaction was lasted for 12h.

(6) Some tips should be noted during the preparation of alginate microspheres by crosslinking method as follows: sodium alginate should be trickled dropwise at speed of 2 to 3 drops per second into calcium chloride solution; the distance of needle had better at the height of 8 to 15cm to ensure to obtain irregular microspheres. Microspheres will be flat if the height is too high. Otherwise they will be tailed.

(7) The concentration of sodium alginate related to it viscosity usually ranges from 1 - 3%; microspheres will not be easy to form if its concentration is lower than 1%, otherwise it will be difficult to obtain spherical microspheres.

(8) No. 6 syringe needle was used in this experiment for intuitive observing the formation of SA microspheres. The diameter of No. 6 syringe needle is 0. 5mm. Alginate microspheres with the diameter of about 0. 5 - 1mm could be visible to our naked eyes due to high swelling property of alginate in the water (about 500 folds). The obtained microspheres will be shrunk into about 0. 5mm after drying. Smaller diameter of needles or other method of preparation can be used to get smaller microspheres.

2. Preparation of Microcapsules

(1) According to the different producing methods, gelatin is classified into type A and type B, isoelectric point of type A gelatin is pH 7 - 9, isoelectric point of type B is pH 4. 8 - 5. 2.

(2) Water in the course of operating should be distilled water or nonionic water in order to avoid interfering coacervation.

(3) Preparing microcapsules with complex coacervation, pay attention to the following points:

Sulfadimerazine powder should be grounded to pass the sieve of 80 meshes for easier encapsulation. It is necessary to drop gradually when we adjust pH with 10% acetic acid solution, especially approaching to about pH 4. It is necessary to sample and observe microencapsulated state by microscope. When we drop the temperature near the freezing point, microcapsules are easy to adhere to each other, so do not stop stirring and add proper quantity water to dilute it.

(4) Preparing with simple coacervation, pay attention to some key points such as:

Gelatin is emulsifying agent of chrismaline emulsion, its emulsifying ability is poor, emulsify chrismaline and 60ml gelatin solution 1 - 2min in emulsion or tissue blender, then obtain the uniform emulsion.

60% sodium sulfate solution has a high concentration, when reduce the temperature, it is easy to crystallize, so cover and keep the temperature at 50℃ to use after preparation (sodium sulfate is the crystal containing 10 molecules crystalized water).

After coacervating and microencapsulating, keep stirring, calculate immediately concentration of sodium sulfate diluted solution. If use polycoagulant sodium sulfate, distilled water in emulsion is 60ml, sodium sulfate concentration in system is (60% × 21ml)/81ml, plus 1.5% again, that is, diluted solution is 17.1% sodium sulfate solution, its volume is more than 3 times (300ml) the system, temperature of the solution is 15℃, the shape can be kept well. If the diluted solution concentration is much high or low, microcapsules will be adhere to form block or dissolve.

Add diluted solution after taking shape, dilute, wash repeatedly with diluted solution, discard the above cleaning solution only, it is not necessary to filter in order to removeuncoacervating gelatin and avoid gelatin forming adhesive agent when adding solidification agent. Filter until dry the solidificated microcapsules, then add excipient to granulate, or suspend in distilled water and lay up statically, wait to use.

(5) Methyl aldehyde make gelatin in microcapsule film degenerate and solidify. The quantity of methyl aldehyde will influence the degenerating extent of gelatin and releasing rate of drug.

(6) Use 5% sodium hydroxide solution to adjust pH up to 7 – 8, strengthen the cross – linking effect between methyl aldehyde and gelatin, diminute pore among reticular structure of gelatin to increase heat stability.

(7) Measure microcapsules size: microcapsules diameter and size distribution were measured through optic microscope. Operating procedures as follows: take a few of wet microcapsules, add distilled water to disperse, take cover glass (precaution: remove air bubble completely), apply microscope with a scale ruler ocular to measure 600 microcapsules, and count on sizes. Or take photos for microcapsules in the visual field before measure and count.

Questions

1. What kind of polymer can be used to prepare microspheres by emulsion method?

2. What are the main factors influenced the particle size of microsphere? What is purpose of controlling the particle size of microsphere for clinical application?

3. To draw the shape of microcapsules prepared in simple and complex coacervation separately and explain the mechanism of microencapsulating.

4. Try to analyze the factors influencing microcapsules diameter.

5. Try to analyze the factors influencing drug release from microcapsules.

6. Try to describe similarities and differences between microspheres and microcapsules.

实验 19　纳米乳及其软胶囊剂的制备

【目的与要求】

1. **掌握**　纳米乳的基本处方组成和制备方法。软胶囊剂的制备方法。

2. **熟悉**　绘制相图的基本方法。

3. **了解**　纳米乳的质量评价方法。

【基本概念与实验原理】

纳米乳在《中国药典》定义归属为微粒给药系统，是将药物溶于脂肪油/植物油中，通常经磷脂乳化分散于水相中形成粒径 50 ~ 100nm 的 O/W 型微粒制剂。但纳米乳广义是指由表面活性剂、油、助表面活性剂及水按适当比例自发形成的一种透明或半透明的、低黏度、各向同性且热力学稳定的分散体系，可有 3 种基本类型，即 W/O 型纳米乳、O/W 型纳米乳和双连续型纳米乳。另外，其表面活性剂除磷脂外，吐温、聚氧乙烯蓖麻油、泊洛沙姆等均可应用；纳米乳区别于普通乳剂和亚微乳制备的关键是表面活性剂的用量以及必须使用助表面活性剂。

纳米乳作为新型药物载体，其优势在于：热力学和动力学稳定，可热压灭菌或过滤除菌；增溶能力强，可增溶不同类型药物；有利于促进药物的体内吸收，提高其生物利用度；可一定程度上提高药物的稳定性；根据需要可达到缓释或靶向的目的。

自乳化系统是指由油相、表面活性剂、助表面活性剂等组成的均匀透明的分散体系，在胃肠道内温和搅拌下即可自发形成 O/W 型乳剂。如果自发形成 O/W 型纳米乳，则称为自纳米乳化系统或自微乳化系统。目前软胶囊剂的使用日趋广泛，其是指将一定量的液体原料药物直接包封，或将固体原料药物溶解或分散在适宜的辅料中制备成溶液、混悬液、乳状液或半固体，密封于软质囊材中的胶囊剂。由此，纳米乳、自乳化或自微乳化系统均可进一步制成软胶囊，工艺简单、使用方便，其亦可压制成片剂等其他剂型。

纳米乳的处方组成包括油、水、乳化剂和助乳化剂等。相图研究是确定纳米乳处方的有效方法，通过伪三元相图确定纳米乳区域，筛选最佳配方组成范围，再根据预定设计目的，确定适宜的处方。采用滴水法可制备 O/W 型纳米乳的相图，即将表面活性剂与辅助表面活性剂按一定质量混合均匀，混合物在室温下分别加入不同质量比的油相，例如 5%、10%、15%、20%、30%、40%、50% 和 60% 的油，涡旋混匀后向澄清液滴加蒸馏水，涡旋或搅拌，然后再充分平衡，观察到体系变成肉眼可见的微乳液、粗乳液或凝胶，并辅以适当方法验证。通常以表面活性剂和助表面活性剂为一组，同油相、水相作为伪三元相图的三个顶点，每一条边表示相应两组分的比例关系，即为纳米乳的伪三元相图（图 19－1）。从相图中可确定形成 O/W 型纳米乳的区域，再根据其他预设性质选择理想的组分比率。在非离子型表面活性剂为基础的纳米乳中，药物对 O/W 型纳米乳区域的范围影响不大。

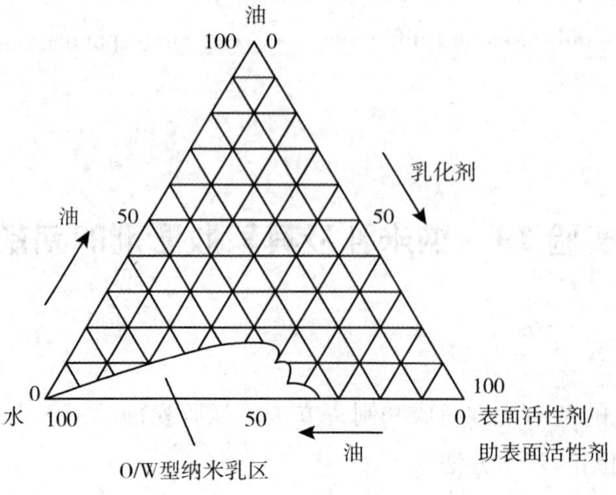

图 19－1　纳米乳相图

【仪器与材料】

1. 仪器　电子分析天平，旋涡混合器，恒温水浴，玻璃棒，烧杯，量筒，称量纸，EP管托，镊子，刮刀，200μl 移液枪，1ml 移液枪，塑料滴管，玻璃滴管，20ml 具塞西林瓶，2ml EP 管，10ml 量筒，10ml 量瓶，50ml 量瓶，1ml 移液管，紫外分光光度计，智能实验软胶囊机，激光粒度分析仪等。

2. 材料　聚氧乙烯（35）蓖麻油，聚氧乙烯（40）氢化蓖麻油，油酸乙酯，尼莫地平，环孢素，无水乙醇，1,2－丙二醇，油酸山梨坦（司盘 80），中链三酰甘油（MCT），明胶，甘油，山梨醇。

【实验内容】

一、尼莫地平纳米乳的制备

尼莫地平是第二代二氢吡啶类钙离子拮抗剂，主要用于缺血性脑血管病和轻、中度高血压病等。尼莫地平的水溶性差、口服生物利用度低，将其制成纳米乳可达到增溶和提高其口服吸收的目的。

1. 处方

尼莫地平	10mg
聚氧乙烯（35）蓖麻油	600mg
无水乙醇	250mg
油酸乙酯	150mg
蒸馏水	4ml

2. 制备工艺　精密称取处方量的尼莫地平置于2ml EP 管中，加入无水乙醇，涡旋使药物溶解后，转移至 20ml 具塞西林瓶中，分别加入聚氧乙烯（35）蓖麻油、油酸乙酯，使用玻璃棒搅拌，涡旋混合均匀，得到澄清透明的尼莫地平纳米乳分散相；再加入 4ml 蒸馏水，涡旋混匀即得。

3. 质量评价　纳米乳制备完毕后，要对其进行质量评价，目前要求控制的主要项目如下。

（1）外观　观察纳米乳的外观，包括透明度、流动性等。

（2）粒径及分布　取纳米乳适量，经蒸馏水稀释 5～10 倍，采用激光粒径分析仪测定纳米乳粒径、分布以及 Zeta 电位。

（3）包封率　取适量纳米乳，3000r/min 离心 15min，取上清液适量，使用无水乙醇稀释 500 倍，涡旋混合 5min，采用紫外分光光度计于 236nm 处测定吸光度，根据尼莫地平标准曲线计算纳米乳的药物浓度 C，计算包封率。尼莫地平标准曲线制备方案如下：制备 200μg/ml 的尼莫地平贮备液，使用 1ml 移液管移取贮备液，制备 2μg/ml、4μg/ml、8μg/ml、12μg/ml、16μg/ml 的尼莫地平无水乙醇稀释液。基线校正后，以无水乙醇为空白，在 236nm 记录各尼莫地平标准品稀释液的吸光度。以吸光度 A 对浓度 C_i 作图，进行线性回归分析。

$$包封率 = \frac{C \times V \times X}{M} \times 100\%$$

式中 C 表示测得稀释后的纳米乳药物浓度；X 表示稀释倍数；V 表示纳米乳体积；M 表示初始药物投料质量。

二、环孢素自纳米乳化软胶囊

环孢素是一种免疫抑制剂，因为其疏水性强，不易吸收，故口服生物利用度低。将其制成纳米乳可增加其口服吸收，提高环孢素生物利用度。另外，环孢素自纳米乳软胶囊服用后，能够在体内自发形成纳米乳，促进药物的吸收，使用更方便。

1. 处方

内容物处方

环孢素	125g
1,2－丙二醇	125g
聚氧乙烯（40）氢化蓖麻油	190g
油酸山梨坦	300g
中链三酰甘油（MCT）	260g

胶液处方

明胶	4000g
甘油	1000g
山梨醇	500g
蒸馏水	4250g

2. 制备工艺

内容物制备：将处方量环孢素、1,2－丙二醇、聚氧乙烯（40）氢化蓖麻油、油酸山梨坦和中链三酰甘油（MCT）均匀混合，37℃磁力搅拌使药物完全溶解，得澄明溶液，作为软胶囊内容物备用。

胶液制备：取处方量明胶，置于蒸馏水中溶胀后，60℃保温溶解；加入甘油和山梨醇，混合均匀，静置脱泡，过筛后保温备用。

软胶囊制备：将内容物和胶液经旋转式模压机压制成软胶囊，每粒软胶囊含内容物 0.2g，用乙醇洗去表面油层，24～32℃干燥，即得。

3. 质量评价

（1）外观　软胶囊外观应整洁，不得有黏结、变形、渗漏或囊壳破裂现象，并应无异臭。

（2）粒径及分布　取纳米乳内容物适量，经 0.1mol/L 盐酸溶液稀释 20～50 倍，混匀后，采用激光粒径分析仪测定纳米乳粒径、分布以及 Zeta 电位。

（3）装量差异　按《中国药典》四部通则 <0103> 胶囊剂项下要求，进行装量差异检查，应符合规定。装量差异限度规定如下：平均装量或标示装量 <0.30g，装量差异限度为 ±10%；平均装量或标示装量 ≥ 0.30g，装量差异限度为 ±7.5%。

（4）崩解时限　按《中国药典》四部通则 <0921> 崩解时限检查法进行检查。软胶囊要求在 1h 内全部崩解。

实验指导

一、预习要求

1. 掌握 纳米乳的种类和性质。

2. 熟悉 常用的乳化剂。

3. 预习 列出各实验的步骤及注意事项。

二、操作要点和注意事项

1. 使用涡旋混合器时要注意防止液体溅出。

2. 聚氧乙烯（35）蓖麻油温度低时较为黏稠，加入后可能会黏在具塞西林瓶底部，需使用玻璃棒进行搅拌，使其分散均匀，再加以涡旋震荡。

3. 制备载药纳米乳时，需要注意药物和水相的加入顺利。如果药物可溶于乳化剂或助乳化剂或油相中的任一组分，则先将药物溶解在该组分中，再与其他组分混合；而水相宜最后加入混合。

4. 进行软胶囊重量差异检查时应用乙醚等易挥发性溶剂将囊壳洗净，置通风处使溶剂挥尽，再分别精密称定囊壳重量。

5. 软胶囊的囊壳以明胶为主，因此自纳米乳化系统的配方中丙二醇等溶剂的含量不宜过高，避免引起囊壳变化。

6. 软胶囊久置容易出现漏液问题，可能原因：液体内容物影响囊壳的稳定性，导致明胶水解或变性，或者影响合口过程等；喷体温度不合适；明胶液的浓度过低。

三、思考题

1. 分析本实验中各处方中各种组分的作用。

2. 影响纳米乳稳定性的因素有哪些？

3. 根据哪些条件来判断纳米乳的类型？

4. 纳米乳作为新型给药系统的优势是什么？

5. 纳米乳与自微乳的区别是什么？

6. 自乳化给药系统在药物制剂中有何意义？

Experiment 19 Preparation of Nanoemulsions and Soft Capsules

扫码“学一学”

Objectives and Requirements

1. To master the preparation methods and formulation compositions of nanoemulsions. To master the Manufacturing process of soft capsules.

2. To be familiar with the preparation method of the pseudo – ternary phase diagram.

3. To understand quality evaluation methods of nanoemulsions.

Introduction

Nanoemulsion is classified as a microparticle drug delivery system in the Chinese Pharmacopoeia. The drug dissolved in fatty oil/plant oil is usually emulsified by phospholipids in aqueous phase to form an O/W type microparticle preparation with a particle size of 50 – 100nm. However, broadly speaking, nanoemulsion refers to a transparent or semitransparent, low viscosity, isotropic and thermodynamically stable dispersion system spontaneously formed by surfactant, oil, cosurfactant and water in a proper proportion. There are three types of nanoemulsiosn, namely W/O, O/W and bicontinuous nanoemulsions. Besides phospholipids, surfactants such as Tween, polyoxyethylene castor oil, and poloxamer also can be used. Different from the preparation procedure of emulsion and submicron emulsion, the amount of the surfactant used in nanoemulsion preparation is generally more and the use of cosurfactant is indispensable.

Nanoemulsions possess many advantages including: (1) Nanoemulsions belong to stable systems in thermodynamics and kinetics. It can be sterilized by autoclaving or/and filtration. (2) Nanoemulsions can increase the solubility of drugs. (3) Nanoemulsions can enhance the *in vivo* absorption and bioavailability of drugs. (4) Nanoemulsions can increase the stability of drugs. (5) Nanoemulsions can achieve excellent sustained drug release or targeted drug delivery if necessary.

The self – emulsifying drug delivery system (SEDDS) is an isotropic mixture of oil, surfactant and co – surfactant, which rapidly and spontaneously forms the fine oil – in – water (O/W) emulsions upon mild agitation in the gastrointestinal (GI) track. It is called self – microemulsifying drug delivery system if it spontaneously forms the fine oil – in – water (O/W) nanoemulsions. At present, the use of soft capsules is also becoming more and more extensive. Soft capsules means a certain amount of liquid drugs are directly encapsulated in capsule materials, or the solid drugs are dissolved or dispersed in a suitable auxiliary material to prepare a solution, a suspension, an emulsion or a semi – solid before encapsulated. Thus, the nanoemulsion and self – emulsifying system can be further prepared into soft capsules for an easy use. Besides, they also can be prepared into other dosage forms such as tablets.

Nanoemulsions consist of oil phase, aqueous phase, surfactants and co – surfactant. In order to creen the formulation of O/W nanoemulsions, pseudo – ternaryphase diagrams are constructed using a water titration method at room temperature. For each phase diagram at a specific Km, the ratios of oil to the mixture of surfactant and co – surfactant were varied as 0.5 : 9.5, 1 : 9, 1.5 : 8.5, 2 : 8, 3 : 7, 4 : 6, 5 : 5 or 6 : 4. The mixtures of oil, surfactant and co – surfactant at certain weight ratios are diluted with the water in a drop – wise manner under moderate stirring. After being equilibrated, the mixtures are assessed and determined as being nanoemulsions, crude emulsions or gels. Generally, the pseudo – ternary phase diagrams of nanoemulsions regard surfactant and co – surfactant as a group, with oil and water as three vertices in pseudo – ternary phase diagrams (as shown in Figure 19 – 1). Each edge represents the ratio of the two points. After the identification of O/W nanoemulsion region in the phase diagrams, the nanoemulsion formulations at desired component ratios are selected according to the area of O/W nanoemulsion region. Drugs have few effects on the O/W nanoemulsion region of non – ionic surfactant – based nanoemulsions.

Equipment and Materials

1. Equipment

Electronic analytical balance, vortex mixer, water bath, glass stick, beaker, graduated cylinder,

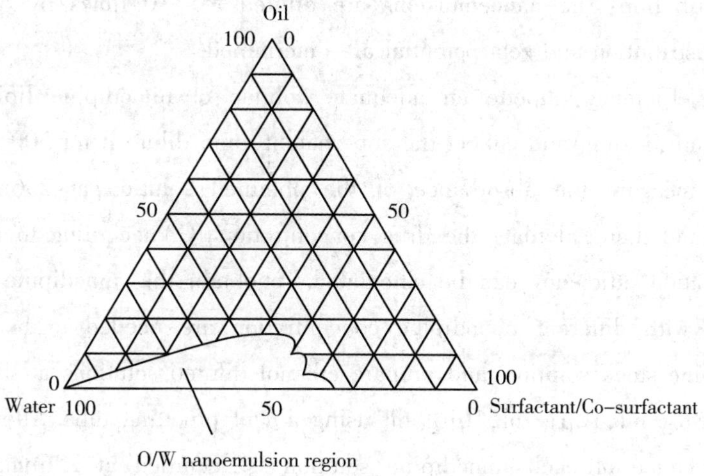

Figure 19 – 1　The phase diagrams of nanoemulsions

weighing paper, EP tube holder, tweezers, scraper, 200μl pipette, 1ml pipette, plastic dropper, glass dropper, 20ml cecillin bottle, 2ml EP tube, 10ml graduated cylinder, 10ml volumetric flask, 50ml volumetric flask, UV spectrophotometer, smart experimental soft capsule machine, particle size apparatus.

2. Materials

Polyoxyl (35) castor oil [Cremophor EL (35)], Polyoxyl (40) hydrogenated castor oil [Cremophor RH (40)], ethyl oleate, nimodipine, ciclosporin, ethanol, 1, 2 – propylene glycol, sorbitan oleate (Span 80), medium chain triglycerides (MCT), gelatin, glycerol, sorbitol.

Experimental Methods

1. Preparation of nimodipine – loaded nanoemulsion

Nimodipine, which is the second generation of dihydro – pyridine calcium channelblocker, is mainly used for the treatment of ischemic cerebrovascular disease, mild and moderate hypertension and so on. The nanoemulsions will improve the water solubility and oral absorption of nimodipine.

(1) Formulation

Nimodipine	10mg
Cremophor EL(35)	600mg
Ethanol	250mg
Ethyl oleate	50mg
Distilled water	4ml

(2) Manufacturing process

Firstly, nimodipine is dissolved in the ethanolin 2ml EP tube by vortex to obtain the solution. Secondly, the solution is transferred into the 20ml secillin. Then, Cremophor EL 35 and ethyl oleate are added in the resulting solution. After mixing, the water is finally added and well mixed.

(3) Quality evaluation

Appearance: The nanoemulsion appearance is observed, including transparency, fluidity and so on.

Size and distribution: The nanoemulsions are diluted 5 - 10 times by distilled water. The particle size, size distribution and zeta potential are determined.

Encapsulation efficiency: Pipette an adequate volume of nimodipine lipid - emulsion for centrifuge (3000r/min, 15min) and collect the supernatant, then dilute it for 500 times with ethanol by vortex. Finally, measure the absorbance of the obtained solution at 236nm using the UV spectrophotometer, and then calculate the drug concentration (C) according to the equation (1). Thus, the encapsulation efficiency can be calculated. To obtain the nimodipine standard curve, a series of solutions with different nimodipine concentration are needed to be prepared. Prepare 200μg/ml nimodipine stock solution, and prepare ethanol diluted solutions at the concentration of 2μg/ml, 4μg/ml, 8μg/ml, 12μg/ml, 16μg/ml using a 1ml pipetting tube. After correction of the baseline, the absorbance of each nimodipine solution is recorded at 236nm. Linear regression analysis is performed by plotting the absorbance A against the concentration C_i.

$$\text{Encapsulation efficiency}(\text{EE}, \%) = \frac{C \times V \times X}{M} \times 100\%$$

C: the detected concentration of the obtained lipid - emulsion product, X: dilution factor, V: the volume of the obtained lipid - emulsion product; M: the feeding amount of drug.

2. Preparation of ciclosporin - loaded self - nanoemulsifying soft capsules

Ciclosporin, an immunosuppressive agent, exhibits low oral bioavailability because of its strong hydrophobicity and poor absorption. The nanoemulsions benefit to improve the oral absorption of ciclosporin. Self - nanoemulsifying soft capsules not only promote the absorption of drugs, but also easier to use.

(1) Formulation

Contents:	
Ciclosporine	125g
1,2 - propylene glycol	125g
Cremophor RH(40)	190g
Sorbitan oleate (Span 80)	300g
Medium chain triglycerides (MCT)	260g
Gel mass:	
Gelatin	4000g
Glycerol	1000g
Sorbitol	500g
Distilled water	4250g

(2) Manufacturing process

Preparation of contents: The ciclosporine, 1,2 - propylene glycol, Cremophor RH(40), span 80 and MCT are well mixed at 37℃, and drugs are totally dissolved in the mixture. The resulting mixture is used as the content of soft capsules.

Preparation of gel mass: The gel mass will provide the soft capsule shell. The gelatin is swelled in the distilled water for a certain time, and then dissolved at 60℃. Next, the glycerol and sorbitol are added into the gelatin solution followed by well mixing. The resulting product is standing to defoam, and then is ready to use after filtration while keeping warm.

Preparation of soft capsules: Ciclosporin - loaded self - nanoemulsifying soft capsules are prepared by the rotary press molding machine. Each soft capsule contains 0.2g content. The soft capsules are washed to take off the oils on their surface by the ethyl alcohol. Finally, products are dried at 24 - 32℃.

(3) Quality evaluation

Appearance: The appearance of soft capsules should be tidy, and soft capsules show no bond, deformation, leakage, rupture and abnormal odor of the capsule shell.

Size and distribution: The nanoemulsion content is diluted 20 - 50 times by 0.1mol/L HCl solution. The particle size, size distribution and zeta potential are determined.

Gross deviation: According to general chapter < 0103 > of ChP, all the soft capsules should comply with the requirements of the test. The limitation of gross deviation in accordance to the following principles: If the average gross or the labeled gross < 0.30g, the limitation of gross deviation is $\pm 10\%$; if the average gross or the labeled gross $\geqslant 0.30$g, the limitation of gross deviation is $\pm 7.5\%$.

Disintegration: According to general chapter < 0921 > of ChP, the soft capsules should disintegrate within 1h.

Experimental Instructions

Requirements for Preview

1. To master the category and characteristics of nanoemulsions.
2. To be familiar with the emulsifiers commonly used.
3. To point out the procedures and precautions according to the experimental teaching material.

Procedures and Precautions

1. Take care when you use the vortex mixer to prevent the liquid spill over.
2. Cremophor EL(35) is viscous when the temperature is low. It may stick to the bottom of the cecillin bottle after the transfer. It needs to be stirred by a glass rod to make it evenly dispersed, and then vortexed.
3. We should pay attention to the adding order of drug and waters phase in preparation of the drug - loaded nanoemulsion. If the drug dissolves in co - surfactants, surfactants or oil phase, the drug should dissolve in these components and then mix with the other components. Finally, the water phase is added.
4. Soft capsule shells were washed by ether or other volatile solvents in the gross deviation test of soft capsules, and then the solvents evaporate completely in fume hood. Finally, soft capsule shells were weighed accurately.
5. Gelatin is the main composition of the soft capsule shell. Therefore, the amount of the propanediol in the formulation of self - nanoemulsifying drug delivery system should be not too high to avoid the change of the capsule shell.

6. Soft capsules are prone to leakage after a long - term storage. The reasons involve in three aspects: (1) The contents effect on the stability of capsule shell, for example, gelatin hydrolysis or denaturation; while they also effect on the procedures of seal, etc. (2) The temperature of the nozzle is not suitable. (3) The concentration of the gelatin solution is too low.

Questions

1. What are the functions of various ingredients in each formulation of this experiment?
2. What are the factors affecting the stability of nanoemulsions?
3. How to determine the type of nanoemulsions.
4. What are the advantages of nanoemulsion as a new drug delivery system?
5. What is the difference between nanoemulsions and self - microemulsions?
6. What is the importance of self - emulsifying drug delivery system in pharmaceutical dosage forms?

实验 20　固体脂质纳米粒的制备

【目的与要求】

1. **掌握**　固体脂质纳米粒的基本制备方法与应用。
2. **熟悉**　固体脂质纳米粒与药物性质的关系。
3. **了解**　常用固体脂质材料及乳化剂的理化性质与应用。

【基本概念与实验原理】

固体脂质纳米粒（solid lipid nanoparticles，SLN）是 20 世纪 90 年代初发展起来的新一代亚微粒给药系统，是指粒径在 10 ~ 1000nm，以毒性低、生物相容性好、生物可降解的固态天然或合成的固体脂质和类脂如三酰甘油、卵磷脂等为药物载体，将药物包裹或夹嵌于脂质内核中制成的固态胶粒给药系统。它综合了传统胶体给药系统如乳剂、脂质体及聚合物纳米粒等的优点，同时避免了它们的一些缺点。SLN 具有良好的生理相容性，能提高药物稳定性，具有缓控释、靶向、长效的作用，对亲脂性药物具有较高的包封率，能用于静脉注射、口服、局部皮肤、肺部、眼部等多种途径给药。

SLN 的关键组分固体脂质为生理相容性好且可降解的天然或合成的脂类分子，主要有脂肪酸（硬脂酸、棕榈酸、癸酸、二十二酸等）、甘油酯（月桂酸甘油酯、棕榈酸甘油酯、单硬脂酸甘油酯等）、蜡质类（鲸蜡醇十六酸酯）和类固醇类（胆固醇等）。而磷脂、胆酸盐、泊洛沙姆、非离子型表面活性剂以及短链醇等常作为 SLN 的乳化剂。

制备 SLN 的方法很多，如高压均质法（high pressure homogenization），是制备 SLN 常用的、可靠而高效的方法。高压均质过程通过空穴效应、撞击效应及剪切效应使物料颗粒尺度达到纳米级。该方法操作简单，易于控制，能避免采用对人体有害的有机溶剂等附加剂，适合于工业大生产。纳米乳 - 超声分散法，通常是将药物制备成纳米乳，然后用带有探头的超声仪进行超声分散，最后获得小而均匀的 SLN。此法通常先将脂质载体加热熔融，然后和药物、乳化剂、辅助乳化剂和同温蒸馏水制成外观透明、热力学稳定的 O/W 型纳米乳液，然后在搅拌条件下将纳米乳液分散于冷水（2～4℃）中，继而进行探头超声，并过微孔滤膜，即可形成SLN。乳化－溶剂挥发法（solvent emulsification－evaporation），是将脂质材料溶解于与水不相混溶的有机溶剂，并在水相中乳化，在减压下有机溶剂蒸发，脂质微粒在水相中沉淀进而形成SLN。此法的优点是避免了在制备过程中与热环境的接触，适用于热敏性药物，但残留的有机溶剂可能产生毒性。薄膜－超声分散法（thin－film and ultrasonic dispersion method），是将脂质和药物溶于适宜的有机溶剂中，减压蒸发除去有机溶剂，形成一层脂质薄膜，然后向其中加入乳化剂溶液，将脂膜充分水化，最后经探针超声分散即得小而均匀的SLN。另外，还有乳化－溶剂扩散法、水相溶剂扩散凝聚法、W/O/W型复乳法、高速搅拌超声法，不同的制备技术和工艺适合于不同性质的药物制备成SLN，有时根据需要也可将两种或多种方法结合使用。

【仪器与材料】

1. 仪器　电子分析天平，恒温磁力搅拌器，高压均质机，探针式超声分散仪，旋转蒸发仪，激光粒度仪、烧杯等。

2. 材料　利多卡因，尼莫地平，单硬脂酸甘油酯，硬脂酸棕榈酸甘油酯，注射用豆磷脂，泊洛沙姆188，聚山梨酯80（吐温80），无水乙醇，蒸馏水，微孔滤膜等。

【实验内容】

一、利多卡因固体脂质纳米粒的制备

1. 处方

利多卡因	100mg
硬脂酸棕榈酸甘油酯（GP）	600mg
2%泊洛沙姆188水溶液	10ml

2. 制备工艺　采用高压匀质法制备利多卡因固体脂质纳米粒。精密称取利多卡因100mg置于烧杯中，加入硬脂酸棕榈酸甘油酯600mg，在80℃下加热熔融，作为油相。取2%泊洛沙姆188溶液10ml，磁力搅拌分散，水浴加热至80℃，作为水相。同温度下将油相滴入水相中，磁力搅拌10min，随后使用高压均质机在10000r/min下剪切10min，制得初乳。再使用高压均质机，在温度80℃、压力1000bar条件下循环3次，自然冷却至室温（25℃），经微孔滤膜过滤，即得利多卡因固体脂质纳米粒。

利多卡因固体脂质纳米粒制备工艺流程图见图20－1。

二、尼莫地平固体脂质纳米粒的制备

1. 处方

尼莫地平	20mg
注射用豆磷脂	100mg
泊洛沙姆188	500mg
聚山梨酯80	100mg
单硬脂酸甘油酯（GMS）	50mg
无水乙醇	2ml
注射用水	加至50ml

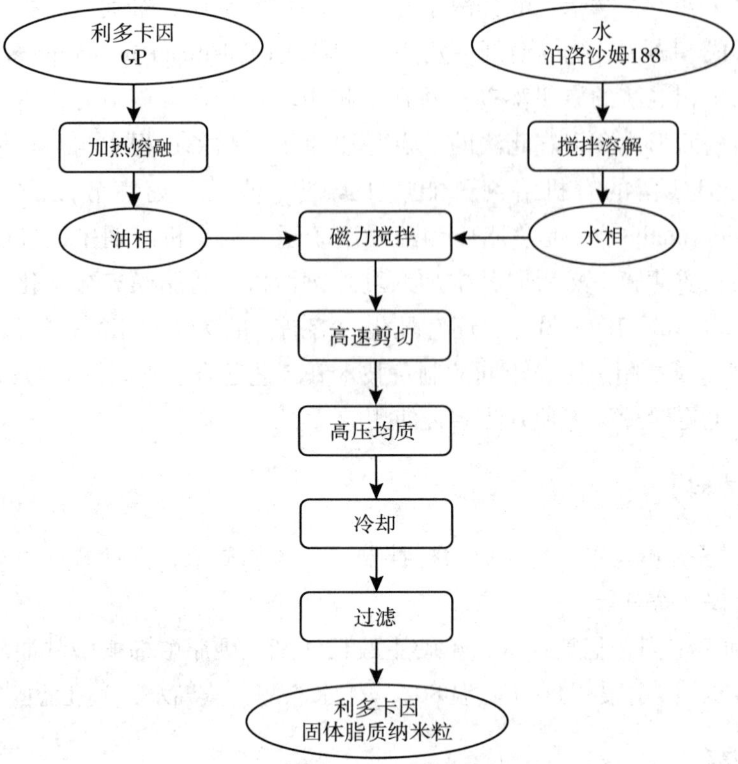

图 20-1　利多卡因固体脂质纳米粒的制备工艺流程图

2. **制备工艺**　采用纳米乳-高压均质分散法制备尼莫地平固体脂质纳米粒。精确称取尼莫地平 20mg，单硬脂酸甘油酯 50mg，聚山梨酯 80 100mg，溶于 2ml 无水乙醇中，加热至 70℃使其溶解，再加入磷脂 100mg 以构成油相。将泊洛沙姆 188 溶于 25ml 蒸馏水中，加热至 70℃，使之完全溶解，构成水相。然后在磁力搅拌（900r/min）下，将油相逐滴加入水相中，70℃搅拌 15min。在磁力搅拌（900r/min）下将纳米乳快速倒入 2~4℃ 的 25ml 冷水中，并继续搅拌 5min。将纳米乳经高压均质仪均质（800bar，1 循环），然后以 0.45μm 微孔滤膜过滤，即得尼莫地平固体脂质纳米粒。整个过程均需要避光操作。

尼莫地平固体脂质纳米粒制备工艺流程图见图 20-2。

三、质量评价

SLN 制备完成后，需对其进行质量评价，具体如下。

1. **粒径及其分布**　取 SLN 样品，使用激光粒度测定仪于室温下测定其粒径及其分布范围。

2. **形态观察**　使用高分辨率的透射电子显微镜（TEM）观察脂质体形貌。

4. **包封率与载药量**　一般采用葡聚糖凝胶色谱法、超速离心法、透析法等分离方法分离包封在 SLN 内和游离的药物，通过测定包封的药物量和游离的药物量，并根据下列公式计算包封率和载药量。

$$包封率(\%)=\frac{\text{SLN 中包封的药物量}}{加入药物总量}\times100\%$$

$$载药量(\%)=\frac{\text{SLN 中包封的药物量}}{\text{SLN 的总质量}}\times100\%$$

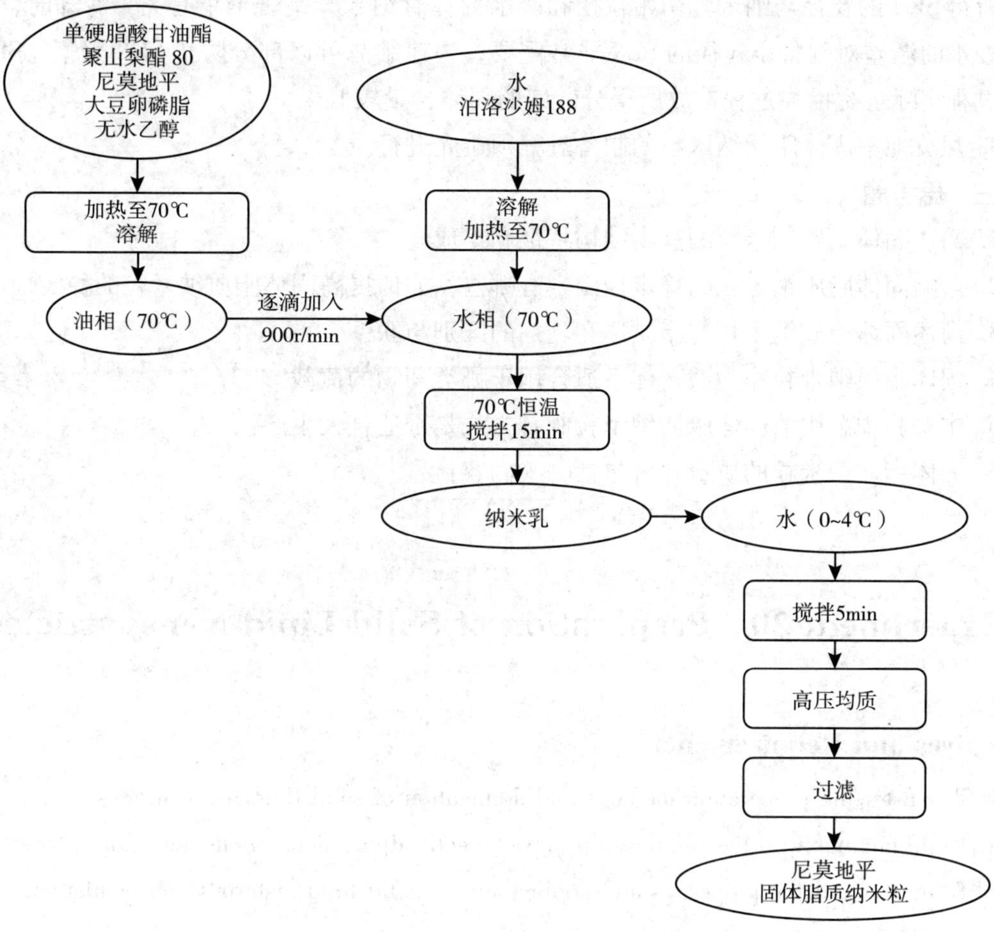

图 20－2　尼莫地平固体脂质纳米粒制备流程图

实验指导

一、预习要求

1. **掌握**　固体脂质纳米粒的不同制备方法。
2. **熟悉**　固体脂质纳米粒的处方组成。
3. **了解**　固体脂质纳米粒的各种载体材料。

二、操作要点和注意事项

1. 高压均质法制备 SLN 分为高温高压均质法和冷却高压均质法两种。高温高压均质法是将含有药物的脂质分散在高温表面活性剂溶液中，并形成纳米乳，然后在脂质熔点以上进行高压均质，最后降温形成 SLN。冷却高压均质法是将固体脂质与液氮或干冰混合研磨，从而获得粒径约为 50～100μm 的固体脂质粉末，然后将固体脂质粉末分散在表面活性剂溶液中，在低于脂质熔点 5～10℃下进行高压均质，使固体脂质粉末形成 SLN。采用高温高压均质法制得的 SLN 粒径小且分布窄，但长时间高温处理可能导致药物发生降解；而采用冷却高压均质法时，药物暴露于热环境的时间短，适用于对温度极敏感的药物，所得的 SLN 颗粒粒径较大且分布广。

2. 纳米乳－高压均质法制备 SLN 通常是将药物制备成外观透明、热力学稳定的 O/W 型纳米乳，然后在搅拌下将纳米乳液分散于冷水继而经高压均质和微孔滤膜过滤获得 SLN。

该法所得 SLN 的粒径与纳米乳初始粒径和冷水稀释时纳米乳是否聚集有关。冷却时，纳米乳与冷水的温差对制备小粒径的 SLN 非常重要，快速结晶可以部分防止 SLN 聚集。SLN 的固化过程实际也是稀释过程，故所得分散液的固体含量较低。

3. 尼莫地平固体脂质纳米粒的制备过程须避光进行。

三、思考题

1. 简述固体脂质纳米粒的基本结构特征和组成。
2. 影响固体脂质纳米粒的稳定性因素有哪些？如何提高固体脂质纳米粒的稳定性？
3. 简述固体脂质纳米粒与脂质体和乳剂的区别与联系。
4. 固体脂质纳米粒作为载药体系适合用于哪类药物的荷载？
5. 本实验中采用的固体脂质纳米粒制备方法是否适合大生产？
6. 固体脂质纳米粒的质量评价包括哪些内容？

Experiment 20　Preparation of Solid Lipid Nanoparticles

Objectives and Requirements

1. To master the preparation methods and application of solid lipid nanoparticles.
2. To be familiar with the relationship between solid lipid nanoparticles and drug properties.
3. To understand the properties and applications of solid lipid materials and emulsifier.

Introduction

Solid lipid nanoparticles(SLN) were developed at 1990s as a new generation of nano – drug delivery system. The particle size of SLN is about 10 – 1000nm. Natural or synthetic solid lipid such as triglyceride or lecithin, are used as carrier based on their low toxicity and good biocompatibility. Drug is encapsulated in the solid lipid core of SLN. SLN combines the advantages of traditional colloidal drug delivery systems such as emulsions, liposomes and polymeric nanoparticles and avoids their disadvantages. It has high entrapment efficiency for lipophilic drugs and can improve drug stability. In addition, SLN possesses the capacity of sustained release, targeting delivery, and long circulating effect. Besides, it can be made into different kinds of dosage forms for intravenous administration, oral administration, percutaneous administration, lung administration, ophthalmic administration and so on. And, there are suitable methods for industrial production of SNL.

The solid matrixin SLN is natural or synthetic biodegradable lipid with ideal physiological compatibility, including fatty acids(stearic acid, palmitic acid, capric acid, twenty – two acid, etc.), glycerol ester(lauric acid glyceride, palmitic acid glyceride, glycerol monostearate, etc), wax tired (cetyl palmitate, etc.) and steroids(cholesterol, etc.). Besides, phospholipids, bile salts, tyloxapol, nonionic surfactant solution and short chain alcohols are often used as emulsifier.

Many method shave been employed to prepare SLN. The high pressure homogenization is the most commonly used and efficient method. The high pressure homogenization process makes the size of material particles reach nanometer level through cavitation effect, impact effect and shear effect. This method is simple, easy to control, and can avoid the use of harmful organic solvents and other additives, which is suitable for industrial product. Nanoemulsion – ultrasonic dispersion method is combined with the nanoemulsion preparation and the ultrasonic dispersion. In this method, usually the lipids are heated to melt firstly and act as oil phase. Next, the medicine, emulsifying agent, auxiliary emulsifier and warm water are applied to make it into a stable O/W type nanoemulsion with transparent appearance. Then, the O/W type nanoemulsion is added in cold water (2 – 4℃) under stirring, dispersed by the ultrasonic probe for a certain period of time and filtered through microporous membrane. Finally, the SLN dispersion system is formed. The method of solvent emulsification – evaporation is to emulsify the lipid material and water – incompatible organic solvent in water. The nanoparticles dispersion of lipid particles in aqueous media is formed with the evaporating of organic solvent under reduced pressure. This method has advantages of avoiding thermal environment in preparation process, thus suitable for heat – sensitive medicine. But the residual organic solvent may produce toxicity. In the thin – film and ultrasonic dispersion method, lipid and drug are dissolved in a suitable organic solvent, and the organic solvent was removed to form a layer of lipid film by vacuum rotary evaporation. Next, the emulsifier solution is added into the lipid film. After ultrasonic dispersion, the small and uniform SLN is obtained. In addition, other ways to prepare SLNs are also used, such as solvent diffusion method, aqueous phase solvent diffusion method, nanoemulsion method, W/O/W type complex emulsion method, high speed stirring ultrasonic method, different preparation technology. These processes are suitable for different drugs according to its properties and sometimes combination with two methods is used when needed.

Equipment and Materials

1. Equipment

Electronic balance, rotary evaporator with water bath, constant temperature magnetic mixer, high pressure homogenizer, high shear emulsifying machine, high pressure milk mixer, ultrasonic dispersion, TOPSIZER laser scattered particle analyzer (OMEC), etc.

2. Materials

Lidocaine, nimodipine, glycerol monostearate, glyceryl palmitostearate, poloxamer 188, polysorbate 80 (Tween 80), soya lecithin (for injection), anhydrous ethanol, distilled water, microporous filter membrane.

Experimental Methods

1. Preparation of lidocaine loaded solid lipid nanoparticles

(1) Formulation

Lidocaine	100mg
Glyceryl palmitostearate	600mg
2% Poloxamer 188	10ml

(2) Manufacturing process

The lidocaine loaded SLN is prepared by high pressure homogenization method. Lidocaine (100mg) and glyceryl palmitostearate (600mg) as the oil phase are heated to melt at 80℃ in the beaker. 10ml of 2% Poloxamer 188 solution as the water phase is heated up to 80℃ in the beaker. Then, the oil phase is added to water phase at 80℃ with stirring for 10min. Next, the emulsion is sheared at a high speed about 10000 rpm for 10min. After that, the emulsion is homogenized by the high pressure homogenization machine for 3 cycles with 1000 bar at 80℃. The final preparation is obtained after cooling to room temperature(25℃) and filtered with microporous cellulose membrane.

The scheme for the preparation of lidocaine loaded SLN is shown in Figure 20 - 1.

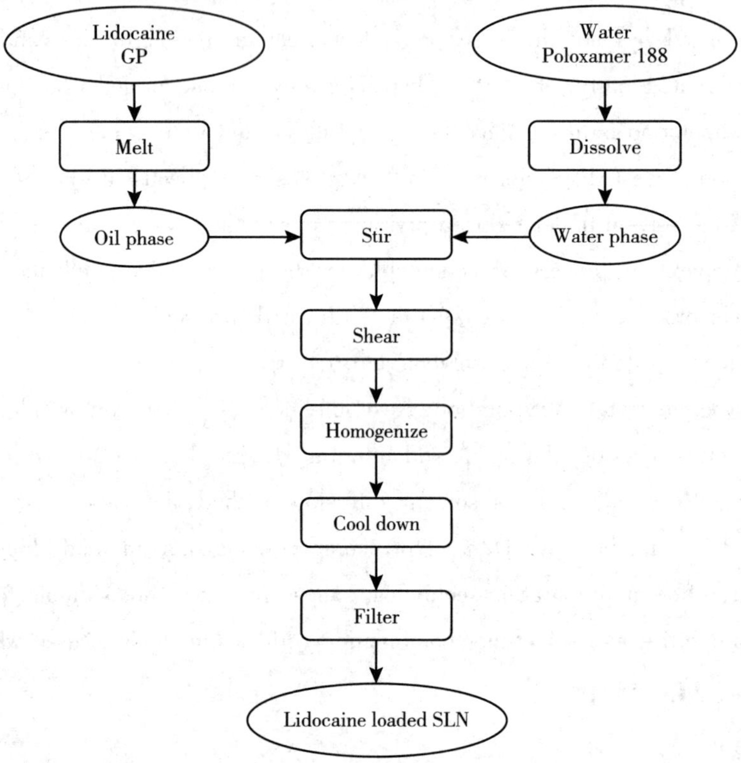

Figure 20 - 1 The scheme of the preparation of lidocaine loaded SLN

2. Preparation of nimodipine loaded solid lipid nanoparticles

(1) Formulation

Nimodipine	20mg
Glyceryl monostearate(GMS)	50mg
Polysorbate 80	100mg
Anhydrous ethanol	2ml
Soya lecithin for injection	100mg
Poloxamer188	500mg
Water for injection	100ml

(2) Manufacturing process

Thenimodipine loaded SLN is prepared by nanoemulsion combined with the high pressure homogenization method. According to the prescription, nimodipine (20mg), glyceryl monostearate (50mg) and Polysorbate 80(100mg) are dissolved in 2ml anhydrous ethanol at 70℃, and then the soya lecithin is added by turns. The mixture solution is acted as oil phase. Poloxamer188(500mg) is dissolved in 25ml of water at 70℃ and acted as water phase. The oil phase is added to the water phase drop by drop at 900r/min stirring, and then the nanoemulsion is keeped stirring for 15min at 70℃. Next, the nanoemulsion is quickly poured into 75ml of cold water at 2 – 4℃ with stirring for 5min. Finally, the nanoemulsion are homogenized with high pressure homogenizer at 800bar for 1 cycles, and then filtrated by 0.45μm microporous membrane to get nimodipine loaded SLN. The procedure should keep away from light.

The scheme for the preparation of nimodipine – loaded SLN is shown in Figure 20 – 2.

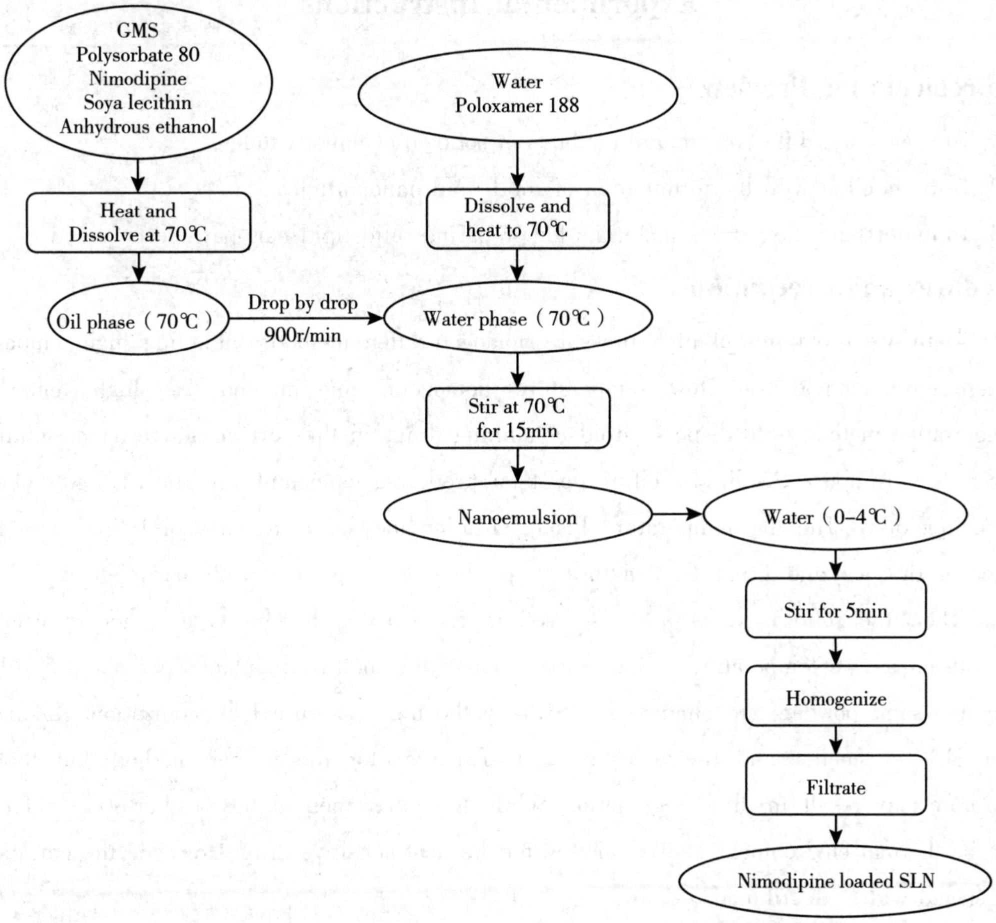

Figure 20 – 2　The scheme of the preparation of nimodipine loaded SLN

3. Quality evaluation

The characteristics of SLN are evaluated as follows:

(1) Particle size and distribution

The particle size and distribution of SLNs are measured using TOPSIZER laser scattered particle analyzer (OMEC) at room temperature.

(2) Morphology observation

Morphology of SLNs is observed using high – resolution transmission electron microscope (TEM).

(3) Loading amount and entrapment efficiency

Usually, free drug and drug loaded in SLN are separated with dextran gel method, centrifugation method, or dialysis method, and are measured respectively. The encapsulation efficiency and drug loading are calculated based on the following equations.

$$\text{Encapsulation efficiency}(\%) = \frac{\text{the weight of encapsulated drug in SLN}}{\text{the total weight of drug added}} \times 100\%$$

$$\text{Drug Loading}(\%) = \frac{\text{the weight of encapsulated drug in SLN}}{\text{the total weight of SNL}} \times 100\%$$

Experimental Instructions

Requirements for Preview

1. To master the different prepare methods of solid lipid nanoparticles.
2. To be familiar with the formulation of solid lipid nanoparticles.
3. To understand the various materials for preparing solid lipid nanoparticles.

Procedures and Precautions

1. There are two kinds of high pressure homogenization methods including high temperature homogenization method and low temperature homogenization method. The high temperature homogenization method is to disperse lipid containing drugs in the surface active agent solution at high temperature above the lipid melting point for preparing nanoemulsion. The SLN was obtained after cooling down. The low temperature homogenization method is to mix solid lipid with liquid nitrogen or dry ice and grind the mixture to produce lipid powder with particle size of 50 – 100μm. Then, the solid powders are dispersed in the surfactant solution and homogenized into nanoemulsion as the temperature is lower than that of the melting point of lipid about 5 – 10℃. Finally, the solid powders are change into SLN by the high pressure homogenization. The particle size of SLN is smaller and the distribution is narrower for the former method, but the high temperature may result in drug degradation. While the latter method has a shorter time for drug under the thermal environment and is suitable for the heat sensitive drug. However, the particle size is larger and widely distributed.

2. For nanoemulsion – high pressure homogenization method, firstly, a transparent and thermodynamic stable O/W type nanoemulsion is prepared. Then, the nanoemulsion is dispersed in cold water and homogenized. The particle size of the obtained nanoparticles was related to the particle size of nanoemulsion and the aggregation of nanoemulsion when diluted. The temperature between nanoemulsion and water when cooling is very important for preparing SLN with small particle size. Fast crystallization will avoid particle aggregation partly. The solidation process of SLN is also the dilution process, which would lead to low solid content of SLN.

3. The preparation process of nimodipine loaded SLN should avoid light.

Questions

1. What is the basic structural characteristics and composition of solid lipid nanoparticles?
2. Which factors would affect the stability of SLN? How to improve the stability of SLN?
3. What is the difference of between solid lipid nanoparticles, liposomes and nanoparticles?

4. What kind of drug is suitable to apply the SLN drug delivery system?
5. Is the preparation method of SLN used in this experiment suitable for industrial production?
6. What does the quality evaluation of SLN include?

实验21　脂质体的制备

【目的与要求】

1. **掌握**　脂质体的基本结构和特征。
2. **熟悉**　脂质体的基本制备方法。
3. **了解**　脂质体的质量评价指标及方法。

【基本概念与实验原理】

脂质体系指药物被类脂双分子层包封成的微小泡。脂质体有单室与多室之分。小单室脂质体的粒径一般为20～80nm，大单室脂质体的粒径在0.1～1μm，多室脂质体的粒径在1～5μm。通常小单室脂质体也称纳米脂质体。

药物被包封于脂质体中，可改善药物的吸收、减少药物的代谢、延长药物的生物半衰期及降低药物的毒性。脂质体既可以负载疏水性药物，亦可负载水溶性药物。疏水性药物一般负载于脂质双分子层中间，而水溶性药物一般负载于脂质体中间的水相以及脂质双分子层之间的水相中。

脂质体常用的制备方法：注入法、薄膜分散法、超声波分散法、逆相蒸发法、冷冻干燥法等。在脂质体制备过程中，若为非极性药物，则先与磷脂、胆固醇混合后，溶于有机溶剂中，当形成脂质体时，药物包封在双分子层中；当包封的药物是极性药物时，则先溶于水相中，当形成脂质体时，药物包封在水相隔室中。影响脂质体中药物包封率的因素主要有：①类脂质膜材料的投料比；②脂质体电荷的影响；③脂质体粒径大小的影响；④药物溶解度的影响；⑤制备容器的影响。

尼莫地平为钙通道阻滞药，用于预防和治疗由于蛛网膜下隙出血后脑血管痉挛引起的缺血性神经损伤以及老年性脑功能损伤、偏头痛、突发性耳聋等。尼莫地平亲脂性强，不溶于水，溶于乙醇和三氯甲烷，目前临床上应用的尼莫地平注射液中含有23.7%（*V/V*）乙醇，这可能对酒精中毒或酒精代谢受损的患者有害。将尼莫地平制成脂质体有望提高尼莫地平的安全性，从而提高临床治疗效果。

胰岛素是治疗糖尿病的首选药，目前治疗糖尿病以注射为主，但长期频繁的注射给患者无论在身体还是心理上都带来极大的痛苦。口服给药途径是患者比较乐于接受的给药途径，将胰岛素以脂质体包封，利用脂质体的生物膜特性和药物转换能力，可极大提高其口服生物利用度和患者用药顺应性。

【仪器与材料】

1. **仪器**　水浴旋转蒸发仪，水循环真空泵，振荡器，超声波恒温水浴，探针式超声仪，高压均质机，水浴超声仪，激光粒度测定仪，电子分析天平，温度计，茄形瓶（型号24#），试管，烧杯等。

2. 材料 尼莫地平，胰岛素，大豆磷脂，胆固醇，三氯甲烷，乙醇，乙醚，氯化钠，pH7.4磷酸盐缓冲液（137mmol/L NaCl，2.6mmol/L KCl，6.4mmol/L $Na_2HPO_4 \cdot 12H_2O$，1.4mmol/L NaH_2PO_4），注射用水等。

【实验内容】

一、薄膜分散法制备尼莫地平脂质体

1. 处方

尼莫地平	5mg
大豆磷脂	250mg
胆固醇	25mg
注射用水	10ml

2. 制备工艺 尼莫地平脂质体制备流程图见图21－1。

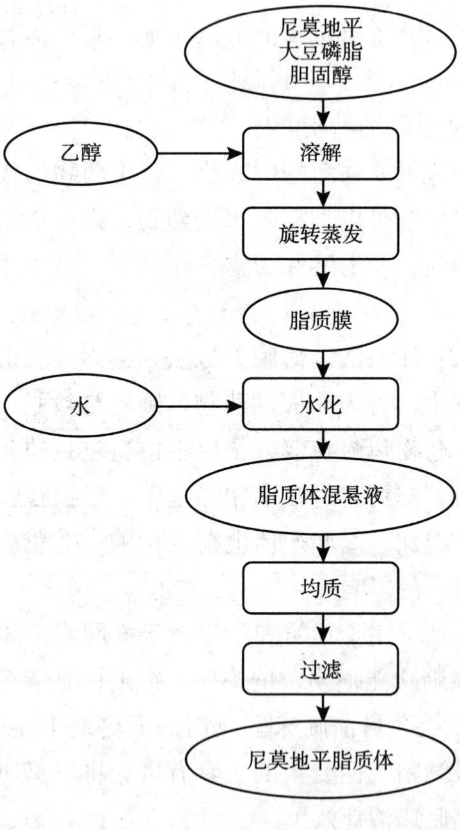

图21－1 尼莫地平脂质体的制备工艺流程图

精确称取尼莫地平5mg、大豆磷脂250mg和胆固醇25mg置于茄形瓶中，然后加入乙醇4ml使上述物质溶解。经减压蒸发除去溶剂（水浴温度37±1℃），使上述物质以薄膜状均匀地沉积于茄形瓶内壁。接着在茄形瓶中加入注射用水10ml，在旋转蒸发仪上旋转水化0.5h（水浴温度37±1℃）。将脂质体混悬液经高压均质仪在800bar下循环均质5次，所得尼莫地平脂质体用0.22μm微孔滤膜过滤。

二、逆相蒸发法制备胰岛素脂质体

1. 处方

胰岛素	4mg
大豆磷脂	200mg
胆固醇	25mg
0.01mol/L HCl 溶液	0.5ml
磷酸盐缓冲液（pH7.4）	4.5ml

2. 制备工艺　精密称取胆固醇 25mg、大豆磷脂 200mg 置于茄形瓶中，然后加入乙醚 10ml 溶解上述物质。另精密称取胰岛素 4mg，溶于 0.5ml 的 0.01mol/L HCl 溶液中，再加入 4.5ml 磷酸盐缓冲液（pH7.4）中，然后与乙醚液混合，振摇，经水浴超声乳化，所得乳液在旋转蒸发仪上减压除去有机溶剂（20℃），直至得到乳状脂质体混悬液。将该脂质体混悬液涡旋振摇 15min，然后用探针式超声仪在冰水浴中超声处理 1min，即得胰岛素脂质体。

三、质量评价

脂质体制备完成后，对其进行质量评价，具体如下。

1. 粒径及其分布　取脂质体样品，使用激光粒度测定仪于室温下测定其粒径及粒径分布。

2. 形态观察　使用高分辨率的透射电子显微镜观察脂质体形貌。

3. 包封率与载药量　一般采用葡聚糖凝胶色谱法、超速离心法、透析法等分离方法分离包封在脂质体内和游离的药物，通过测定包封的药物量和游离的药物量，并根据下列公式计算包封率和载药量。

$$包封率(\%)=\frac{脂质体中包封的药物量}{加入药物总量}\times 100\%$$

$$载药量(\%)=\frac{脂质体中包封的药物量}{脂质体的总质量}\times 100\%$$

实验指导

一、预习要求

1. 掌握　脂质体的常用材料及基本结构，复习脂质体相关知识。

2. 熟悉　脂质体的常用制备工艺。

3. 了解　脂质体的质量评价方法。

二、操作要点和注意事项

1. 脂质体的制备方法应根据药物的性质以及该脂质体的用途和要求进行选择。

2. 用薄膜分散法制备含药脂质体时，应注意正确称量，按规定控制温度，并将溶剂蒸发除尽。另外，控制好旋转蒸发仪的旋转速度和真空度，以便成膜均匀。

3. 用逆相蒸发法制备含药脂质体时，应注意乳化要充分、水浴温度和真空度要控制得当。

4. 使用旋转蒸发仪进行减压蒸发时，要防止水循环真空泵的水倒灌。

5. 脂质体制备完毕后，要对其进行质量评价，目前要求控制的主要项目有：①粒径及分布、Zeta 电位、形态；②包封率、载药量和渗漏；③药物的含量测定；④有害有机溶剂的限量检查；⑤药物体内分布测定等。

三、思考题

1. 简述脂质体的基本组成和结构特征。

2. 影响脂质体稳定性的因素有哪些？如何提高脂质体的稳定性？

3. 影响脂质体包封率的主要因素有哪些？

4. 脂质体与固体脂质纳米粒和乳剂的区别与联系是什么？

5. 脂质体的制备工艺有哪些？哪些制备工艺可在脂质体大生产中运用？

6. 如何评价脂质体的质量？

Experiment 21 Preparation of Liposomes

Objectives and Requirements

1. To master the basic structures and characteristics of liposomes.

2. To be familiar with the preparation procedures of liposomes.

3. To understand the quality evaluations of liposomes.

Introduction

Liposomes are tiny bubbles (vesicles), made out of the same material as a cell membrane. Liposomes can be filled with drugs, and used to deliver drugs for cancer and other diseases. Liposomes are usually made of phospholipids and cholesterol. According to the structure and the number of lipid bilayer, the major types of liposomes are separated into small unilamellar liposome vesicle (SUV, with one lipid bilayer), the large unilamellar vesicle (LUV) and the multilamellar vesicle (MLV, with several lamellar phase lipid bilayers). The particle size of SUV is in the range of 20 – 80nm, as well as LUV 0.1 – 1μm and MLV 1 – 5μm. SUV is also named as nano – liposomes.

Liposomes have been used to improve the therapeutic index of new or established drugs by modifying drug absorption, reducing metabolism, prolonging biological half – life or reducing toxicity. The unique feature of liposomes is their ability to compartmentalize and solubilize both hydrophilic and hydrophobic materials by nature. Hydrophobic drugs place themselves inside the bilayer of the liposome and hydrophilic drugs are entrapped within the aqueous core or at the bilayer interface.

The preparation techniques of liposome are listed as follows: infusion, film dispersion, ultrasonic dis persion, reverse phase evaporation, freezing drying method, etc. During the preparation of liposomes, for non – polar drug it should be firstly mixed with phospholipid and cholesterol and then dissolve in organic solvent. When the liposome is formatted, the non – polar drug will encapsulated in the molecular bilayer; if the drug encapsulated is polar, it should be firstly dissolved in the water phase, when the liposome is formatted, drug will be encapsulated in water phase chambers. Some factors would affect the encapsulation efficiency of drug, including: (1) the feed ratio of lipid materials; (2) the surface charge of liposomes; (3) the particle size of liposomes; (4) the solubility of drug; (5) the vessel used for preparation.

Nimodipine is a calcium channel blocker. It is used to prevent and treat ischemic nerve damage caused by cerebral vasospasm after subarachnoid hemorrhage, as well as senile brain damage, migraine, and sudden deafness. However, nimodipine is lipophilic, insoluble in water, but soluble in ethanol and chloroform. The current clinical nimodipine injection contains 23.7% (V/V) ethanol, which may be harmful to patients with alcoholism or alcohol metabolism. The preparation of nimodipine into liposomes is expected to improve the safety, thereby improving the clinical therapeutic effect.

Insulin is the drug used to control blood sugar in people with diabetes. In clinical, insulin injections are commonly used. However, continuous injections bring suffering to patients. Oral administration is a better choice. Insulin is a kind of protein drug, which is apt to be destroyed by enzyme in the gastrointestinal tract with poor absorption. When insulin is encapsulated in liposomes, liposomes can sufficiently protect insulin from enzymatic attack and improve the oral bioavailability.

Equipment and Materials

1. Equipment

Rotary evaporator with water bath, hydrologic cycle vacuum pump, shaker, ultrasonic bath, high pressure homogenizer, probe ultrasonifier, TOPSIZER laser scattered particle analyzer (OMEC), electronic analytical balance, thermometer, pyriform flask, test tube, etc.

2. Materials

Nimodipine, porcine insulin, soy lecithin, cholesterol, chloroform, ethanol, ether, sodium chloride, pH7.4 phosphate buffered saline (137mmol/L NaCl, 2.6mmol/L KCl, 6.4mmol/L $Na_2HPO_4 \cdot 12H_2O$, 1.4mmol/L NaH_2PO_4), water for injection.

Experimental Methods

1. Nimodipine - loaded liposomes prepared by film dispersion method

(1) Formulation

Nimodipine	5mg
Soya lecithin	250mg
Cholesterol	25mg
Water for injection	10ml

(2) Manufacturing process

A mixture of soya lecithin, cholesterol and nimodipine are dissolved in 4ml ethanol and dried under evaporation in a rotary evaporator at 37℃. The lipid film is further dried in vacuum for 1h to remove the solvent completely. Then, the resulting lipid film is hydrated with 10ml water for injection in a rotary evaporator until ivory - white liposome suspension is successfully formed, and then the ivory - white liposome suspensions are homogenized with water bath ultrasonic instrument for 2min. after that the liposome suspensions are homogenized with high pressure homogenizer at 800bar for 5 cycles. The liposome suspensions are preserved in light - resistant, tightly closed containers and stored at 4℃.

The flow graph for the preparation of nimodipine – loaded liposomes is shown in Figure 21 – 1.

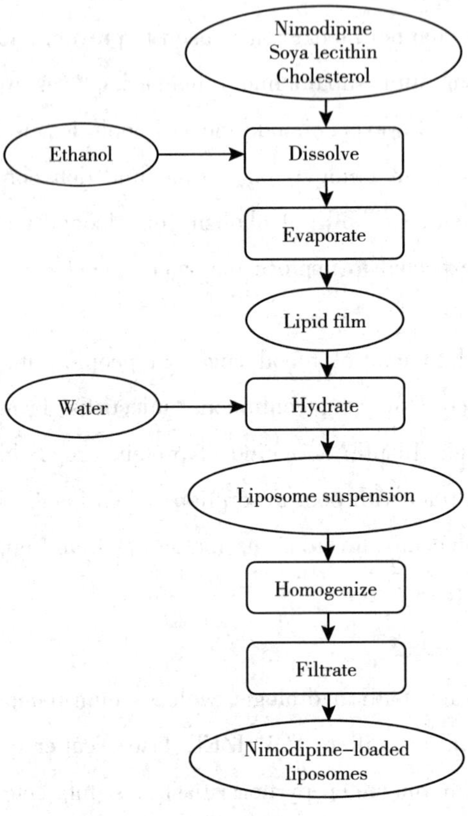

Figure 21 – 1 The flow graph for the preparation of nimodipine – loaded liposomes

2. Insulin – loaded liposomes prepared by reverse phase evaporation

(1) Formulation

Insulin	4mg
Soy lecithin	200mg
Cholesterol	25mg
0.01mol/L HCl	0.5ml
Phosphate buffered saline (pH7.4)	4.5ml

(2) Manufacturing process

A total lipid mixture of 225mg (soy lecithin/cholesterol in the weight ratios of 8 : 1) is dissolved in 10ml of ether in pyriform flask. 4mg of insulin is dissolved in 0.5ml of 0.01mol/L HCl, and 4.5ml of phosphate buffered saline is added. The resulting water phase is added to the flask, then dispersed with a shaker at room temperature, and emulsified with a bath – type ultrasonifier. The ether is evaporated using a rotary evaporator in 20℃ water bath under reduced pressure. The resulting liposomal dispersions are vortex – mixed for 15min to form the liposomal suspensions, and then homogenized with probe – type ultrasonifier in ice bath for 1min. The liposomal suspensions are preserved in light – resistant, tightly closed containers and stored at 4℃.

3. Quality evaluation

The characteristics of liposome are evaluated as follows:

(1) Particlesize and distribution

The particle size and distribution of lipsomes are measured using TOPSIZER laser scattered particle analyzer (OMEC) at room temperature.

(2) Morphology observation

Morphology of the liposomes is observed using high - resolution transmission electron microscope (TEM).

(3) Loading amount and entrapment efficiency

Usually, free drug and liposomes are separated with dextran gel method, centrifugation method, or dialysis method, and are measured respectively. The encapsulation efficiency and drug loading amount are calculated based on the following equations.

$$\text{Encapsulation efficiency}(\%) = \frac{\text{the weight of encapsulated drug in liposome}}{\text{the total weight of drug added}} \times 100\%$$

$$\text{Drug Loading}(\%) = \frac{\text{the weight of encapsulated drug in liposome}}{\text{the total weight of liposome}} \times 100\%$$

Experimental Instructions

Requirements for Preview

1. To master the widely used materials and basic structures of liposomes and to preview the theory of liposome.

2. To be familiar with the methods used for preparation of liposomes.

3. To understand the methods for quality evaluations of liposomes.

Procedures and Precautions

1. The preparation method of liposomes is selected depending on the characteristics of drug, and the requirements for the particle size.

2. When liposomes are prepared by film dispersion method, more attention should be focused on the following: first, all materials should be weighted correctly; second, the temperature should be controlled in a suitable range; third, organic solvent should be completely removed. In addition, rotate speed and vacuum degree of rotary evaporator have an effect on the formation of even film.

3. When liposomes are prepared by reverse phase evaporation, more attention should be focused on the following: first, the mixture of oil and water should be emulsified fully; second, the temperature of water bath and vacuum should be controlled accurately.

4. When evaporating the solvent with rotary evaporator under reduced pressure, the refluence of water should be avoided in hydrologic cycle vacuum pump.

5. The characteristics of liposome are evaluated as follows: particle size and its distribution, zeta potential, morphology, entrapment efficiency, loading amount, in vitro release, leakage rate, determination of drug content, residue of toxic organic solvent, in vivo distribution of drug etc.

Questions

1. What is the basic structural characteristics and composition of liposomes?

2. Which factors would affect the stability of liposomes? How to improve the stability of liposomes?

3. Which factors have an influence on the entrapment efficiency of liposomes?

4. What is the difference of between liposome, solid lipid nanoparticle, and emulsion?

5. What are the preparation techniques of liposomes? Is the preparation method of liposomes used in this experiment suitable for industrial production?

6. What does the quality evaluation of liposomes include?

第六部分　高端仪器设备的操作

实验 22　冷冻干燥机的操作与维护

【目的与要求】

1. **掌握**　冷冻干燥的原理及冷冻干燥设备的标准操作规程和常规维护程序。
2. **熟悉**　影响冻干产品质量的因素及用于冻干产品的常用辅料。
3. **了解**　冷冻干燥设备的组成部分及功能。

【基本概念与实验原理】

真空冷冻干燥简称冻干，是将湿物料或溶液在较低的温度下冻结成固态，然后在真空下使其中的水分不经液态直接升华成气态，使物料脱水的干燥技术。冷冻干燥的基本原理是基于水的三态变化。水有固态、液态和气态，三种相态既可以相互转换又可以共存。当水在三相点时，水、冰、水蒸气三者可共存且相互平衡。在高真空状态下，利用升华原理，使预先冻结的物料中的水分，不经过冰的融化，直接以冰态升华为水蒸气被除去，从而达到冷冻干燥的目的。

图 22－1 为本实验所用 LABCONCO FreeZone 12L 型冷冻干燥机外观图。

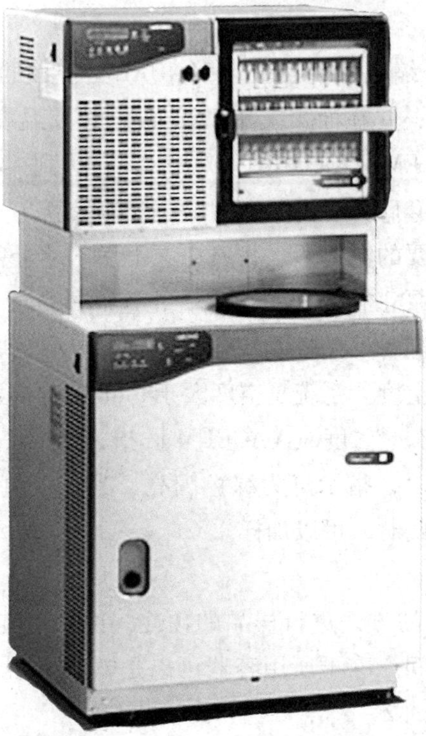

图 22－1　冷冻干燥机（LABCONCO FreeZone 12L）外观图

【仪器与材料】

1. **仪器** 冷冻干燥机（LABCONCO FreeZone 12L）。

2. **材料** 预冻物料（10%甘露醇溶液，每一瓶5ml西林瓶中含甘露醇水溶液1ml）。

【操作与维护规程】

冷冻干燥设备的标准操作规程如下。

1. 开机

（1）将电源开关打开（On）。

（2）自动运行

①按下AUTO按键，自动运行程序开始启动。AUTO键上面的指示灯点亮，表明压缩机正在工作。冷阱温度开始下降，并在面板上用LCD数码管及温度指示灯显示冷阱实际温度及温度波形图。当冷阱温度（COLLECTOR TEMPERATURE,℃）没有达到-40℃时，冷阱温度指示灯为黄色，并相应顺序点亮，以表示10，0，-10，-20，-30℃；当冷阱温度达到-40℃后，冷阱温度指示灯变为绿色。

②当冷阱温度达到-40℃后，真空泵自动启动，面板上的真空泵指示灯点亮，表明真空泵正在工作。装配有止逆阀的冻干机，当按下AUTO键后，真空泵即开始启动，止逆阀处于关闭状态，止逆阀指示灯点亮。当冷阱温度达到-40℃后，止逆阀打开。系统真空度开始下降，并在面板上用LCD数码管及真空度指示灯显示系统实际真空度。系统实际真空度大于5mBar时，显示“high”，当系统真空度为2~0.450mBar时，系统真空度（VACUUM）指示灯为黄色，并相应顺序点亮，以表示2，1，0.8，0.6，0.450 mBar，当系统真空度低于0.450 mBar接近0.120 mBar时，指示灯为绿色闪亮，当系统真空度达到及低于0.120mBar时，指示灯为稳定的绿色。此时，可以加样。

（3）手动运行

①按下MANUAL键，压缩机开始启动。MANUAL键上面的指示灯点亮，表明压缩机正在工作。冷阱温度开始下降，并在面板上用LCD数码管及温度指示灯显示冷阱实际温度。当冷阱温度（COLLECTOR TEMPERATURE,℃）还没有达到-40℃时，冷阱温度指示灯为黄色；当冷阱温度达到-40℃后，冷阱温度指示灯变为绿色。

②当冷阱温度达到所需要的温度后，按真空泵开关，真空泵开始启动，VACUUM键上面的指示灯点亮，表明真空泵正在工作。装配有止逆阀的冻干机，当按下VACUUM键后，真空泵即开始启动，止逆阀同时处于打开状态，止逆阀指示灯熄灭。系统真空度开始下降，并在面板上显示系统实际真空度。系统真空度大于5mBar时，显示“high”，当系统真空度为2~0.450mBar时，系统真空度（VACUUM）指示灯为黄色，当系统真空度低于0.450mBar接近0.120mBar时，指示灯为绿色闪亮，当系统真空度达到及低于0.120mBar时，指示灯为稳定的绿色。此时，可以加样。

2. 加样及冻干

（1）推荐使用旋转冷冻的方法进行样品的预冷，以尽可能地增大预冻样品的表面积，提高冻干效率，缩短冻干时间。冻干所用容器可以是安瓿、血浆瓶或广口冻干瓶。容器的大小至少应是所盛样品体积的2~3倍。

（2）将预冷好的样品接到样品阀，转动样品阀上的旋钮到“VAC”位置（斜面朝向冻干瓶方向）。

（3）当系统真空度重新恢复到0.120mBar时，再加另一个样品，以保证足够低的冷阱温度和系统真空度，防止预冻样品溶化。

（4）当冻干瓶外表面不再有冰霜并用手握住冻干瓶不再有凉的感觉时，样品就接近干燥了。此时，再冻干几小时即可结束冻干。

（5）打开一个样品瓶阀门（斜面朝向阀门进气孔方向），卸掉真空（如需要的话，还可在阀门的进气孔上通入惰性气体）。取下此冻干瓶。

（6）如果是用安瓿冻干的话，可直接在阀门上用火炬密封。

注意：千万不要烧到阀门，最好在阀门与火矩之间加入防火材料。

3. 关机

（1）打开一个样品瓶阀门，卸掉真空，并关闭“VAC”键。

（2）按AUTO或MAN键，关掉制冷压缩机。此时，AUTO或MAN键上面的指示灯熄灭。

（3）取下所有冻干瓶。

（4）关掉电源开关。

（5）打开冷阱盖，拔出冷阱排液管，拔掉冷阱排液管塞，并将冷阱排液管放置到适当的容器内。

（6）若有“Defrost”功能的，亦可快速解冻，按面板上的除霜按键（Defrost），此时，除霜按键上面的指示灯点亮。待冷阱内的冰完全融化后，再按面板上的除霜按键，关掉除霜，此时，除霜按键上面的指示灯熄灭。

（7）将冷阱内擦拭干净。

（8）将冷阱排液管塞重新装好，并将冷阱排液管放回到原来位置。

4. 日常维护保养

（1）通过真空泵上的油窗，检查真空泵油的状况及油标高度。如果油标低于下限，应补充真空泵油。如果真空泵内进入较多的水分而造成真空泵油成浑浊状，换油。如果真空泵内进入较少的水分，拧开真空泵气震阀，排干真空泵油中的潮气。

（2）用软布、海棉或麂皮沾中性、非研磨作用的肥皂水或洗涤剂擦拭有机玻璃盖，冻干机前面板及侧板。必要时，可用喷水枪或刷子刷洗。但千万不要用溶剂，因为溶剂会损坏仪器表面涂层。

（3）用带刷子的吸尘器吸走制冷压缩机前散热器上的灰尘，以保证良好的通风散热性能。如果冻干系统在粉尘较多的环境中工作，需要增加吸尘的次数。

实验指导

一、预习要求

1. 掌握　冷冻干燥的定义。

2. 熟悉　注射用无菌粉末的制备工艺流程及质量要求。

3. 了解　冷冻干燥过程中出现的异常现象及处理方法。

二、操作要点及注意事项

1. 冻干操作前，需检查真空泵中真空油量。

2. 冻干样品中不能含有酸及有机溶剂。

3. 冻干样品液层不宜过厚，厚度不宜超过1.5cm。

4. 本仪器制冷系统严禁频繁启动。当制冷压缩机被关掉后，至少要间隔15分钟后才能重新启动制冷压缩机。

5. 冻干是在低温下实现干燥的，适合不稳定药物尤其是蛋白类药物的干燥和保存，但是有些药物在冻干或后续储存过程中不稳定，需要加入一些辅料增加药物的稳定性，即冻干保护剂。

6. 冻干过程参数对冻干产品十分关键，冻干过程中样品温度不合适，容易出现样品塌陷等现象，产品水分含量也会对产品稳定性产生一定影响。

7. 在预冻过程中，样品溶液可能会出现结晶现象（蛋白类药物没有结晶现象，其他药物根据性质及浓度），样品浓度高，预冻速率慢更容易出现结晶现象。如甘露醇在处方中仅作为填充剂，这时希望甘露醇在预冻阶段结晶，样品可以在较高温度干燥，缩短冻干周期；这时药物以无定形形态包裹在甘露醇外部，甘露醇没有冻干保护剂作用。

8. 冻干处方同冻干工艺一样重要，如果冻干处方不佳，即使优化工艺也不能达到冻干要求。

三、思考题

1. 简述冷冻干燥的原理。
2. 冷冻干燥产品中，常用的冻干保护剂有哪些？
3. 简述注射用无菌冻干粉末的制备工艺。
4. 试分析冻干成品中出现喷瓶现象的原因及解决方法。
5. 同注射液相比，冻干制剂有哪些优势？
6. 试分析冷冻干燥产品含量不均匀或含量偏低的原因。

扫码“学一学”

Experiment 22　Operation and Maintenance of Freeze Dryer

Objectives and Requirements

1. To master the principle of the freeze drying and the standard operating procedure and general maintenance of freeze dryer.

2. To be familiar with the influence of lyophilized product and the excipients for freeze drying.

3. To understand the basic structure of the freeze dryer and their functions.

Introduction

The principle of freeze - drying is based on the tri - state change of water. Water has solid, liquid and gaseous phase. They can convert to each other and can both coexist. Under high vacuum, we can use the principle of sublimation to remove the water of the previously frozen material in the water. The ice without melting can be directly sublimated, so as to achieve the purpose of freeze - drying.

Figure 22 - 1 is the photo of LABCONCO FreeZone 12L freeze dryer used in this experiment.

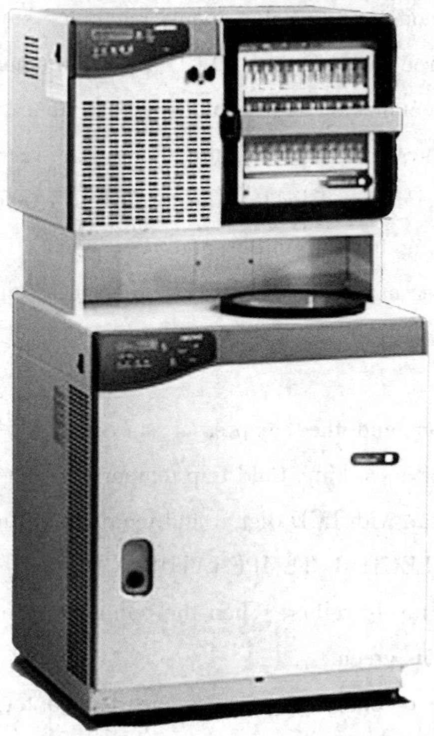

Figure 22 – 1　The photo of freeze dryer(LABCONCO FreeZone 12L)

Equipment and Materials

1. Equipment

Freeze dryer(LABCONCO FreeZone 12L).

2. Materials

The previously frozen material (10% mannitol solution, 1ml of mannitol solution in 5ml penicillin bottle).

Procedure

1. Power

(1) Turn on the power switch(On).

(2) Automatic operation.

①Press AUTO button, the program automatically started. The indicator light above AUTO button lights, indicating that the compressor is working. The temperature of the cold trap begins to drop, and it will show the actual temperature and the temperature waveforms of the cold trap with LCD digital indicator and temperature indicator light on the panel. When the cold trap temperature (collector temperature, ℃) does not reach –40℃, the cold trap temperature of the light is yellow, and the corresponding sequence of lights to represent 10, 0, –10, –20, –30℃; When the temperature of cold trap reach –40℃, the cold trap temperature light turns green.

②When the temperature of cold trap reaches –40℃, the vacuum pump starts automatically and the vacuum indicator on the front panel is light, indicating that the vacuum pump is working. When you press the AUTO button of the lyophilizer fitted with non – return valve, the vacuum pump starts, the check valve is in a closed state, and the check valve indicator lights. When the temperature of cold trap reaches –40℃, the non – return valve opens. Vacuum system begans to decline, and it will be displayed to the actual degree of vacuum with LCD digital tube and vacuum level indicator on the panel. When the degree of vacuum system is actually greater than 5mBar, it will display "high". When the vacuum degree of system reaches 2 to 0. 450mBar, vacuum system (VACUUM) light is yellow, and the corresponding sequence of lights indicates 2, 1, 0. 8, 0. 6, 0. 450mBar. When the vacuum degree of system is approaching to 0. 450mBar and less than 0. 120 mBar, the indicator flashes green. When the vacuum degree of system reaches less than 0. 120mBar, the light is solid green. At this point, you can add the sample.

(3) Manual operation

①Press MANUAL button, and the compressor starts. MANUAL button above the indicator light, indicating the compressor is working. Cold trap temperature begins to drop, and it will show the actual temperature of a cold trap with LCD digital and temperature indicator on the panel. When the cold trap temperature (COLLECTOR TEMPERATURE, ℃) has not yet reached – 40℃, the temperature indicator of cold trap is yellow. When the temperature of cold trap reaches –40℃, the cold trap temperature light turns green.

②When the temperature of cold trap reaches the desired temperature, we should press the vacuum switch, pump starts, and VACUUM button indicator above lights indicating the vacuum pump is working. When you press the VACUUM button, the vacuum pump starts, the check valve is in a opened state, and the check valve indicator does not light. Vacuum system begans to decline, and it will be displayed to the actual degree of vacuum on the panel. When the degree of vacuum system is actually greater than 5mBar, it will display "high". When the vacuum degree of system reaches 2 to 0. 450mBar, vacuum system (VACUUM) light is yellow. When the vacuum degree of system is approaching to 0. 450mBar and less than 0. 120mBar, the indicator flashes green. When the vacuum degree of the system reaches less than 0. 120mBar, the light is solid green. At this point, you can add the sample.

2. Samples adding and freeze drying

(1) Recommend using a rotary freezing precooled sample, to increase the surface area of the pre – freezing samples, to improve lyophilized efficiency and reduce drying time. The container can be freeze – dried ampoules, lyophilized plasma bottles or wide mouth bottles. The size of the container should be at least 2 to 3 times the volume containing the sample.

(2) The pre – cooling sample is connected to the sample valve, turning the knob of the sample valve to "vac" position (slant toward the direction of lyophilized bottle).

(3) When the vacuum system is 0. 120 mBar, we should add another sample, in order to ensure a sufficiently low temperature cold trap and vacuum system to prevent pre – freeze samples dissolved.

(4) When lyophilized bottle has no frost and holding the outer surface is no longer lyophilized cool feeling, the sample will be close to drying up. At this time, it just needs a few hours to end lyophilized.

(5) Open a vial valve (slant toward the direction of the valve inlet port), and remove the

vacuum(if desired, also on the air intake valve of an inert gas). Remove these lyophilized bottles.

(6) If you are using ampoules to freeze - dry, we can directly use the torch to the valve seal.

Note: Do not burn valves. Fire protection material is preferably added between the valve and the torch.

3. Shutdown

(1) Open a vial valve, remove vacuum and close the "VAC" button.

(2) Press AUTO or MAN key to turn off the refrigeration compressor. In this case, the light indicator above AUTO or MAN button does not light.

(3) Remove all lyophilized bottles.

(4) Turn off the power switch.

(5) Open the cold trap cover, pull out the drain pipe of cold trap, unplug the cold trap drain plug and place the drain of cold trap tube into an appropriate container.

(6) If it has "Defrost" function, it can also be thawed quickly. When we press the defrost button (Defrost) on the panel, the defrost button above the indicator lights.

(7) Wipe clean inside of the cold trap.

(8) Reinstall the drain plug of cold trap and put the drain tube of cold trap back to its original position.

4. General Maintenance

(1) Check the oil condition and its volume in the vacuum pump through the oil window on the vacuum pump. If the oil volume is below the lower limit, the oil should be supplemented. If the vacuum pump oil becomes turbid, turn on the air shock valve of the vacuum pump or change the oil.

(2) Wipe the polymethyl methacrylate cover, front panel and side panel of freeze dryer using soft cloth, sponge or suede stained with neutral, non - abrasive soap water or detergent. If necessary, water syringe or brush can be used. Solvents are forbidden to use, because solvents will damage the coating on the surface of the instrument.

(3) Clean dust in the front radiator of the refrigeration compressor with a vacuum cleaner to ensure good ventilation and heat dissipation performance. If the freeze - drying system works in a dusty environment, the number of vacuuming needs to be increased.

Experimental Instructions

Requirements for Preview

1. To master the definition of the freeze drying.

2. To be familiar with the manufacture process and quality control of sterile powder for injection.

3. To understand the problems during the freeze drying process and their reasons.

Procedures and Precautions

1. Before the freeze - drying process, heck the oil level in the vacuum pump.

2. It is required that the freeze drying sample is an aqueous solution, free of organic solvents

such as ethanol and acid.

3. The thickness of the freeze drying sample is supposed to be no more than 1.5cm.

4. When the machine is powered off, the interval time before the next start must be more than 15min.

5. Freeze drying is a low – temperature process, as a technique for stabilization of labile drugs, including proteins. Even when the labile drug survives the freeze – drying process without degradation, the resulting product is rarely found perfectly stable during long – term storage. Lyoprotectants are added for stability during the freeze – drying process as well as to provide storage stability.

6. Optimization of the freezing process may be critical, control of product temperature during drying is critical for products that tend to suffer cake collapse during primary drying, and control of residual moisture is nearly always critical for storage stability.

7. In the case of protein drugs, the drug does not crystallize, but other solute components may (or may not) crystallize, depending on their nature and concentration, other formulation components, and the details of the freezing process. High initial concentrations and slow freezing tend to favor crystallization. For example, if mannitol is intended only as a bulking agent, and is not expected to play a role in stabilization of the drug, crystallization is desirable as crystalline mannitol can easily be freeze dried at high temperatures to give an elegant product, meaning a short freeze – drying cycle and freedom from product defects such as collapse. Here, the drug form is that of an amorphous coating on the crystalline mannitol, with stability properties normally close to that of a system freeze dried without the mannitol.

8. Formulation and process are interrelated: A bad formulation can be nearly impossible to freeze dry, and even with a well – designed formulation.

Questions

1. Describe the Principle of freeze drying.

2. Illustrate some kinds of commonly used lyoprotectants in the freezing drying products and their function?

3. Describe manufacture process and quality control of sterile powder for injection.

4. Analyze the reason of spray bottle during the freezing drying process and the resolvent.

5. What are the advantages of lyophilized preparations compared with injections?

6. Analyze the reason when the content uniformity of the freeze – dried products is unqualified.

实验23　高压均质机的标准操作规程

【目的与要求】

1. **掌握**　高压均质机的工作原理。高压均质机的标准操作规程。

2. **熟悉**　影响均质过程的参数。

3. 了解　高压均质机的主要部件及其功能。

【实验原理】

高压均质机系指依靠高压往复泵为动力传递与输送物料的设备，物料被送到工作阀区后，由于高压而产生的剪切、撞击、空穴等作用，使物料被细化与匀化。高压均质机主要由传动系统、均质阀与柱塞泵等构成，主要功能包括细化与匀化物料、改善产品稳定性与降低产品黏度等，在食品、生命科学与制药等领域均有广泛应用。目前，在制药领域，高压均质机主要用于制备各种微粒制剂如脂质体、纳米乳、脂质纳米粒等。高压均质的主要特点包括：在高压条件下依靠物料间的强烈碰撞产生细化作用；依靠外部能量定量输送物料，动能消耗大；不适用于黏度过高的物料。

均质是由柱塞泵和均质阀共同作用使物料在均质阀区发生细化和均匀混合的过程（图 23－1）。均质原理是：物料通过柱塞泵吸入并加压，在柱塞作用下进入压力大小可调节的阀组中，经过特定宽度的限流缝隙（工作区）后，瞬间失压的物料以极高的流速（1000～1500 m/s）喷出，碰撞在阀组件之一的碰撞环上，产生 3 种效应。空穴效应，被柱塞压缩的物料内积聚了极高的能量，通过限流缝隙时瞬间失压，造成高能释放引起空穴爆炸，致使物料强烈粉碎细化；撞击效应，物料通过限流缝隙时以上述极高的速度撞击到特制的碰撞环上，造成物料粉碎；剪切效应，高速物料通过阀腔通道和限流缝隙时产生强烈的剪切。

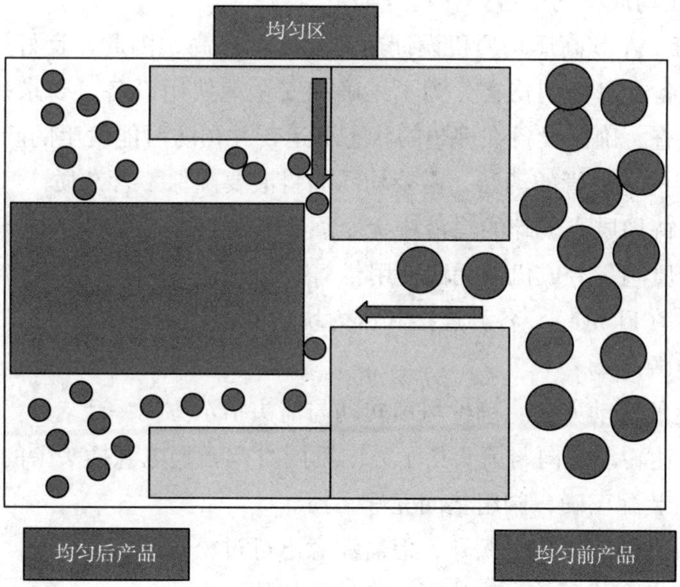

图 23－1　高压均质机工作原理图

本实验采用 ATS 高压均质机进行样品制备，设备示意图见图 23－2。AH－2010 型高压均质机的相关参数：流量 5～10L/h，最高使用压力 2000bar，机器冲程数 140 次/分，最大产品黏度 2000cP，最高产品温度 90℃，最高蒸汽温度 121℃。

【仪器与材料】

AH－2010 型 ATS 高压均质机，烧杯（250ml）。

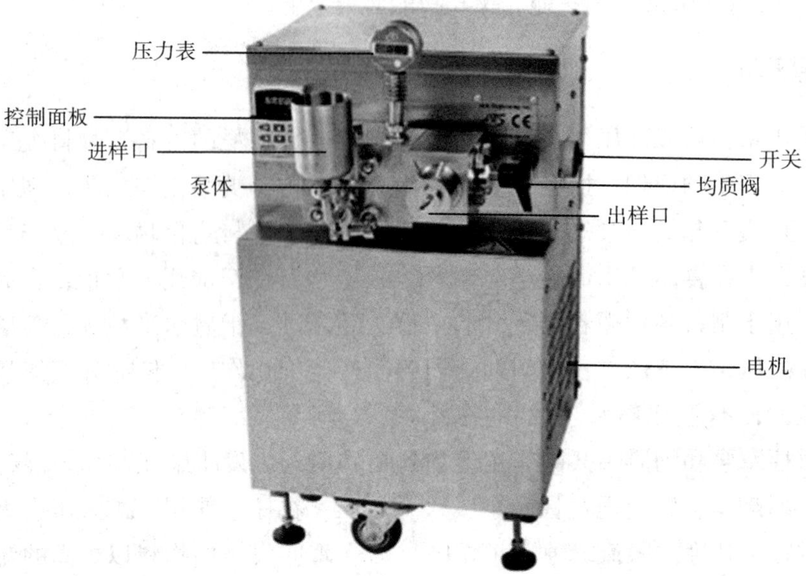

图 23 - 2　ATS - 2010 高压均质机示意图

【标准操作规程】

AH - 2010 高压均质机的标准操作规程如下。

1. 开机前检查　ATS 高压均质机设计达到的压力很高，因此，良好的操作习惯可以预防和避免人员和设备本身受到伤害。为了正确和安全地使用设备，要求操作人员对设备进行定期的必需的检查，确保设备在理想的状态下运转并预防可能发生的问题。

（1）保证机器的进料管的清洁，需要均质的料液要确保不含杂质。

注意：要确保待均质或破碎的料液中无金属颗粒；在料液中若有金属颗粒存在，会严重损伤进料阀和均质阀，造成机器无法使用。

（2）确认法兰（Flange），各种连接和压力块上的螺栓完全锁紧。

（3）接通主电源。

（4）检查马达的转动方向，确保风扇转动与箭头指示方向一致。

注意：如果马达转动方向与箭头指示方向不同时，调整电源插头上的接线。

（5）检查阀组装配正确，阀组垫圈完好无损。

（6）确定均质阀的手轮完全松开，但需注意不可过松。

（7）按下压力表上的开关，确认压力表显示的数值为零。

（8）定期检查密封圈和柱塞密封，确保无泄漏。

2. 开机

（1）往进料斗中加入清水。

（2）排出进料弯管中的空气。

（3）检查均质阀手轮是否完全松开。

（4）接通电源，转动机身右侧开关至“1”开机键，按面板上“ON”设备即可开始运行。

（5）按面板上的▲或▼键，调节泵的频率来调节流出速度，要求出料均匀连续，无异常的噪音。

注意：如果开机30 s后，出料口无料液排出，说明有气堵现象，可用排气杆插入进料斗中进行排气处理，直至出料均匀连续。如排气后仍然无料液排出，可能是均质管路堵塞，需要拆卸均质阀和固体陶瓷柱塞部分进行清洗。

3. 压力调节

（1）压力升高 调节均质阀的压力，缓慢顺时针转动手轮，压力缓慢稳定升高至所需总压力。建议压力升高幅度：100bar/10s。

注意：当压力升高时，设备传动声也随之升高；压力减小，传动声也随之减小，此为正常现象。

（2）排放压力 排放均质阀压力：缓慢逆时针转动手轮，压力缓慢、稳定地降低至零。停止转动手轮。

注意：手轮转动到压力为零即可停止，不可转动到过松的位置。

4. 均质操作

（1）料斗中加入清水，开机，调节频率。

（2）调节均质压力到所需工作压力。

（3）当清水流到料斗底部时，往料斗中加入物料。

（4）在机器均质过程中，操作人员要随时关注料斗中的存料量，及时补料，最后一次循环结束后，调节压力为零，并排出设备内部所有物料。

5. 仪器清洗及保养

（1）均质结束后，加料斗中加入清水，开机，无压力运行，清洗均质机料斗及管路直至干净。

（2）往料斗中加入75%乙醇，开机，无压力运行，清洗均质机料斗及管路直至干净。最后按面板上“OFF”按钮关机，料斗中加入约2/3的75%乙醇，保鲜膜密封。

（3）转动机身右侧开关至“—”关闭电源。

实验指导

一、预习要求

1. 掌握 高压均质法制备脂质体、脂肪乳剂、固体脂质纳米粒等的过程。

2. 熟悉 微粒制剂的特点与作用。

3. 了解 均质参数对脂质体、脂肪乳剂、固体脂质纳米粒等质量的影响。

二、操作要点与注意事项

1. 任何物料在进入均质机进行均质之前，必须经60～100目滤网过滤，避免颗粒杂质（如铁屑、玻璃碎片等）进入均质机磨损机器的进料阀座和均质阀。

2. 均质机禁止在无物料的情况下长时间运行。

3. 均质机严禁在均质阀手柄旋紧的情况下开机，突然的过载负荷会严重损伤马达。

4. 均质机使用固体陶瓷柱塞，与柱塞接触的物料温差变化不得超过70℃，否则可能造成柱塞断裂。物料的温度增加或降低的幅度不得大于每分钟5℃（特别在机器灭菌操作时）。

三、思考题

1. 简述高压均质机的基本组成和工作原理。

2. 高压均质过程影响脂质体、脂肪乳等微纳米制剂质量的主要因素有哪些?
3. 简述高压均质仪操作过程。
4. 高压均质仪的操作要点与注意事项有哪些?
5. 简述高压均质仪的保养与维护过程。
6. 简述高压均质仪在制药领域中的应用。

Experiment 23 Standard Operation Procedure of High – pressure Homogenizer

Objectives and Requirements

1. To master the principle of the high – pressure homogenization. To master the standard operating procedure of the machines.

2. To be familiar with the factors affecting the homogenization process.

3. To understand some main parts of the machine and their functions.

Introduction

High – pressure homogenizer is a machine that can deliver the materials to homogenizing gap with the help of high pressure reciprocating pump, and allows the materials to be microsized and homogenized via the cavitation, impingement, shear stresses, etc produced by high pressure, consisting of driving system, homogenizing valve and plunger pump, etc. It is mainly used to microsize and homogenize the liquid materials, improve the product stability, reduce the product viscosity and so on, widely being used in food, life sciences and pharmaceutical fields. In pharmaceutical field, it is extensively used to produce mirco/nanoparticle preparations such as liposomes, nanoemulsions, lipid nanoparticles, etc. Its predominant features include: (1) The microsizing relies on the impingement of materials under high pressure condition; (2) The delivery of material into the homogenizing gap is depend on the external energy and the energy consumption is large; (3) The suitability for high viscosity material is poor.

Homogenizationis a process that allows the material to be broken into pieces and mixed uniformly in the homogeneous valve with the help of both plunger pump and homogenizing valve (see Figure 23 – 1).

Theory of homogenization:

Material is inhaled through the plunger pump with pressure impact. With the help of the plunger effect, it enters the valve groups within which the pressure is adjustable, passes through limiting gap (work area) with specific width; after that, due to instantaneous loss of pressure, the material ejects with extremely high speed of one thousand to half one thousands meters per second and crashes onto the collision ring within one of the valve group, thereby producing three effects (Figure 23 – 1): hole effect, the high energy which is accumulated within the material by plunger compression, because of the sudden decrease of pressure as passes through the limiting gap, would result in high powder release and resultant hole explosion, thus leading to the fact that the material is strongly crushed into pieces; impact effect, when passing through the limiting gap, the material is smashed and refined after hitting the special impact ring with extremely high speed; shear effect, strong shearing effect is produced when the material is passing the valve chamber channel and limiting gap with the high speed.

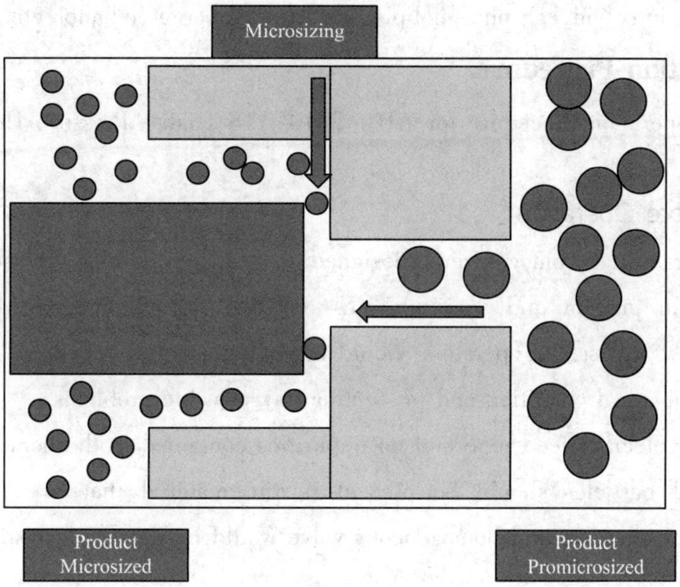

Figure 23 – 1 Diagram of high – pressure homogenization mechanism

In this experiment, the lipid – emulsions will be prepared using High – Pressure Homogenizer, which its diagram and control system are displayed in Figure 23 – 2. Parameters of AH – 2010 ATS High – Pressure Homogenizer are listed below: capacity, 5 – 10L/h; maximum operating pressure, 2000bar; stroke of equipment, 140 times/min; maximum viscosity, 2000cP; maximum temperature of the product, 90℃; maximum temperature of the steam, 121℃.

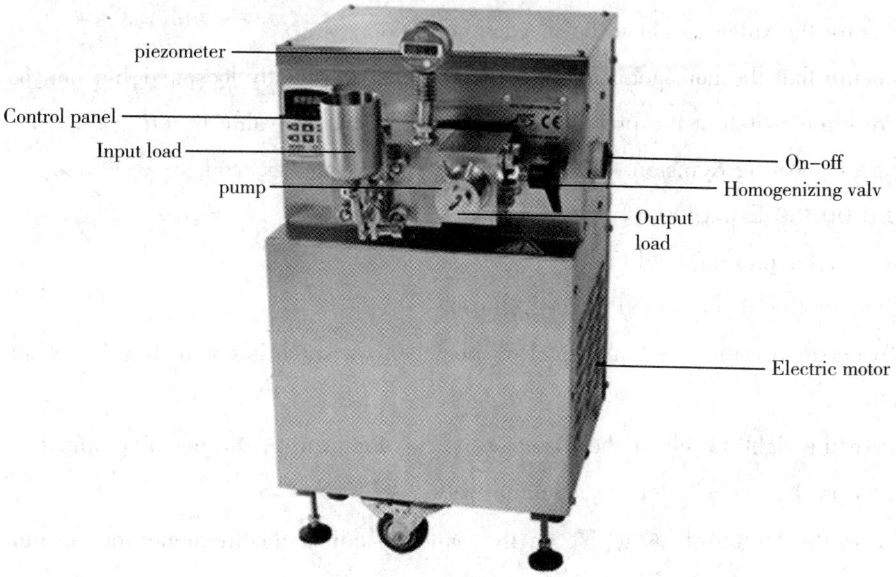

Figure 23 – 2 ATS high – pressure homogenizer

Equipment and Materials

1. Equipment

AH – 2010 ATS homogenizer (ATS Engineering Inc. , Canada), beakers (50ml and 250ml), electronic balance, high – speed ultra – turrax blender.

2. Materials

Soybean oil for injection, egg phospholipid, water for injection, ethanol, etc.

Standard Operation Procedure

The standard operation procedure for AH – 2010 ATS High – Pressure Homogenizer is listed below:

1. Check Before Operation

ATS high – pressured homogenizeris designed to reach very high pressure, therefore, good operational habit can prevent and avoid injuries & harm to device itself. In order to use this equipment accurately and safely, operators should make regular and necessary inspection, ensuring the machine works in ideal condition and preventing any possible problems.

(1) Ensure the clean of feed pipe and no impurities contained in the homogeneous material.

Note: no metal particles should be present in the material that needs homogenization or breaking; otherwise, feed valve and homogeneous valve would be damaged, resulting in the machine stopping working.

(2) Confirm that the bolts in the Flange, all connecting and pressure mass are totally locked.

(3) Connect the power line to the plug and main power supply.

(4) Check the rotational direction of the motor and ensure that fan rotates in the direction of the arrow.

Note: If the direction of the motor is not consistent with the direction of the arrow, please adjust the connection of the power plug.

(5) Check the correct of manifolds assembly; if not, manifolds must be reassembled.

(6) Ensure the valve gasket to be in good condition.

(7) Ensure that the homogenizing valve hand wheel are totally loosened, but not too loosen.

(8) Press the switch of the pressure gauge and confirm the value is zero.

(9) Check the ring & piston seal periodically to make it leak – off.

2. Turn on the Equipment

(1) Add water into the feed cup.

(2) Remove the air presented in feed elbow.

(3) To make sure that the handwheel on homogenizer valve is completely loose before turning on the machine.

(4) Turn the right switch of the fuselage to "1" for turn on the machine, and then press the "ON" button on the panel to let the machine work.

(5) Press the button of ▲或▼ on the panel to adjust the frequency of the pump and the outflow speed. The discharge should be well – distributed and continuous without abnormal noise.

Note: If there is no material fluid is output from the outlet after you turn on the equipment for

30 s, it indicates that air – blocking exists in the pressure mass. If so, the exhaust rod can be inserted into the feed hopper for removing the gas until the discharge is uniform and continuous. If the above procedure can not work, you should disassemble the homogenizing valve and the solid ceramic plunger for cleaning.

3. Pressure Adjustment

(1) Pressure increase

Rotate handle clockwise slowly to increase the pressure to the required pressure with recommended speed of 100bar/10s.

Remarks: It is a normal phenomenon that the noise is increased or decreased for pressure increase or reduction.

(2) Pressure release

Rotate handle widdershins slowly until the pressure is decreased to zero, and then stop rotating.

Attention: Stop rotating as the pressure is zero, and do not rotate to too loose position.

4. Operation Procedure

(1) Add water into the feed cup, and then turn on the machine and adjust the frequency of pump.

(2) Adjust the pressure to the requirement.

(3) Place the material into the feed cup as water flows to the bottom of the cup.

(4) In the homogenization process, operator should pay attention to the volume of material in feed cup and feed the material in time. After the last cycles, release the pressure and discharge all materials, then adjust the frequency of pump to zero.

5. Instrument cleaning and maintenance

(1) When operating finished, add fresh water to the hopper, adjust the frequency of pump and run without pressure for cleaning the homogenizer hopper and pipeline until it is clean.

(2) Add 75% ethanol to the hopper, turn on the machine and adjust the frequency of pump and run without pressure for cleaning the homogenizer hopper and pipeline until it is clean. After that press the "OFF" button on the panel to shut down, and then add about 75% ethanol in the hopper, and seal the plastic wrap.

(3) Turn the right switch of the fuselage to "—" to turn off the power.

Experiment Instructions

Requirements for Preview

1. To be familiar with the preparation of liposome, lipid – emulsions and solid lipid nanoparticle with high – pressure homogenization procedures.

2. To preview and be familiar with the properties and functions of micro (nano) preparations.

3. To understand the homogenization parameters on the quality of liposome, lipid – emulsions and solid lipid nanoparticle.

Procedures and Precautions

1. To avoid the breaking of the inlet valve and homogenizing valve, the sample should be

filtered through 60 to 100 meshes to remove the particles of impurities (such as iron, glass, etc.) before it is placed into homogenizer to homogenize.

2. It is forbidden to operate the machine for a long time if there is no material.

3. Do not turn on homogenizer as handle is tightened because sudden overload capacity will damage the motor.

4. Solid ceramic plunger is used for homogenizer. Therefore, temperature changes of product contacting with the plunger cannot be over 70℃; otherwise, the plunger may rupture. The range of temperature changes of the sample should not be over 5℃, especially under the sterilization operation.

Questions

1. Briefly describe the basic composition and working principle of the high pressure homogenizer?

2. What are the main factors affecting the quality of micro – nano preparations such as liposome and lipid – emulsion in the high pressure homogenization process?

3. Briefly describe the operation of the high pressure homogenizer?

4. What are the operating points and precautions of the high pressure homogenizer?

5. Briefly describe the maintenance process of the high pressure homogenizer?

6. Briefly describe the application of high pressure homogenizers in the pharmaceutical industry?

实验 24　激光粒度仪的标准操作规程

【目的和要求】

1. 掌握　激光粒度仪的标准操作规程。
2. 熟悉　激光粒度仪的测定原理及意义。
3. 了解　激光粒度仪主要部件及其功能。

【实验原理】

一束平行光在传播过程中遇到障碍物颗粒，光波会发生散射（衍射）偏转，偏转的角度与颗粒的大小相关，散射（衍射）现象可以通过“Mie 散射理论”来描述。颗粒粒径越大，光波偏转的角度越小；颗粒粒径越小，光波偏转角度越大（图 24－1）。激光粒度仪就是利用颗粒对光的散射现象，根据散射光能的分布推算被测颗粒的粒度分布。目前激光粒度仪应用遍及化工、机械、建材、能源、医药等领域。TOPSIZER 型激光粒度仪系统主要由测量单元、循环进样系统、电脑系统（测试软件）以及相关附件组成，量程为 0.02～2000μm，适合相应量程范围内的纳米药物、固体、乳剂和混悬液的粒度测定。

（A）　　（B）

图 24－1　激光粒度仪原理示意图

【仪器与材料】

1. **仪器**　激光粒度测定仪（TOPSIZER 型，欧美克），1000ml 烧杯。

2. **材料**　脂肪乳。

【标准操作规程】

TOPSIZER 激光粒度仪的标准操作规程如下。

1. **仪器主机预热**　打开激光粒度仪主机电源开关预热 30min。

2. **打开粒度仪测试软件**　鼠标左键双击桌面上软件图标，进入到软件的主界面，此时仪器会自动进行通讯连接，软件最下方一行会显示仪器的连接状态和进样器窗口的连接状态。如出现连接错误，单击菜单上“工具”，“端口”，然后选择合适端口。

3. **新建报告并进入测试界面**　点击“新建”图标，建立一个新的空白报告。然后点击“手动”图标，进入手动测量操作界面。

进入手动操作界面之后，循环进样器开动水循环，并检查仪器背景的初始状态。

（1）总光强不小于 50%。

（2）散射光强随着探测器序列号的增加依次递减。

（3）理想状态下，1 号探测器的散射光强不超过 200，波动幅度小于 40。

（4）背景随时间的波动很小。

每次打开软件后，系统会先进行背景对中，在参数设置中选择自动对中（在“选项”—“测量”把“手动对中”的勾去掉），则仪器会自动对中。

4. **设置测量参数**　点击左下角“选项”图标在“测量选项”中设置测量参数。

（1）在“物质”选项里选择或建立样品参数

①选择样品参数：选定左边“可用的样品物质列表”中需要用的参数“移动”到右边列表，单击“确定”；或选定右边“常用物质列表”中需要用的参数，“确定”。

②建立样品参数：点击“样品物质列表”窗中“添加”按钮，在弹出的窗口中编辑样品参数，单击“确定”。

③修改已有样品参数：在“样品物质列表”窗中右边“常用物质列表”中选择需要用的参数，点击“修改”按钮，在弹出的窗口中修改成需要用的样品参数，单击“确定”。

（2）在“结果计算”的“模型”中设置数据计算模型（一般样品默认“通用”—“常规”）

（3）在“结果计算”“高级”中使用默认即可。

（4）在“测量”选项中设置测量时间（15s）、遮光比（1% ~20%）、对中；在“对中”一项选择手动对中或者自动对中（把勾去掉）均可。在“高级选项”—“测量”设置样品遮光比。

(5) 在“测量循环”中设置测量次数，一般设3次，测量之间延迟一般10s。

(6) 在“报告格式”中设置所需的报告数据：D10、D25、D50、D75、D100，从小到大。

参数设置完毕，点击“确定”返回信号窗界面。

(7) 点击左下角“文档”按钮编辑样品名称、编号、测试条件等，单击“确定”。

特别强调：在这些设置项目中，会影响测试结果就是“物质”页面中的折射率、吸收率和计算模型。所以在设置时，尤为要注意这些项目的设置是否正确。

5. 测量 在烧杯中加入800ml蒸馏水。设置泵速（1500～2500r/min），打开循环进样器。点击“开始”，等系统自动扣除背景，出现“加入样品”提示后，将样品加入到进样池中，等到软件中遮光比蓝色柱条进入绿色区域（遮光比在5%～20%较为适宜），单击“开始”后，进入测试阶段，测试结束，测试报告会显示在软件的右边。

6. 仪器清洗 测量完成后，就对循环系统进行清洗。在清洗过程中保持测量显示窗口打开，在测量背景状态下，观察背景是否恢复到测样之前的良好状态。否则应继续清洗。

7. 报告 报告如果需要打印，请在电脑上安装好打印机程序直接打印。可在报告打印预览中，把报告输出为PDF、Excel、Word等几种报告形式。

实验指导

一、预习要求

1. 掌握 激光粒度仪测量粒度基本流程。

2. 熟悉 激光粒度仪测量粒度的基本原理。

3. 了解 激光粒度仪的基本组成。

二、操作要点及注意事项

1. 每次测量下一个样品前均需要清洗烧杯和进样系统。

2. 如果进样系统有气泡，测试结果总会出现不存在的“大颗粒”。为了避免气泡的影响，可将介质在使用前脱气处理，可关闭循环进样器，待气泡排出液面后再次开启循环，还可降低测量时的泵速。

3. 如果测量窗口遭到污染，可排干水，然后打开测量窗口进行清洗（清洗窗口的方法：先冲洗窗口玻璃内表面，去除较大颗粒；使用镜头纸或无屑的面巾纸，横向擦拭，直至其洁净。玻璃外表面用洗耳球吹去灰尘即可。非必要，请不要将玻璃从金属边框中取出）。

4. 实验结束后还原所使用附件。

三、思考题

1. 简述光散射和粒度间的关系。

2. 激光粒度仪测量颗粒尺寸的原理是什么？

3. 简述影响激光粒度仪测定准确性的因素。

4. 简述多分散系数的概念及在粒径测定过程中的意义。

5. 颗粒粒度测定的常用方法有哪些？

6. 简述激光粒度仪在制药行业中的应用。

Experiment 24　Standard Operation Procedure of the Laser Particle Size Analyzer

Objectives and Requirements

1. To master the standard operating procedures of the laser particle size analyzer.

2. To be familiar with the principles of the laser particle size analyzer.

3. To understand the main parts of the equipment and their functions.

Introduction

A bundle of parallel light encounters obstacle particles during propagation, and the light wave is deflected (diffracted). The angle of deflection is related to the size of the particle. The scattering (diffraction) phenomenon can be described by the "Mie scattering theory". (Figure 24 – 1) The larger the particle size, the smaller the angle of deflection of the light wave; the smaller the particle size, the larger the angle of deflection of the light wave. The laser particle size analyzer uses the scattering phenomenon of particles to light, and estimates the particle size and distribution according to the distribution of scattered light energy. At present, the application of laser particle size analyzer covers various fields of modern industry such as chemical industry, machinery, building materials, energy and medicine. The TOPSIZER laser particle size analyzer is mainly composed of measuring unit, loop sampling system, computer system (test software) and related accessories. The suitable range of TOPSIZER laser particle size analyzer is from 0.02 to 2000μm, which could be applied to measure the particle size and distribution nano – medicine, solids, emulsions and suspensions.

Figure 24 – 1　The principle of scattering (diffraction) phenomenon

Equipment and Materials

1. Equipment

Laser particle size analyzer (TOPSIZER, OMEC), 1000ml beaker.

2. Materials

Lipid emulsion.

Standard Operation Procedure

Standard Operation Procedure of TOPSIZER laser particle size analyzer:

1. warmed up

Turn on the power switch and warm up for 30minutes.

2. Open the particle size analyzer test software

Double – click the software icon 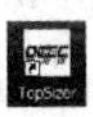 on the desktop to enter the main interface of the software. At this time, the instrument will automatically connect the communication. The bottom line of the software will display the connection status of the instrument and the injector window. In the event of a connection error, click "Tools", "Ports" on the menu and select the appropriate port.

3. Create a new report and enter the test interface

Click the "New" icon  to create a new blank report. Then click the "Manual" icon  to enter the interface of manual measurement.

After entering the interface of manual operation, start the loop injector and the water cycle, then check the initial state of the instrument background.

(1) The total light intensity is not less than 50%.

(2) The scattered light intensity decreases in turn as the detector serial number increases.

(3) Under ideal conditions, the scattered light intensity of the No. 1 detector does not exceed 200, and the fluctuation amplitude is less than 40.

(4) The background has little fluctuation with time.

Each time the software is opened, the system will perform background alignment first, and select automatic alignment in the parameter settings (in the "Options" - "Measurement" to remove the "Manual Centering"), the instrument will automatically center.

4. Set the measurement parameters

Click the "Options" icon  in the lower left corner to set the measurement parameters in "Measurement Options".

(1) Select or establish sample parameters in the "Material" option

①Select sample parameters: select the parameter "Move" in the "Available Sample Material List" on the left to the right list, then click "OK"; or select the parameter in the "Common Material List" on the right, then click "OK".

②Create sample parameters: click the "Add" button in the "Sample Substance List" window, and edit the sample parameters in the pop - up window, click "OK".

③Modify the existing sample parameters: select the required parameters in the "Common Material List" on the right side of the "Sample Substance List" window, click the "Modify" button, and modify the sample parameters to be used in the pop - up window, click "OK".

(2) Set the data calculation model in the "model" of "Result Calculation" (general sample default "general" - "normal").

(3) Use the default in "Result Calculation" - "Advanced"

(4) Set the measurement time (15 seconds), shading ratio (1% - 20%), and centering in the "Measurement" option; select manual centering or automatic centering (to remove the hook) in the "Centering" item. Set the sample shading ratio in "Advanced Options" - "Measurement".

(5) Set the number of measurements in the "measurement cycle", generally set 3 times, and the delay between measurements is generally 10 seconds.

(6) Set the required report data in "Report Format": D10, D25, D50, D75, D100, from small to large. After the parameters are set, click "OK" to return to the signal window interface.

(7) Click the "Document" button in the lower left corner to edit the sample name, number, test conditions, etc., click "OK".

Special emphasis: in these setup projects, the test results will be affected by the refractive index, absorption rate and calculation model in the "Materials" page. Therefore, when setting up, it is especially important to pay attention to whether the settings of these items are correct.

5. Measurement

Add 800ml of distilled water to the beaker as the injection pool. Set the pump speed(1500r/min ~ 2500r/min) and open the loop injector. Click "Start", wait for the system to automatically deduct the background, and after the "Add Sample" prompt appears, add the sample to the injection pool, and wait until the software blocks the blue bar into the green area(the shading ratio is between 5% and 20%). Clicking the "Start" button, wait for test, and the test report will be displayed on the right side of the software.

6. Instrument cleaning

After the measurement is completed, the circulation system should be cleaned. Keep the measurement display window open during the cleaning process. In the state of measurement background, observe whether the background returns to the good state. Otherwise continue to clean.

7. Report

If the report needs to be printed, please install the printer program on the computer and print directly. In the report print preview, the report is output as PDF, Excel, Word and other report forms.

Experiment Instructions

Requirements for Preview

1. To master the basic procedure using the equipment to determineparticle size.
2. To be familiar with the basic principle of laser particle size measurement of particle size.
3. To know the basic components of the laser particle size analyzer.

Procedures and Precautions

1. The beaker and sample system need to be cleaned before each measurement.
2. If there is a bubble in the injection system, the test result will always appear as a "large particle" that does not exist. In order to avoid the influence of air bubbles, the medium can be degassed before use; the circulating sampler can be closed until the air bubbles are discharged from the liquid surface; the pump speed during measurement can be reduced.
3. If the measurement window is contaminated, drain the water and open the measurement window for cleaning. (Method to clean the window: firstly rinse the inner surface of the window glass to remove larger particles; use lens paper or chipless tissue, wipe it horizontally until it is clean. Use the ear washing bulb to blow off the dust on the outer surface of the glass. Please do not remove the glass from the metal frame.)
4. Restore the attached accessories after the experiment.

Questions

1. Briefly describe the relationship between light scattering and particle size?
2. What is the principle of laser particle size measurement of particle size?

3. Briefly describe the factors that affect the accuracy of the laser particle size analyzer?

4. Briefly describe the concept of polydispersity coefficient and its significance in the process of particle size determination.

5. What are the common methods for particle size determination?

6. Briefly describe the application of laser particle size analyzers in the pharmaceutical industry.